PRACTICAL BEDSIDE
ECHOCARDIOGRAPHY CASES
An Atlas for Mobile Devices

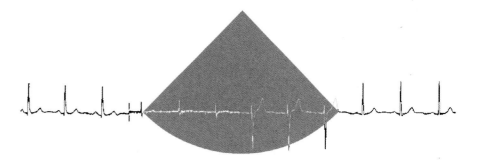

PRACTICAL BEDSIDE
ECHOCARDIOGRAPHY CASES
An Atlas for Mobile Devices

Daniel M. Shindler, MD

Professor of Medicine
Rutgers—Robert Wood Johnson Medical School
New Brunswick, New Jersey

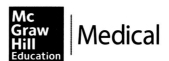

New York Chicago San Francisco Athens London Madrid Mexico City
Milan New Delhi Singapore Sydney Toronto

Practical Bedside Echocardiography Cases: An Atlas for Mobile Devices, 1 ed.

1 2 3 4 5 6 7 8 9   QVS/QVS   19 18 17 16 15 14

ISBN 978-0-07-181265-8
MHID 0-07-181265-2

This book was set in New Century Schoolbook by Aptara, Inc.
The editors were Christine Diedrich and Christie Naglieri.
The production supervisor was Catherine Saggese.
Quad Graphics was the printer and binder.

This book is printed on acid-free paper.

Library of Congress Cataloging-in-Publication Data

Shindler, Daniel, author.
  Practical bedside echocardiography cases : an atlas for mobile devices / Daniel Shindler.
      p. ; cm.
    ISBN 978-0-07-181265-8 (soft cover : alk. paper)—ISBN 0-07-181265-2 (soft cover : alk. paper)
    I. Title.
    [DNLM: 1. Echocardiography—methods—Atlases.   2. Echocardiography—methods—Case Reports.   3. Point-of-Care Systems—Atlases.   4. Point-of-Care Systems—Case Reports. WG 17]

  RC683.5.U5
  616.1′207543–dc23
                                                                                2013032869

McGraw-Hill Education books are available at special quantity discounts to use as premiums and sales promotions or for use in corporate training programs. To contact a representative, please visit the Contact Us pages at www.mhprofessional.com.

This book is dedicated to my wife and collaborator—Dr. Olga Shindler.

The book would not be possible without you.

Echocardiographic imaging is a mainstay of cardiac diagnosis. The following topics are immediately useful to clinicians at various stages of training and practice. There are questions to challenge the knowledge of the reader. The questions are followed by an explanation of the practical value of the topic, and these discussions answer the questions. Illustrations and text are supplemented by numerous animations that can be opened with a QR code reader using a smartphone or a tablet computer with Internet access.

Whenever possible, multiple variations on a theme are provided to illustrate the echocardiographic spectrum of the abnormalities being discussed.

Bedside findings and the electrocardiogram are considered an integral part of the practice of echocardiography. They are incorporated into the discussions where applicable.

References are provided with focus on freely available full-text articles. They are identified in the text with an open book icon [[pdf]] indicating that they are freely obtainable as PDF files.

There are references that point the reader to full-text cardiac physical diagnosis articles that are useful at the bedside. Some references are annotated to further explain their utility. Some were chosen for their comprehensive illustration of cardiac pathology as it relates to echocardiographic imaging. Some are classic "must-have" echocardiography articles.

The open text articles comprise a virtual evidence-based textbook. The articles can be easily located on the Internet in the PDF file format—by using a search engine such as PubMed, Google, or Bing.

This book utilizes QR codes to provide instant access to hundreds of video loops and echo images. Many QR code readers are free and can be downloaded to your mobile device from the App Store or Play Store on your device. The QR app uses the mobile device's camera to scan the QR graphic. It subsequently downloads the echo images or videos to the mobile device for display.

The QR codes included in this book point to an Internet address where video loops and echo images are located. You may point and click using your QR code reader to access these images, or you may type in the Internet address directly to your mobile device web browser. An index of video loops and Internet addresses is provided at the end of this book for your convenience. All files are located at www.mhprofessional.com/echoatlas.

CHAPTER 1

CORONARY ARTERY DISEASE

OVERVIEW OF THE ROLE OF ECHOCARDIOGRAPHY IN CORONARY ARTERY DISEASE

" *Look locally—interpret globally.* "

Regional left ventricular wall motion analysis is the cornerstone of echocardiographic imaging in coronary artery disease. Regional left ventricular wall motion abnormalities are indicators of myocardial ischemia during a stress test. Regional left ventricular wall motion abnormalities are present in acute myocardial infarction. In addition to localizing myocardial infarction, echocardiography serves to diagnose *complications* of infarction. Anterior myocardial infarction can be complicated by an apical left ventricular aneurysm. Inferior myocardial infarction can be complicated by mitral regurgitation. Pulmonary edema and a new murmur, in a patient with myocardial infarction, may indicate either papillary muscle rupture or ventricular septal rupture. Echocardiography helps to identify these critical complications. Right ventricular infarction is an important complication of inferior myocardial infarction, and echocardiography is used for diagnosis and subsequent management. The electrocardiogram (ECG) is utilized in conjunction with the echocardiogram in *all* patients with coronary artery disease.

There is an extensive section on wall motion analysis at the end of this book.

QR 1.1: Ventricular septal rupture complicating acute myocardial infarction. The patient did not survive despite surgical repair.

QR 1.2: Large basal inferior left ventricular wall aneurysm. The large size of this aneurysmal dilatation of the basal inferior wall is unusual after inferior myocardial infarction. It can be associated with ventricular septal rupture. In some cases, there may be a question as to whether it is a true aneurysm, or a pseudoaneurysm.

QR 1.3: Akinesis of the basal and mid-inferior left ventricular wall. Calcifications of mitral chordae and papillary muscles suggest that this is an old inferior infarction. The incidentally noted false tendon close to the apex may rarely cause a murmur. In this patient, mitral regurgitation is a more likely cause of an apical systolic murmur.

QR 1.4: Akinesis of the basal and mid-inferior left ventricular wall. Calcifications of mitral chordae. Possible thrombus overlying some of the akinetic basal inferior wall close to the mitral annulus.

QR 1.5: Thinning, akinesis, and increased echogenicity of the interventricular septum due to an old anterior myocardial infarction. There is systolic left ventricular dysfunction and biatrial enlargement. There is apical tethering of the mitral valve, with localized calcification at the papillary muscle tip. Note: There is no secundum atrial septal defect. The thin membrane of the intact fossa ovalis simply does not reflect any ultrasound back at the transducer.

QR 1.6: Absence of myocardial thickening at the mid-portion of the interventricular septum.

QR 1.7: Thinning of the apical walls.

ROLE OF ECHOCARDIOGRAPHY IN MYOCARDIAL INFARCTION

QUESTION:

What is the role of echocardiography in acute ST elevation myocardial infarction (STEMI)?

A. Make the decision for initiating treatment.

B. Exclude alternative diagnoses.

C. Diagnose complications.

D. Both B and C, but not A.

The decision for initiating treatment in acute STEMI is made quickly and is based on the ECG and on the cardiac symptoms. The echocardiogram serves to help exclude alternative diagnoses for the cause of chest pain, such as aortic dissection or pericarditis. The echocardiogram can also help diagnose complications of myocardial infarction such as papillary muscle rupture, or ventricular septal rupture.

ANSWER: D

CORONARY ARTERY DISEASE VERSUS DIFFUSE ST SEGMENT ELEVATION

QUESTION: **Which disorder affects the left ventricle, or the 12 leads of the ECG, as a *focal* (rather than diffuse) process? More than one answer may be correct.**

A. Myocarditis.

B. Pericarditis.

C. Myocardial infarction.

D. Myocardial ischemia induced during stress echocardiography.

The role of echocardiography in coronary artery disease centers on *regional* wall motion analysis of the left ventricle. Both the ECG and the echocardiogram serve to localize the affected territory in coronary artery disease. In contrast, the ECG of pericarditis and myocarditis shows *diffuse* ST segment abnormalities. The echocardiogram helps to distinguish between myocarditis and pericarditis. There should be diffuse left ventricular motion abnormalities and left ventricular cavity dilatation on the echocardiogram of patients with myocarditis. There should be a pericardial effusion on the echocardiogram of patients with pericarditis.

• PRACTICAL NOTE: Pericarditis and myocarditis are not mutually exclusive. Elevated troponins in pericarditis may indicate coexisting myocarditis.

REFERENCES: Wang K, Asinger RW, Marriott HJ. ST-segment elevation in conditions other than acute myocardial infarction. *New Engl J Med.* 2003;349:2128–2135.

Riera AR, Uchida AH, Schapachnik E, et al. Early repolarization variant: epidemiological aspects, mechanism, and differential diagnosis. *Cardiol J.* 2008; 15:4–16.

ANSWER: C and D

ECHOCARDIOGRAPHIC WALL MOTION ANALYSIS COMPARED WITH THE ECG IN CORONARY ARTERY DISEASE

QUESTION:

What information is NOT immediately provided by the ECG in patients with coronary artery disease when compared with echocardiographic left ventricular wall motion analysis?

A. Infarction.

B. Injury.

C. Ischemia.

D. Aneurysm.

The electrocardiographic hallmark of myocardial infarction is the Q wave. The electrocardiographic hallmark of myocardial *injury* is ST segment elevation. The electrocardiographic hallmark of myocardial *ischemia* is ST segment depression. Echocardiography can demonstrate the presence of myocardial ischemia during a stress test as a new left ventricular wall motion abnormality.

Acute myocardial injury in a patient with chest pain and ST segment elevation (in two contiguous leads) is treated emergently without waiting for an echocardiogram (or for cardiac enzyme results). The echocardiogram (when performed) will confirm the diagnosis by showing left ventricular wall motion abnormalities.

Aneurysm can complicate myocardial infarction. ECG makes the diagnosis after the fact—the ECG sign of aneurysm is *persistent* (more than 30 days) ST segment elevation. The echocardiogram can *readily* demonstrate the aneurysm.

GOOD NEWS: Patients with myocardial enzyme elevations indicating myocardial infarction do not always develop regional echocardiographic wall motion abnormalities. Usually, this denotes a small infarct. Absence of regional wall motion abnormalities under these circumstances is typically associated with a better prognosis.

REFERENCE:

Dubnow MH, Burchell HB, Titus JL. Postinfarction ventricular aneurysm. A clinico-morphologic and electrocardiographic study of 80 cases. *Am Heart J.* 1965;70:753–760. *Utility of persistent ST segment elevation for more than a month following myocardial infarction as an indicator of left ventricular aneurysm.*

ANSWER: D

REGIONAL WALL MOTION AND MYOCARDIAL SEGMENTS

66   *The left ventricular walls are analyzed by dividing them*   **99**
into basal, mid-ventricular, and apical segments.

QUESTION: **Which segment of the left ventricle is most likely to simulate prior myocardial infarction in a *normal* person?**

A. Apical lateral.

B. Basal inferior.

C. Basal septal.

D. Apical cap.

Regional left ventricular wall motion abnormalities are usually reliable indicators of coronary artery disease.

However, the echocardiogram of a normal person may sometimes show a regional wall motion abnormality such as can be seen following inferior myocardial infarction.

QR 1.8: Abnormal "scooped" basal inferior wall shown in the two-chamber apical view. As a result, there is apical tethering of the mitral valve. The consequent decrease in the coaptive surface between the mitral leaflets results in mitral regurgitation and eventual left atrial enlargement.

QR 1.9: Abnormal basal inferior left ventricular wall motion.

BAD NEWS: Of all the left ventricular walls, the *basal inferior wall* is the most prone to erroneous interpretation. Echocardiography is considered highly specific (rarely wrong when abnormal) for the diagnosis of myocardial ischemia. The basal inferior wall can be an exception to this rule.

This is particularly evident in patients with left ventricular hypertrophy. The hypertrophy may spare the basal inferior left ventricular wall, and the relatively thin basal inferior wall may simulate a prior inferior myocardial infarction. Prominent "septal" Q waves on the ECG (due to the hypertrophy) may further confound the clinical picture by being discordant with the echocardiographic appearance.

The basal septum retains its normal thickness and motion in the *normal* patient. The apical lateral left ventricular wall will not be falsely abnormal but may often be difficult to image. Contrast enhancement will help. The apical cap is analyzed for motion, rather than for presence or absence of thickening. It will *not* be falsely abnormal.

QR 1.10: Abnormal basal and mid-inferior left ventricular wall motion in a patient with known inferior myocardial infarction. The motion of the basal and mid-interventricular septum was also abnormal.

QR 1.11: Basal inferior myocardial infarction that extends to the basal lateral wall.

QR 1.12: Short axis—normal wall motion.

ANSWER: B

Table 1 Pitfalls in the display, and wall motion analysis, of the parasternal and apical long axis views.

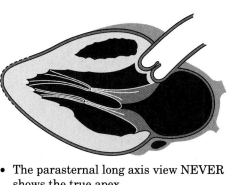

- The parasternal long axis view NEVER shows the true apex.
- The thickness and wall motion of the basal and mid left ventricular segments should be comparable in the parasternal and apical images.
- The apical long axis view can be misleading when it is foreshortened – because it then fails to show the true apex.
- The thickness of the normal true apex should not be greater than the thickness of the normal basal and mid left ventricular segments.
- The "inferior" wall is actually the inferolateral wall, and it corresponds to circumflex coronary artery distribution.

BUNDLE BRANCH BLOCK—ECHOCARDIOGRAPHIC IMPLICATIONS

66 *Wall motion analysis is reserved for the "true echocardiographer."* 99

QUESTION: **A 70-year-old diabetic hypertensive patient has a left bundle branch block on the ECG. Which statement is FALSE?**

A. Wall motion analysis may be difficult in patients with bundle branch block.

B. It is important to scrutinize the ECG to note the width of the QRS complex before interpreting left ventricular wall motion.

C. Right and left bundle branch block will have different effects on left ventricular wall motion.

D. Left bundle branch block is never associated with cardiomyopathy.

Left bundle branch block makes nuclear scanning for ischemia challenging. Left bundle branch block is *frequently* associated with cardiomyopathy. All the *other* above statements are true.

FIGURE 1.1

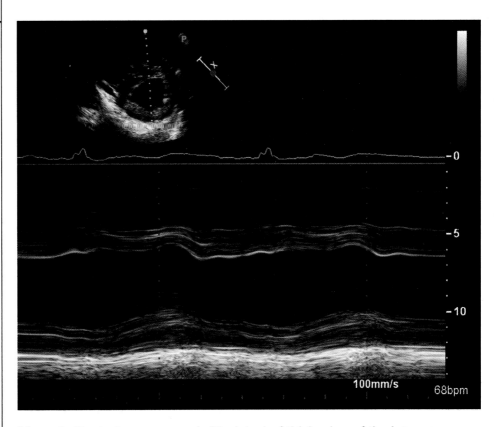

M-mode illustrates presence (with delay) of thickening of the interventricular septum.

New quantitative echocardiographic technologies that measure regional myocardial velocities promise to make interpretation of myocardial wall motion easier (even for the experienced interpreter).

QR 1.13: Dilated cardiomyopathy with left bundle branch block on the ECG and no thickening of the interventricular septum.

REFERENCES:

Mor-Avi V, Lang RM, Badano LP, et al. Current and evolving echocardiographic techniques for the quantitative evaluation of cardiac mechanics: ASE/EAE consensus statement on methodology and indications endorsed by the Japanese Society of Echocardiography. *Eur J Echocardiogr.* 2011;12:167–205.

Urheim S, Edvardsen T, Torp H, et al. Myocardial strain by Doppler echocardiography: validation of a new method to quantify regional myocardial function. *Circulation.* 2000;102:1158–1164.

ANSWER: D

Table 2 Pitfalls in the display, and wall motion analysis, of the apical views.

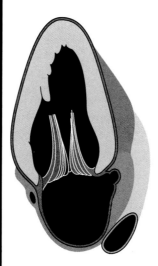
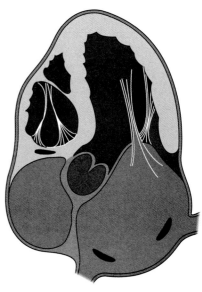

- A thick apical segment may indicate a foreshortened view.
- Scanning tip: An acoustic standoff and/or contrast injection – may be useful when the true apex is too close to the transducer.

ECG LEAD V1 IN INFERIOR MYOCARDIAL INFARCTION

" Before analyzing wall motion on an echocardiogram, it is always "
worthwhile to review the electrocardiogram and to know about rare
disorders that may affect the ECG.

QUESTION: **What are the causes of tall R waves on the ECG in lead V1?**

A. Posterior extension of inferior myocardial infarction.

B. Right ventricular hypertrophy.

C. Duchenne muscular dystrophy.

D. Dextrocardia.

E. Wolff-Parkinson-White syndrome.

F. Ventricular tachycardia.

G. Normal variant in the young.

H. All of the above.

Tall R waves in V1 may simply be an extension of inferior Q waves.
They may also signal the presence of other, rare, perhaps previously
undiagnosed abnormalities with different echocardiographic and electrocardiographic implications. The presence of Q waves in leads II, III,
and aVF will easily establish the presence of prior inferior myocardial
infarction. This is frequently much easier to do on the ECG than on
the wall motion analysis of the echocardiogram.

FIGURE 1.2

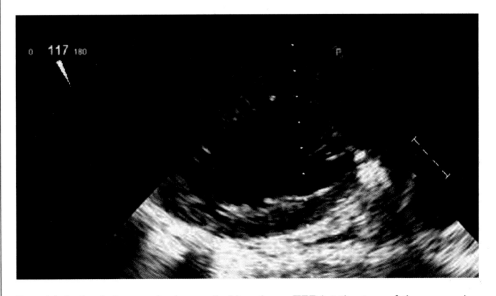

Basal inferior left ventricular wall akinesis on TEE (at the top of the screen).

QR 1.14: Right coronary artery—parasternal short axis view.

REFERENCE:

Casas RE, Marriott HJ, Glancy DL. Value of leads V7–V9 in diagnosing posterior wall acute myocardial infarction and other causes of tall R waves in V1–V2. *Am J Cardiol.* 1997;80:508–509. *Left posterolateral chest leads (V7, V8, V9) helped distinguish the multiple causes of tall R waves in V1 and/or V2, diagnosed true posterior myocardial infarction when standard leads did not, and identified the presence or absence of posterior injury in patients with inferior infarction.*

ANSWER: H

Table 3 Pitfalls in the display, and wall motion analysis of the short axis views.

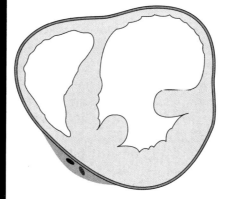
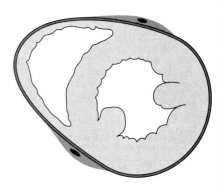

- Short axis images should be round, not oval.
- A tangential off angle tomographic view affects the segmental wall motion interpretation of both the anterior and inferior walls.

WALL MOTION ANALYSIS ON A STRESS ECHOCARDIOGRAM

  " *I just bought a two-story house.* **"**
I got one story before and another story after I bought it.

How many stories can the left ventricular wall tell you during a stress echo?

A. Normal at rest, normal with stress.

B. Normal at rest, abnormal with stress.

C. Abnormal at rest, improved at low-level stress, abnormal again at peak stress.

D. Abnormal at rest, fails to improve with stress.

Regional wall motion analysis is accomplished by a stepwise comparison of resting and stress images. The images are synchronized and displayed side by side on the same screen.

Interpretation

A is negative for ischemia.

B is positive for ischemia.

C is a biphasic response that indicates abnormal but viable myocardium.

D is an indication of abnormal nonviable scarred myocardium.

QR 1.15: Abnormal inferior left ventricular akinesis at rest that failed to improve with stress, indicating nonviable myocardium.

QR 1.16a: Distal left anterior descending (LAD) coronary artery obstruction with apical inferior and apical septal scar.

QR 1.16b: Distal left anterior descending (LAD) coronary artery obstruction with apical inferior and apical septal scar.

REFERENCES:

Lancellotti P, Hoffer EP, Pierard LA. Detection and clinical usefulness of a biphasic response during exercise echocardiography early after myocardial infarction. *J Am Coll Cardiol.* 2003;41:1142–1147. *A biphasic response predicts reversible ischemic myocardial dysfunction.*

Quiñones MA, Verani MS, Haichin RM, et al. Exercise echocardiography versus 201Tl single-photon emission computed tomography in evaluation of coronary artery disease. Analysis of 292 patients. *Circulation.* 1992;85:1026–1031.

RIGHT VENTRICULAR INFARCTION

QUESTION:

A patient with acute inferior myocardial infarction on ECG is found to have jugular venous distention. The lungs are clear to auscultation. Chest X-ray shows a normal cardiac silhouette with clear lung fields. Which of the following is true?

A. The echocardiogram may show hypokinesis of the basal and mid-right ventricular free wall.

B. The apical right ventricular wall may appear hyperdynamic.

C. The echocardiographic report may suggest the possibility of pulmonary embolism.

D. All of the above (A, B, and C).

E. The standard 12-lead ECG has no value in the diagnosis.

Echocardiographic Features of Right Ventricular Infarction

Hypokinesis or akinesis of the basal and mid-right ventricular free wall, with a hyperdynamic apical right ventricular wall, constitutes an echocardiographic sign first described by McConnell in patients with acute pulmonary embolism. The same echocardiographic appearance was subsequently described in some patients with right ventricular infarction.

There are other possible echocardiographic findings in right ventricular infarction. There may be right ventricular dilatation. The systolic excursion of the tricuspid annulus may be decreased due to right ventricular dysfunction. The interatrial septum may be abnormally displaced, bulging toward the left atrium. Abnormal late diastolic compliance of the right ventricle may be manifested on echo as late diastolic flow reversal in the hepatic veins (following atrial contraction). The velocity of pulmonic regurgitation may decrease rapidly in late diastole for the same reason.

QR 1.17a: Dilated hypokinetic right ventricle in a patient with acute inferior myocardial infarction. Thin and akinetic right ventricular free wall. Basal inferoseptal left ventricular wall akinesis (due to the same infarction). Flattening of the interventricular septum in diastole. D-shaped left ventricle in diastole. The interventricular septum moves toward the left ventricle in systole indicating right ventricular pressure (not volume) overload.

QR 1.17b: Dilated hypokinetic right ventricle in a patient with acute inferior myocardial infarction. Thin and akinetic right ventricular free wall. Basal inferoseptal left ventricular wall akinesis (due to the same infarction). Flattening of the interventricular septum in diastole. D-shaped left ventricle in diastole. The interventricular septum moves toward the left ventricle in systole indicating right ventricular pressure (not volume) overload.

QR 1.18: Inferoseptal left ventricular wall hypokinesis extending to the adjacent right ventricular wall.

QR 1.19: Diffuse right ventricular dysfunction with preserved wall thickness.

QR 1.20: Akinetic infundibular right ventricular free wall.

REFERENCE:

McConnell MV, Solomon SD, Rayan ME, et al. Regional right ventricular dysfunction detected by echocardiography in acute pulmonary embolism. *Am J Cardiol.* 1996;78:469–473. *The right ventricular apex is spared.*

Electrocardiography of Right Ventricular Infarction

All patients with acute inferior myocardial infarction should have an ECG that includes right-sided leads to look for ST segment elevation in lead V4R (on the right side of the chest—electrically over the right ventricle). Although the ECG in lead V4R is very sensitive, it does not quantitate the severity of right ventricular involvement, and the findings are transient.

The standard 12-lead ECG of patients with right ventricular infarction may show ST segment elevation in V1 at the same time as the

ST segments are elevated in leads II, III, and aVF. ECG Caveat: ST segment elevation in V1 during acute inferior *left* ventricular infarction indicates that the *right* ventricle is affected.

REFERENCES:

Kinch JW, Ryan TJ. Right ventricular infarction. *New Engl J Med.* 1994;330:1211–1217. *Review article.*

Jacobs AK, Leopold JA, Bates E, et al. Cardiogenic shock caused by right ventricular infarction: a report from the SHOCK registry. *J Am Coll Cardiol.* 2003;41:1273–1279. *Mortality is unexpectedly high.*

Dell'Italia LJ, Starling MR, O'Rourke RA. Physical examination for exclusion of hemodynamically important right ventricular infarction. *Ann Intern Med.* 1983;99:608–611. *Look for jugular venous distention with a Kussmaul sign.*

ANSWER: D

THE ANTERIOR LEFT VENTRICULAR WALL

QUESTION:

Which myocardial segment is NOT affected by LAD occlusion?

A. Apical inferior.

B. Basal inferior.

C. Apical lateral.

D. Basal septal.

Anterior myocardial infarction occurs in the distribution of the left anterior descending artery (LAD a.k.a. the widow maker). Consequently, echocardiographic wall motion abnormalities can be found in the anterior left ventricular wall. The abnormalities can extend to the interventricular septum because the LAD sends branches (perforators) to the septum. The LAD also wraps around the left ventricular apex and continues to the apical inferior wall.

QR 1.21: Unusually prominent coronary artery.

REFERENCE:

 Angelini P, Velasco JA, Flamm S. Coronary anomalies: incidence, pathophysiology, and clinical relevance. *Circulation.* 2002;105:2449–2454.

ANSWER: B

WALL MOTION ANALYSIS OF THE LAD ARTERY TERRITORY

❝ *Distance makes the heart go under.* **❞**

The counterintuitive aspect of wall motion analysis of anterior myocardial infarction stems from the fact that the LAD artery *wraps around* the apex. The most *distal* and therefore the most vulnerable territory can be the apical *inferior* wall. In the apical two-chamber view, it is possible to determine whether the wall motion abnormality at the apical inferior wall is due to right coronary or left coronary disease.

Anterior myocardial infarction can be complicated by an apical left ventricular aneurysm. Echocardiography can detect some, but not all of the consequences of a left ventricular aneurysm. Apical left ventricular thrombus is one such consequence. The thrombus "seals" the aneurysm but thromboembolism may occur. The other two clinical consequences are left heart failure and ventricular arrhythmias.

QR 1.22a: Normal left main. Stenosis should be suspected when there is turbulent color flow.

QR 1.22b: Normal left main. Stenosis should be suspected when there is turbulent color flow.

QR 1.23: Akinesis of the mid and the apical anterior left ventricular wall. Note: Small pericardial effusion, mitral annular, and chordal calcification.

QR 1.24a: Akinesis of the mid and the apical anterior left ventricular wall—extending to the apical inferior wall.

QR 1.24b: Akinesis of the mid and the apical anterior left ventricular wall—extending to the apical inferior wall.

QR 1.25: Contrast enhanced akinesis of the mid and of the apical anterior left ventricular wall—extending to the apical inferior wall.

QR 1.26: Anterior myocardial infarction. Note: The parasternal long axis view does not display the actual left ventricular apex. Only the base and the mid-portion of the left ventricle are shown.

LEFT VENTRICULAR ANEURYSM

QUESTION:

Which is NOT a complication of apical left ventricular aneurysm following myocardial infarction?

A. Rupture.

B. Ventricular arrhythmias.

C. Congestive heart failure.

D. Thromboembolism.

E. All of the above can complicate apical left ventricular aneurysm.

It is a misconception that an apical left ventricular aneurysm is complicated by rupture. A "ruptured aneurysm" is actually called a pseudoaneurysm. This is a distinct entity with a different natural history. It requires urgent surgical intervention.

A pseudoaneurysm does not evolve from a true aneurysm. An aneurysm is a bulge. A pseudoaneurysm is a hole. Aneurysm only has three complications: thromboembolism, arrhythmias, and systolic left ventricular dysfunction (manifested as heart failure).

Imaging Tip to Improve Echocardiographic Diagnosis of an Apical Aneurysm

• An aneurysm may be too close to the transducer in some patients.
• Aside from using contrast ventriculography, an acoustic standoff can be made by overfilling an intravenous solution bag so that it is stretched and free of air bubbles.
• Some of the near-field artifacts that make the echocardiographic examination of an apical aneurysm difficult will be removed by interposing the bag between the transducer and the skin.
• Harmonic imaging dramatically reduces ultrasound artifacts due to the standoff.

QR 1.27: Apical left ventricular aneurysm.

QR 1.28: Apical left ventricular aneurysm with a hazy apical artifact. Thrombus was ruled out using contrast.

QR 1.29a: Walled off rupture of the basal inferior left ventricular wall with a circumferential pericardial effusion.

QR 1.29b: Walled off rupture of the basal inferior left ventricular wall with a circumferential pericardial effusion.

QR 1.29c: Walled off rupture of the basal inferior left ventricular wall with a circumferential pericardial effusion.

REFERENCES:

 Catherwood E, Mintz GS, Kotler MN, et al. Two-dimensional echocardiographic recognition of left ventricular pseudoaneurysm. *Circulation.* 1980;62:294–303.

 Hurst CO, Fine G, Keyes JW. Pseudoaneurysm of the heart. Report of a case and review of literature. *Circulation.* 1963;28:427–436.

Frances C, Romero A, Grady D. Left ventricular pseudoaneurysm. *J Am Coll Cardiol.* 1998;32:557–561. *Clinical findings in 290 patients.*

Oliva PB, Hammill SC, Edwards WD. Cardiac rupture, a clinically predictable complication of acute myocardial infarction: Report of 70 cases with clinicopathologic correlations. *J Am Coll Cardiol.* 1993;22:720–726. *Rupture is often preceded by warning signs and symptoms that should prompt a bedside echocardiogram.*

ANSWER: A

LEFT VENTRICULAR THROMBUS

Which of the following is likely to have contributed to the decreasing incidence of left ventricular thrombus following myocardial infarction?

A. Reperfusion therapy with thrombolytic agents.

B. Percutaneous coronary intervention (PCI).

C. The common use of antiplatelet agents during the course of acute myocardial infarction.

D. A and B only.

E. A and B and C.

Thrombus develops in areas of akinesis where there is nonviable myocardium. It has a predilection for the left ventricular apex. Thrombus may develop as early as a few hours after onset of infarction with a peak incidence at 3 days. It can occur as late as a few weeks after myocardial infarction.

Restoration of myocardial contractility and limiting the extent of myocardial damage seems to be the key to reducing the incidence of this important complication of myocardial infarction. Both thrombolysis and PCI reduce the incidence of left ventricular thrombus. The use of antiplatelet therapy alone is unlikely to affect the incidence. Warfarin is started when echocardiography reveals the presence of a thrombus.

The most important complication of thrombus is the possibility of an embolism and consequent stroke. Anticoagulation with warfarin appears useful in preventing this complication, whereas antiplatelet therapy does not. The likelihood of embolism is highest in the first 2 weeks after acute myocardial infarction, and it decreases over the next 6 weeks. After that the thrombus becomes adherent to the wall with endothelialization, and the likelihood of embolism decreases.

Thrombus mobility is an ominous echocardiographic finding. Over time, the appearance may go back-and-forth between a mural and a protruding thrombus. The echocardiographic appearance of a thrombus is that of a mass. The fact that there is underlying wall motion abnormality separates it from other possibilities such as a tumor or an artifact. The apical location makes endocarditis highly unlikely.

The underlying wall motion abnormality, combined with a mass (that may or may not protrude into the cavity), is the echocardiographic hallmark of a thrombus. It must be distinguished from other findings such as a false tendon or abnormally trabeculated myocardium. The latter is especially common in patients with left ventricular hypertrophy.

FIGURE 1.3

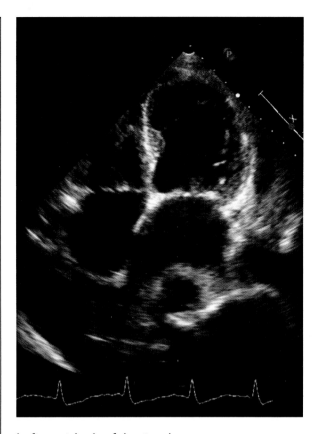

Left ventricular false tendon.

QR 1.30: Apical left ventricular thrombus. Diffusely hypokinetic left ventricle. Dilated left atrial appendage.

QR 1.31a: Apical left ventricular aneurysm with superimposed thrombus.

QR 1.31b: Apical left ventricular aneurysm with superimposed thrombus.

QR 1.31c: Apical left ventricular aneurysm with superimposed thrombus.

QR 1.31d: Apical left ventricular aneurysm with superimposed thrombus.

QR 1.31e: Apical left ventricular aneurysm with superimposed thrombus.

QR 1.31f: Apical left ventricular aneurysm with superimposed thrombus.

QR 1.31g: Apical left ventricular aneurysm with superimposed thrombus.

QR 1.31h: Apical left ventricular aneurysm with superimposed thrombus.

QR 1.31i: Apical left ventricular aneurysm with superimposed thrombus.

QR 1.31j: Apical left ventricular aneurysm with superimposed thrombus.

QR 1.31k: Apical left ventricular aneurysm with superimposed thrombus.

QR 1.32a: Apical left ventricular thrombus.

QR 1.32b: Apical left ventricular thrombus.

QR 1.32c: Apical left ventricular thrombus.

QR 1.33: Apical left ventricular thrombus intentionally outlined by color Doppler.

QR 1.34a: Left ventricular thrombus found from the parasternal window.

QR 1.34b: Left ventricular thrombus found from the parasternal window.

QR 1.35a: Right ventricular apical thrombus.

QR 1.35b: Right ventricular apical thrombus.

REFERENCES:

 Delewi R, Zijlstra F, Piek JJ. Left ventricular thrombus formation after acute myocardial infarction. *Heart.* 2012;98:1743–1749.

 Haugland JM, Asinger RW, Mikell FL, et al. Embolic potential of left ventricular thrombi detected by two-dimensional echocardiography. *Circulation.* 1984;70:588–598. *Thrombus mobility and protrusion can help in the identification of embolic potential.*

ANSWER: D

POSTERIOR MYOCARDIAL INFARCTION—UTILITY OF ECHOCARDIOGRAPHY

QUESTION:

Which modality helps with the diagnosis of a "true-transmural" posterior myocardial infarction?

A. Echocardiography.

B. Additional ECG leads.

C. Both.

STEMI indicates transmural injury. Minutes count. Time is muscle. The elevated ST segments of STEMI correspond to an area of myocardium where blood flow has stopped due to a closed coronary artery.

There is urgent need to reperfuse the myocardium by PCI, or by thrombolysis (to open the closed artery). Conversely, non-ST elevation myocardial infarction (NSTEMI) warrants initial stabilization with medical therapy. Thrombolysis or PCI may, or may not, be necessary, depending on clinical risk stratification.

Transmural myocardial infarction of the posterior left ventricular wall falls into STEMI category. It is due to a *closed* coronary artery and requires urgent PCI or thrombolysis. Unfortunately, the standard 12-lead ECG is misleading in this case. It will be interpreted as NSTEMI because the posterior wall ST segment elevation presents as a "mirror image" ST *depression* in leads V1 and V2.

Posterior ECG leads in leads V7, V8, and V9 will show ST segment elevation. The echocardiogram will help make the diagnosis by showing left ventricular wall motion abnormalities in a region *other than* the anterior wall. The wall motion abnormalities typically involve the circumflex coronary artery territory.

QR 1.36: Inferior left ventricular wall akinesis. *Normal* anterior wall motion. The patient had ST segment depression in leads V1 and V2. Coronary angiography showed total occlusion of a large circumflex coronary artery. The wall motion abnormalities also involved the lateral left ventricular wall (not seen in this view).

REFERENCE: Matetzky S, Freimark D, Feinberg MS, et al. Acute myocardial infarction with isolated ST-segment elevation in posterior chest leads V7–9: "hidden" ST-segment elevations revealing acute posterior infarction. *J Am Coll Cardiol.* 1999;34:748–753. *Wall motion abnormality of the circumflex territory was present in 97%. Mitral regurgitation was present in 69%.*

ANSWER: C

ROLE OF ECHOCARDIOGRAPHY IN CARDIOGENIC SHOCK

QUESTION: **What is the role of echocardiography in cardiogenic shock?**

A. Evaluate the most common cause.

B. Identify rare alternative causes.

C. Help prevent therapeutic mistakes.

D. All of the above.

The most common cause of cardiogenic shock is severe left ventricular dysfunction. Alternative causes (identifiable with echocardiography) include ventricular septal rupture, papillary muscle rupture, left ventricular free wall rupture, right ventricular infarction, and aortic dissection.

Echocardiographic evaluation of volume status, filling pressures, valvular disease, pericardial disease, right ventricular function, and pulmonary artery pressures helps guide therapeutic decisions. The therapeutic goals are early revascularization and avoidance of iatrogenic pitfalls.

Iatrogenic Causes of Cardiogenic Shock

Echocardiography may help avoid making some of the wrong therapeutic decisions below.

1. Excessive diuresis during acute myocardial infarction.
2. Excessive or inadequate fluid administration during the therapy of right ventricular infarction.

3. Inappropriate intravenous nitroglycerin and/or beta-blocker administration in susceptible patients.

QR 1.37: Flail mitral chordae. Dilated left ventricle and left atrium. Inferior wall infarction. Calcified aortic valve. Pleural effusion.

QR 1.38: Papillary muscle rupture.

QR 1.39a: Ventricular septal rupture complicating acute myocardial infarction.

QR 1.39b: Ventricular septal rupture complicating acute myocardial infarction.

QR 1.39c: Ventricular septal rupture complicating acute myocardial infarction.

QR 1.39d: Ventricular septal rupture complicating acute myocardial infarction.

QR 1.39e: Ventricular septal rupture complicating acute myocardial infarction.

QR 1.39f: Ventricular septal rupture complicating acute myocardial infarction.

QR 1.40a: Failed attempt to patch ventricular septal rupture in a patient with cardiogenic shock.

QR 1.40b: Failed attempt to patch ventricular septal rupture in a patient with cardiogenic shock.

REFERENCES:

 Picard MH, Davidoff R, Sleeper LA, et al; SHOCK Trial. Should we emergently revascularize Occluded Coronaries for cardiogenic shock. Echocardiographic predictors of survival and response to early revascularization in cardiogenic shock. *Circulation.* 2003;107:279–284.

Reynolds HR, Hochman JS. Cardiogenic shock: current concepts and improving outcomes. *Circulation.* 2008;117:686–697.

Figueras J, Alcalde O, Barrabes JA, et al. Changes in hospital mortality rates in 425 patients with acute ST-elevation myocardial infarction and cardiac rupture over a 30-year period. *Circulation.* 2008;118:2783–2789.

Lopez-Sendon J, Gonzalez A, Lopez de Sa E, et al. Diagnosis of subacute ventricular wall rupture after acute myocardial infarction: sensitivity and specificity of clinical, hemodynamic and echocardiographic criteria. *J Am Coll Cardiol.* 1992;19:1145–1153. *Clinical findings: syncope, recurrent chest pain, hypotension, electromechanical dissociation, cardiac tamponade, pericardial effusion, high acoustic intrapericardial echoes, right atrial and right ventricular wall compression.*

ANSWER: D

POSTINFARCTION LEFT VENTRICULAR OUTFLOW OBSTRUCTION

66 *This is a medically treatable cause of cardiogenic shock.* **99**

QUESTION: **What are the clinical and echocardiographic findings of postinfarction left ventricular outflow obstruction?**

A. New systolic murmur that increases with the Valsalva maneuver.

B. Apical left ventricular aneurysm.

C. Basal to mid-ventricular septal hypertrophy (adjacent to the area of apical infarction).

D. Dynamic left ventricular outflow obstruction.

Patients with acute anterior myocardial infarction may develop cardiogenic shock due to new onset of dynamic left ventricular outflow obstruction. There is usually a long-standing history of hypertension and a small body mass index. This is a rare, but treatable, cause of cardiogenic shock. There is a systolic murmur that gets louder during the strain phase of the Valsalva maneuver.

FIGURE 1.4

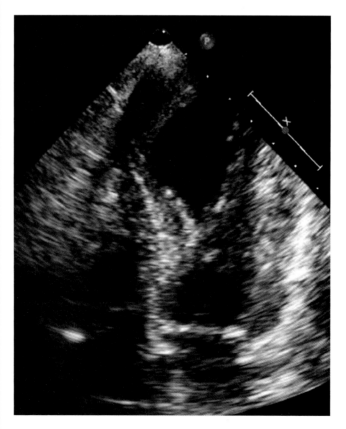

Mid left ventricular systolic cavity obliteration in a patient with an apical aneurysm and superimposed apical thrombus.

The (sometimes rapidly changing) hemodynamic echocardiographic findings are used in making decisions about medical therapy. After-load reduction with angiotensin-converting enzyme inhibitors, or the use of intravenous nitroglycerin, may make the hemodynamics *worse*. Beta-blockers may be beneficial, and echocardiography may be useful in determining the appropriate dose. Vasoconstriction without increasing left ventricular inotropy (using a pure alpha stimulant such as phenylephrine) may sometimes reverse intractable hypotension in the critical care unit.

1.41: Apical left ventricular aneurysm with basal septal hypertrophy.

1.42: Mid left ventricular cavity narrowing in systole. Normal left ventricular wall motion.

1.43: Hypertrophic cardiomyopathy. Mid left ventricular cavity narrowing in systole. Normal left ventricular wall motion.

REFERENCES:

Haley JH, Sinak LJ, Tajik AJ, et al. Dynamic left ventricular outflow tract obstruction in acute coronary syndromes: an important cause of new systolic murmur and cardiogenic shock. *Mayo Clin Proc.* 1999;74:901–906.

Chockalingam A, Tejwani L, Aggarwal K, et al. Dynamic left ventricular outflow tract obstruction in acute myocardial infarction with shock: cause, effect, and coincidence. *Circulation.* 2007;116:e110–e113.

ANSWER: All of the above (we ran out of ink before we could write that as choice E).

CHAPTER 2

PULMONARY DISEASE

ECHOCARDIOGRAPHIC EVALUATION OF CHEST PAIN NOT DUE TO CORONARY ARTERY DISEASE

QUESTION: Which of the following nonischemic causes of chest pain may be better served by a negative blood test than by a negative echocardiogram?

A. Pericarditis.

B. Mitral valve prolapse.

C. Aortic stenosis.

D. Hypertrophic cardiomyopathy.

E. Pulmonary embolism.

F. Aortic dissection.

Pericarditis is diagnosed by the pathognomonic rub and by the electrocardiogram. There may not be pericardial fluid on the initial echocardiogram. Mitral valve prolapse may be diagnosed on auscultation by a click, or by a click followed by a murmur. Echocardiography remains the gold standard. Chest pain in patients with aortic stenosis or hypertrophic cardiomyopathy may indicate associated coronary artery disease. Plasma D-dimer is a derivative of fibrin. A *normal* D-dimer level is highly useful in *excluding* pulmonary embolism and deep venous thrombosis when the pretest probability is low. An *elevated* D-dimer has too many alternative causes to be clinically useful.

REFERENCES: Carrier M, Righini M, Djurabi RK, et al. VIDAS D-dimer in combination with clinical pre-test probability to rule out pulmonary embolism. A systematic review of management outcome studies. *Thromb Haemost.* 2009;101:886–892.

Rathbun SW, Whitsett TL, Vesely SK, et al. Clinical utility of D-dimer in patients with suspected pulmonary embolism and nondiagnostic lung scans or negative CT findings. *Chest.* 2004;125:851–855. *Limited clinical utility of D-dimer for inpatients with clinically suspected pulmonary embolism and non-diagnostic lung scans or negative helical CT.*

ANSWER: E

PULMONARY EMBOLISM

QUESTION:

Transthoracic echocardiography is useful in patients with suspected pulmonary embolism for the following, EXCEPT?

A. Confirmation of diagnosis.

B. Evidence of right ventricular hemodynamic compromise.

C. Pulmonary artery systolic pressure.

D. Paradoxical embolism due to patent foramen ovale.

QR 2.1a: Basal and mid right ventricular free wall akinesis. Hyperdynamic right ventricular apex.

QR 2.1b: Basal and mid right ventricular free wall akinesis. Hyperdynamic right ventricular apex.

QR 2.1c: Basal and mid right ventricular free wall akinesis. Hyperdynamic right ventricular apex.

QR 2.1d: Basal and mid right ventricular free wall akinesis. Hyperdynamic right ventricular apex.

QR 2.1e: Basal and mid right ventricular free wall akinesis. Hyperdynamic right ventricular apex.

QR 2.2: Embolus in the main pulmonary artery.

QR 2.3a: Thrombus in the inferior vena cava.

QR 2.3b: Thrombus in the inferior vena cava.

REFERENCES:

Ribeiro A, Lindmarker P, Johnsson H, et al. Pulmonary embolism: one-year follow-up with echocardiography Doppler and five-year survival analysis. *Circulation*. 1999;99:1325–1330. *Echo can identify patients with persistent right heart dysfunction.*

Pruszczyk P, Torbicki A, Pacho R, et al. Noninvasive diagnosis of suspected severe pulmonary embolism: transesophageal echocardiography vs. spiral CT. *Chest*. 1997;112:722–728.

Kasper W, Geibel A, Tiede N, et al. Distinguishing between acute and subacute massive pulmonary embolism by conventional and Doppler echocardiography. *Br Heart J*. 1993;70:352–356.

Konstantinides S, Geibel A, Kasper W, et al. Patent foramen ovale is an important predictor of adverse outcome in patients with major pulmonary embolism. *Circulation*. 1998;97:1946–1951.

ANSWER: A (you can figure it out by looking at the titles of the references above).

SYSTOLIC PULMONARY ARTERY PRESSURE

QUESTION:

Which auscultatory feature of the second heart sound is LEAST useful in the diagnosis of pulmonary hypertension?

A. Location.

B. Splitting.

C. Radiation.

D. Loudness.

The bedside diagnosis of a loud P2 requires practice and is best honed by correlating auscultatory and echocardiographic findings. The loudness of the second heart sound should be compared by listening at the upper left and at the upper right sternal border. The normal second heart sound can *split* at the upper left sternal border, but it should not be *louder* on the left. A split second heart sound in pulmonary hypertension goes "up the musical scale." A loud P2 may radiate to the apex and to other areas of the chest. The listener should make sure there is no bundle branch block on the ECG to confound these findings.

Systolic pressures in the pulmonary artery are equal to the systolic pressures in the right ventricle when there is no obstruction across the pulmonic valve. This is most easily measured by looking at the velocity of the jet of tricuspid regurgitation. This peak velocity (squared and multiplied by four) indicates the gradient between the right ventricle and the right atrium. By estimating the right atrial pressure, it becomes possible to determine the right ventricular systolic pressure, and (in the absence of pulmonic valve obstruction) the pulmonary artery systolic pressure.

Unfortunately, in patients with pulmonary hypertension the level of right ventricular systolic pressure may not correlate well with prognosis. However, the presence of right ventricular enlargement *is* ominous. The right ventricle is geometrically complex. Right ventricular dimensions are difficult to determine reproducibly by echocardiography, by CT scanning, and by MRI. As the right ventricle becomes dilated, there is eventual loss of tricuspid leaflet opposition. At this point, measurement of right ventricular systolic pressures by Doppler becomes unreliable (just when one needs it the most).

Echocardiographic findings in severe pulmonary hypertension:

1. Dilated right atrium.
2. Dilated right ventricle.
3. Right to left atrial septal displacement.
4. D-shaped short axis left ventricle.

FIGURE 2.1

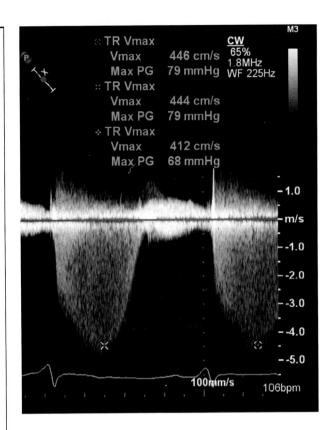

FIGURE 2.2

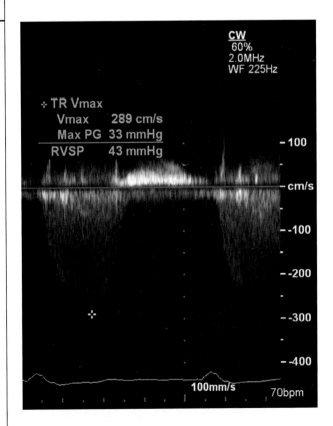

FIGURE 2.3

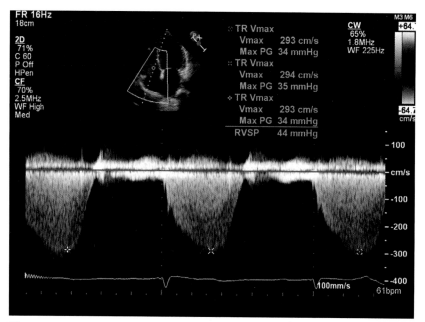

Figures 2.1, 2.2, and 2.3 show various continuous-wave Doppler patterns of tricuspid regurgitation in pulmonary hypertension. The simplified Bernoulli equation is used to calculate the peak systolic pressure gradient between the right ventricle and the right atrium. The right ventricular systolic pressure is calculated by adding this gradient to the estimated right atrial pressure. The peak pulmonary artery pressure is equal to this right ventricular systolic pressure (as long as there is no gradient between the right ventricle and the pulmonary artery).

FIGURE 2.4

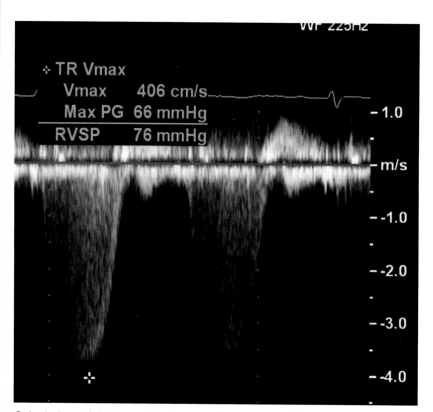

Calculation of right ventricular systolic pressure. Abnormal right ventricular systolic function manifested by delayed acceleration of the tricuspid regurgitation jet.

FIGURE 2.5

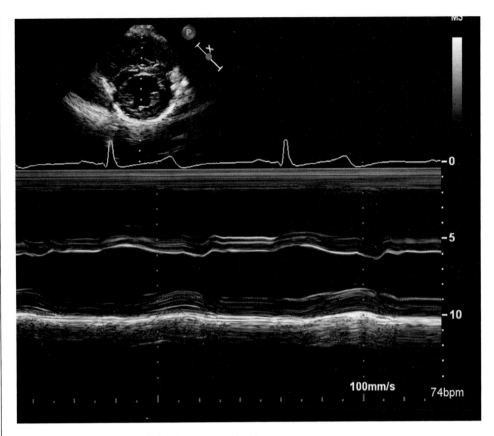

Delayed thickening of the interventricular septum.

FIGURE 2.6

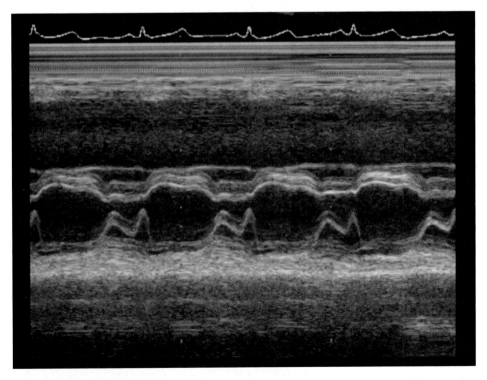

Diastolic displacement of the interventricular septum toward the left ventricle as a result of right ventricular pressure overload in a patient with severe pulmonary hypertension.

FIGURE 2.7

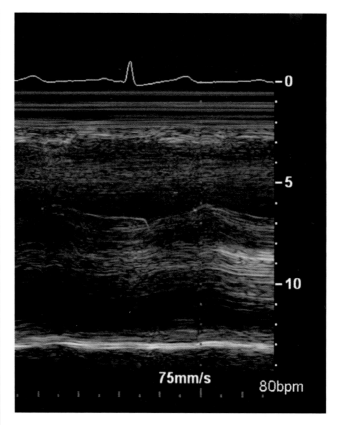

Absent A wave on a pulmonic valve M-mode.

FIGURE 2.8

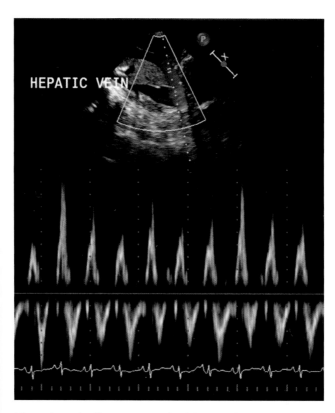

Hepatic vein flow reversal with phasic respiratory changes. Inspection of the jugular pulse revealed prominent 'a' waves.

FIGURE 2.9

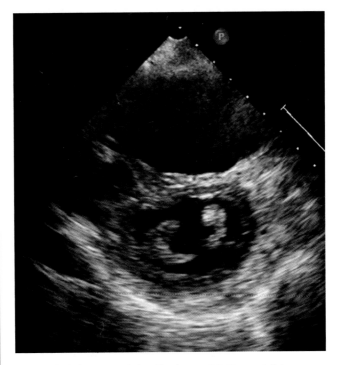

Dilated right ventricle. D-shaped left ventricle.

QR 2.4: Loss of tricuspid leaflet opposition renders Doppler unusable for pressure estimation.

QR 2.5: Right ventricular hypertrophy and dilatation in a patient with severe pulmonary hypertension. The presence of a pericardial effusion has an ominous prognosis in severe pulmonary hypertension.

QR 2.6: Right to left displacement of the interatrial septum in pulmonary hypertension with tricuspid regurgitation.

QR 2.7: Dilated right ventricle. Persistent flattening of the interventricular septum in *systole* indicates right ventricular systolic pressures similar to left ventricular systolic pressures. The left ventricle is unable to push the interventricular septum back into the right ventricular cavity.

QR 2.8: Dilated right ventricular outflow.

QR 2.9: Right ventricular outflow dilatation and hypertrophy.

QR 2.10a: Hypertrophy of the right ventricular free wall.

QR 2.10b: Hypertrophy of the right ventricular free wall.

QR 2.11: Right ventricular hypertrophy. Dilated right atrium. Right to left atrial septal displacement.

QR 2.12a: Thrombus and spontaneous contrast in the inferior vena cava.

QR 2.12b: Thrombus and spontaneous contrast in the inferior vena cava.

QR 2.13a: Changes in the caliber of the inferior vena cava—indicating normal right atrial pressures.

QR 2.13b: Changes in the caliber of the inferior vena cava—indicating normal right atrial pressures.

QR 2.13c: Changes in the caliber of the inferior vena cava—indicating normal right atrial pressures.

QR 2.13d: Changes in the caliber of the inferior vena cava—indicating normal right atrial pressures.

QR 2.14: Elevated right atrial pressure—manifested as minimal collapse of the dilated inferior vena cava on inspiration.

QR 2.15a: Dilated superior vena cava.

QR 2.15b: Dilated superior vena cava.

QR 2.15c: Dilated superior vena cava.

REFERENCES:

Yock PG, Popp RL. Noninvasive estimation of right ventricular systolic pressure by Doppler ultrasound in patients with tricuspid regurgitation. *Circulation.* 1984;70:657–662. *Adding the transtricuspid gradient to the mean right atrial pressure (estimated clinically from the jugular veins) gave predictions of right ventricular systolic pressure that correlated well with catheterization values.*

Lavie CJ, Hebert K, Cassidy M. Prevalence and severity of Doppler-detected valvular regurgitation and estimation of right-sided cardiac pressures in patients with normal two-dimensional echocardiograms. *Chest.* 1993;103:226–231.

Masuyama T, Kodama K, Kitabatake A, et al. Continuous-wave Doppler echocardiographic detection of pulmonary regurgitation and its application to non-invasive estimation of pulmonary artery pressure. *Circulation.* 1986; 74:484–492.

Raffoul H, Guéret P, Diebold B, et al. [The value of recording the pulmonary insufficiency flow by continuous Doppler for the evaluation of systolic pulmonary artery pressure]. *[Article in French] Arch Mal Coeur Vaiss.* 1990;83:1703–1709. *Systolic pulmonary artery pressure was calculated from pulmonary regurgitation as: 3 x early diastolic gradient – 2 x late diastolic gradient + 10 mmHg.*

ANSWER: B

PULMONARY VASCULAR RESISTANCE

"   *Resistance is not futile.*   **"**

Pulmonary vascular resistance cannot be measured directly with echocardiography. As a result, right heart catheterization may become necessary. Resistance is measured as the ratio between pressure difference and cardiac output. Although pulmonary vascular resistance cannot be measured accurately, one should still think about it while interpreting echocardiographic studies by looking at the multiple available echocardiographic measurements of right heart function.

One looks for a consistent pattern, and discrepancies in the multiple measurements are reconciled. Pulmonary artery systolic flow is easily measured with Doppler. The following parameters are obtained from this signal.

1. Duration of systole.
2. Presystolic and postsystolic isovolumic periods.
3. Initial pulmonary artery flow acceleration with time to peak.
4. Presence or absence of mid systolic slowing.

REFERENCES:

Roule V, Labombarda F, Pellissier A, et al. Echocardiographic assessment of pulmonary vascular resistance in pulmonary arterial hypertension. *Cardiovasc Ultrasound*. 2010;8:21.

Mutlak D, Aronson D, Lessick J, et al. Functional tricuspid regurgitation in patients with pulmonary hypertension: is pulmonary artery pressure the only determinant of regurgitation severity? *Chest*. 2009; 135:115–121. *Many patients with pulmonary hypertension do not exhibit significant tricuspid regurgitation.*

Shandas R, Weinberg C, Ivy DD, et al. Development of a noninvasive ultrasound color M-mode means of estimating pulmonary vascular resistance in pediatric pulmonary hypertension: mathematical analysis, in vitro validation, and preliminary clinical studies. *Circulation*. 2001;104:908–913. *Color M-mode velocity of propagation may be useful to identify abnormal pulmonary vascular resistance.*

DIASTOLIC PULMONARY ARTERY PRESSURE

"   *Size does matter.*   **"**

Patients with pulmonary hypertension have elevated diastolic pulmonary artery pressures. The elevated diastolic pulmonary artery pressure increases the amount of regurgitation across the pulmonic valve. Echocardiographic examination reveals a *larger* color flow jet than what is seen in the normal patient with normal pulmonary artery pressures.

The slope of the pulmonic regurgitation jet deceleration velocities reflects the rate of equalization of pressures between the pulmonary artery and the right ventricle. Normally, equalization is slow and the slope is flat. In patients with elevated right ventricular end-diastolic pressures, the slope is steep.

An early diastolic maximum velocity over 3 m per second may be present in some patients with severe systolic left heart failure. This indicates pulmonary diastolic hypertension with an early diastolic gradient of 36 mmHg between the pulmonary artery and the right ventricle. Volume overload of the right ventricle results in chamber dilatation. Right ventricular *chamber dilatation* with pressure overload (severe pulmonary systolic hypertension) is an ominous finding.

FIGURE 2.10

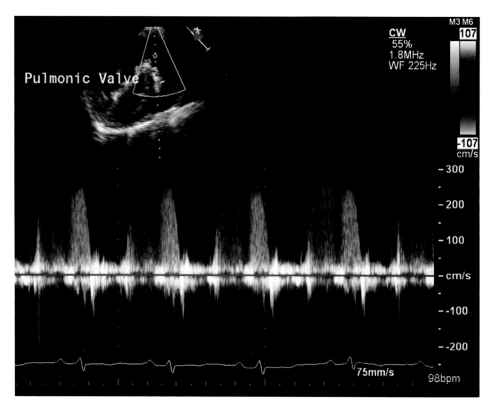

Brief cessation of pulmonic regurgitation following the atrial contraction in pulmonary diastolic hypertension.

FIGURE 2.11

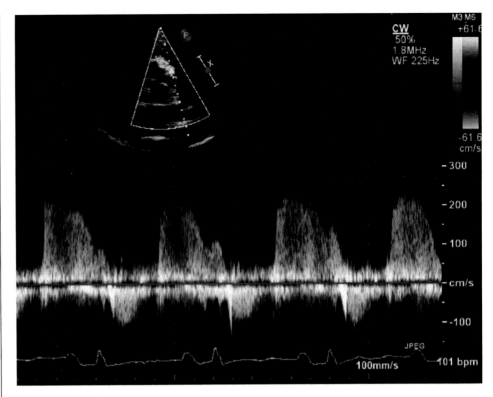

Decreased pulmonary regurgitation following the atrial contraction (shown by using continuous wave Doppler).

FIGURE 2.12

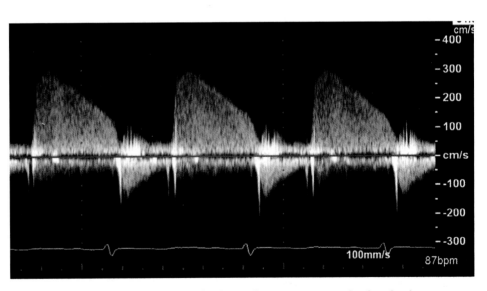

Rapid deceleration of a high-velocity pulmonary regurgitation jet in a patient with diastolic pulmonary hypertension and elevated right ventricular end-diastolic pressure.

QR 2.16: Large pulmonary regurgitation color flow jet.

QR 2.17: Magnified view showing loss of pulmonic leaflet coaptation.

QR 2.18: Right ventricular hypertrophy.

REFERENCE:

Stephen B, Dalal P, Berger M, et al. Noninvasive estimation of pulmonary artery diastolic pressure in patients with tricuspid regurgitation by Doppler echocardiography. *Chest*. 1999;116:73–77. *Because right ventricular and pulmonary artery diastolic pressure is equal at the time of pulmonary valve opening, Doppler echocardiographic estimation of right ventricular pressure at this point provides an estimate of pulmonary artery diastolic pressure. Tricuspid velocity at the time of pulmonary valve opening is measured by superimposing the interval between the onset of the QRS complex on the ECG and the onset of pulmonary flow on the tricuspid regurgitation envelope. The tricuspid gradient at this instant is calculated from the measured tricuspid velocity using the Bernoulli equation.*

ECHOCARDIOGRAPHY OF THE LUNGS

" *Things that you may normally not do with an ultrasound* **"**
transducer, or for that matter, with your ears.

A transducer is applied to the *posterior* chest wall in a patient with congestive heart failure. Which of the two patterns below will be found in this patient?

A. Parallel horizontal lines.

B. Vertical bundles with a narrow base.

Lung comet tail images correlate with extravascular lung water.

 Zanobetti M, Poggioni C, Pini R. Can chest ultrasonography replace standard chest radiography for evaluation of acute dyspnea in the ED? *Chest.* 2011; 139:1140–1147.

 Frassi F, Gargani L, Gligorova S, et al. Clinical and echocardiographic determinants of ultrasound lung comets. *Eur J Echocardiogr.* 2007;8:474–479.

 Lichtenstein DA, Mezière GA. Relevance of lung ultrasound in the diagnosis of acute respiratory failure: the BLUE protocol. *Chest.* 2008;134:117–125.

Lichtenstein DA, Mezière GA, Lagoueyte JF, et al. A-lines and B-lines: lung ultrasound as a bedside tool for predicting pulmonary artery occlusion pressure in the critically ill. *Chest.* 2009;136:1014–1020. *A horizontal artifact indicates a normal lung surface. A comet-tail artifact indicates subpleural interstitial edema.*

Herrnheiser G, Hinson KF. An anatomical explanation of the formation of butterfly shadows. *Thorax.* 1954;9:198–210.

ANSWER: B

EWART SIGN—ECHOCARDIOGRAPHIC VARIATIONS

Pleural fluid can provide an echocardiographic window to the heart from an unusual transducer position.

Examples of unconventional (but sometimes very effective) transducer positions for imaging the heart:

1. The left infrascapular window in a patient with a left pleural effusion.
2. The right axilla in a patient with a right pneumonectomy.

REFERENCES:

Ewart W. Practical aids in the diagnosis of pericardial effusion, in connection with the question as to surgical treatment. *Br Med J.* (London) 1896;1:717–721. *The bedside physical findings are created by compressive atelectasis due to pressure on the lungs by distended pericardium.*

 Maguire R. On palpation and auscultatory percussion. *Br Med J.* 1898;1938: 484–5.

 Yernault JC, Bohadana AB. Chest percussion. *Eur Respir J.* 1995;8:1756–1760.

 Winter R, Smethurst D. Percussion – a new way to diagnose a pneumothorax. *Br J Anaesth.* 1999;83:960–1.

Piccoli M, Trambaiolo P, Salustri A, et al. Bedside diagnosis and follow-up of patients with pleural effusion by a hand-carried ultrasound device early after cardiac surgery. *Chest.* 2005;128:3413–3420.

IMMEDIATE OR DIRECT AUSCULTATION OF THE LUNGS

❝ *The most important part of the cardiac exam is between the ears,* **❞**
not around the ears.

The ear was used as a "sound transducer" before Laennec came around with his newfangled stethoscope in 1816. The ear was applied directly to the body of the patient. (Practice this at home on your significant other.) A thin cloth or tissue can be interposed between the examiner's ear and the patient's skin.

The technique of immediate auscultation may actually *still be useful* for listening to the base of the lungs in the back. We will admit to occasionally becoming a bit overly enthusiastic about some forgotten aspects of the cardiac physical examination.

REFERENCES:

 Benbassat J, Baumal R. Narrative review: should teaching of the respiratory physical examination be restricted only to signs with proven reliability and validity? *J Gen Intern Med*. 2010;25:865–872.

 Sapira JD. About egophony. *Chest*. 1995;108:865–867.

Ginghina C, Beladan CC, Iancu M, et al. Respiratory maneuvers in echocardiography: a review of clinical applications. *Cardiovasc Ultrasound*. 2009;7:42.

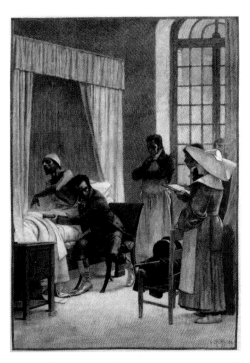

Immediate auscultation of the chest being performed by the inventor of "mediate" (stethoscope) auscultation. Rene Theophile Hyacinthe Laennec (1781–1826), French physician, inventor of the stethoscope in 1816 at the Hopital Necker in Paris, where he was working at the time. Seen here applying his ear directly to the chest of the patient – immediate auscultation. In his left hand is the stethoscope he invented. The image was provided by the Mary Evans Picture Library.

PLATYPNEA—ORTHODEOXIA

" *Dyspnea in the upright position.* **"**

QUESTION: **Which of the following is associated with the rare syndrome of platypnea-orthodeoxia?**

A. Patent foramen ovale.

B. Pericardial disease.

C. Pneumonectomy.

D. Recovery from adult respiratory distress syndrome.

E. Recurrent pulmonary embolism.

F. COPD.

G. Cirrhosis of the liver.

H. Autonomic dysfunction.

Platypnea is a rare symptom of dyspnea in the upright position. It is relieved by assumption of the recumbent position and is the converse of orthopnea. Orthodeoxia, arterial desaturation in the upright position, may also be present. Echocardiography (on a tilt table if possible) is used to look for a patent foramen ovale. Proposed mechanisms for platypnea—orthodeoxia: Postural increased *right-to-left* shunt through a patent foramen ovale.

In the setting of a pericardial effusion—the effusion distorts the architecture of the right atrium when the patient is *standing*; in such a way as to direct the flow of blood returning from the inferior vena cava directly toward a patent foramen ovale.

In patients with underlying lung disease, areas with elevated alveolar pressures may exceed pulmonary arteriolar pressures. As a result, these areas are not perfused. In the upright position, gravitational forces diminish pulmonary arteriolar pressure in the upper lung fields. This also creates small amounts of pulmonary dead space in normal states. An increase in pulmonary dead space when the patient is upright may lead to platypnea.

It can also occur in cirrhosis and in autonomic dysfunction.

REFERENCES:

 Faller M, Kessler R, Chaouat A, et al. Platypnea-orthodeoxia syndrome related to an aortic aneurysm combined with an aneurysm of the atrial septum. *Chest.* 2000;118:553–557.

 Acharya SS, Kartan R. A case of orthodeoxia caused by an atrial septal aneurysm. *Chest.* 2000;118:871–874.

 Ferry TG, Naum CC. Orthodeoxia-platypnea due to diabetic autonomic neuropathy. *Diabetes Care.* 1999;22:857–859.

 Kennedy TC, Knudson RJ. Exercise-aggravated hypoxemia and orthodeoxia in cirrhosis. *Chest.* 1977;72:305–309.

ANSWER: All of the above.

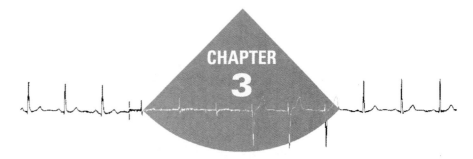

CHAPTER 3

VALVULAR DISEASE

BEDSIDE EVALUATION OF AORTIC STENOSIS

" *Does it look (and sound) like a U or a V?* *"*

QUESTION: **Which statement about the murmur of aortic stenosis is FALSE?**

A. The murmur is invariably audible.

B. Loudness correlates with severity.

C. Late peaking correlates with the Doppler pattern.

D. It can sound musical at the apex.

The murmur of aortic stenosis is typically loud enough to *not* be missed on physical examination. It is best heard at the upper right sternal border and transmits to the neck. Loudness does *not* correlate with severity. The murmur has a crescendo–decrescendo ejection quality that can be confirmed with Doppler. In order to estimate the severity of aortic stenosis on auscultation, one must train the ear to recognize a murmur that is *peaking late* as opposed to a nonobstructive ejection murmur that peaks in early-to-mid systole. The best way to hone this bedside skill is by feedback. The *contour* of the aortic stenosis Doppler signal correlates with the peaking of the murmur. It can be used as feedback to refine the auscultatory impression.

QR 3.1: Aortic stenosis with delayed systolic peaking of both Doppler flow and of the stenosis murmur. Ejection time is prolonged. (The "closing click" in the image is actually a filter saturation artifact.) It serves to time the aortic closure sound in relation to the QRS. There was paradoxical splitting of the second heart sound due to the long left ventricular ejection time. In other words, the pulmonic valve closed earlier than the aortic valve during expiration.

FIGURE 3.1

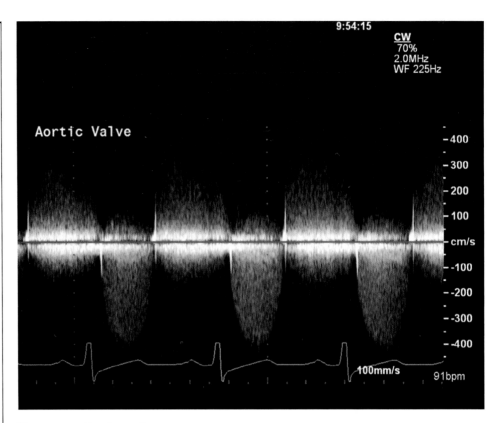

Severe aortic stenosis.

FIGURE 3.2

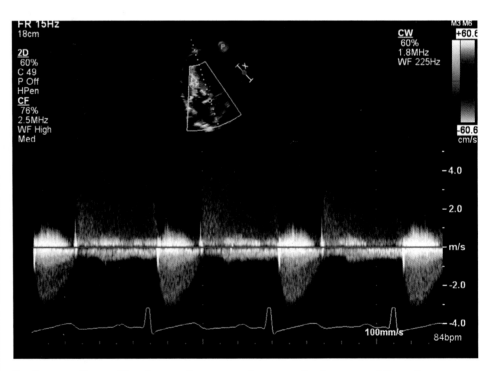

Early systolic peaking in moderate aortic stenosis. Increased flow from aortic regurgitation may contribute to the loudness of the systolic murmur.

REFERENCES:

 Baumgartner H, Hung J, Bermejo J, et al. EAE/ASE. Echocardiographic assessment of valve stenosis: EAE/ASE recommendations for clinical practice. *Eur J Echocardiogr*. 2009;10:1–25.

 Maganti K, Rigolin VH, Sarano ME, et al. Valvular heart disease: diagnosis and management. *Mayo Clin Proc*. 2010;85:483–500.

GALLAVARDIN PHENOMENON

The Gallavardin phenomenon is diagnosed by using color flow Doppler in conjunction with auscultation. It refers to an *auscultatory dissociation* of the aortic stenosis murmur in some patients. The same murmur sounds remarkably different at the apex and at the base. The aortic stenosis murmur in these patients is harsh and noisy (as usual) at the base, but paradoxically soft, blowing, and musical at the apex.

Although an experienced clinician knows that mitral regurgitation is frequently associated with aortic stenosis, the auscultatory impression of *combined* aortic stenosis and mitral regurgitation may be wrong in patients with the Gallavardin phenomenon. Absence of mitral regurgitation on color flow Doppler confirms the presence of the Gallavardin phenomenon in aortic stenosis patients with a musical apical "mitral" murmur.

FIGURE 3.3

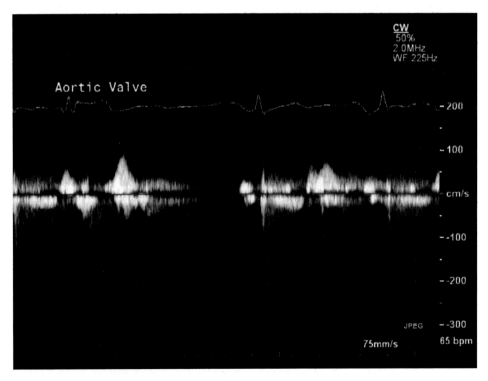

Figures 3.3 and 3.4 show increased Doppler flow velocity in aortic stenosis following a long cardiac cycle. A corresponding increase in the loudness of an aortic stenosis murmur is useful at the bedside to differentiate this murmur from that of mitral regurgitation. In mitral regurgitation, there is no increase in murmur loudness (or Doppler flow velocity) following a long cardiac cycle.

FIGURE 3.4

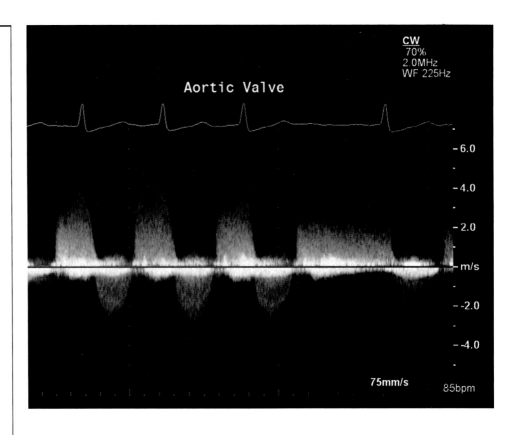

REFERENCES:

Giles TD, Martinez EC, Burch GE. Gallavardin phenomenon in aortic stenosis. A possible mechanism. *Arch Intern Med.* 1974;134:747–749.

Gallavardin L, Pauper-Ravault. Le souffle' du retrecissement aortique puet changer de timbre et devenir dans sa propagation apexienne. *Lyon Med.* 1925:523.

THE AORTIC SECOND HEART SOUND

"   *How to determine at the bedside that A2*   **"**
is decreased or absent?

Over time, in worsening aortic stenosis, the aortic component of the second heart sound (A2) progressively decreases in intensity. It tends to disappear completely in severe aortic stenosis. The pulmonic component of the second heart sound remains audible.

The bedside examination should start with identification of the heart sounds. Murmurs should initially be ignored. One must compare the second heart sound at the *left* upper sternal border with the second heart sound at the *right* upper sternal border. In the absence of pulmonary hypertension, the pulmonic component of the second heart sound is confined to the upper *left* sternal border. At the upper *right* sternal border, the second heart sound should not have components from the pulmonic valve, and should therefore only be influenced by the degree of aortic valve mobility.

FIGURE 3.5

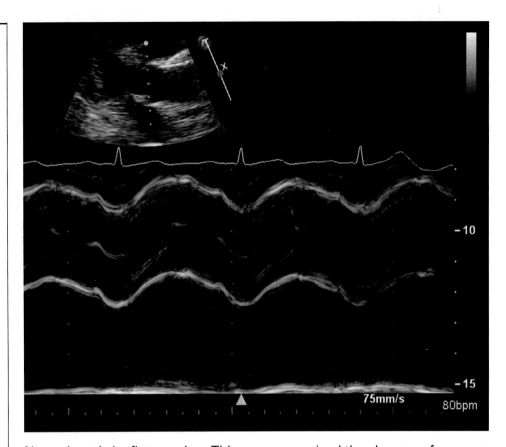

Normal aortic leaflet opening. This appearance (and the absence of a murmur on auscultation) rules *out* significant aortic stenosis. Conversely, the presence of calcified aortic leaflets along with a systolic ejection murmur does not rule *in* the presence of significant aortic stenosis.

FIGURE 3.6

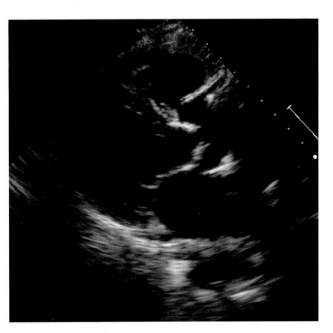

Thick aortic leaflets. Note: Systolic fluttering of the aortic leaflets is somewhat counterintuitive. It is common in healthy pliable leaflets. It is typically absent in thick, rigid leaflets such as these; and therefore, does not correlate with the presence or absence of a murmur.

FIGURE 3.7

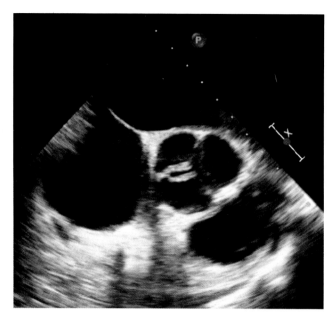

Aortic stenosis with decreased excursion of all three leaflets. The appearance is that of a slit-like orifice. The mobility of all three leaflets is decreased. In this case, the existing leaflet calcification does not create the artifacts that so frequently hinder planimetry of the stenotic aortic valve orifice in other cases.

NOTE: The size of the stenotic orifice can be overestimated if planimetry is inadvertently done in a plane other than the narrowest orifice. Metaphorically, planimetry must be done at the "mouth of the volcano."

QR 3.2: Aortic sclerosis: Patchy aortic leaflet calcifications appear to "hover over" mobile aortic leaflets. The aortic component of the second heart sound was normal in this patient, who presented with a loud systolic murmur.

REFERENCES:

Luisada AA. The second heart sound in normal and abnormal conditions. *Am J Cardiol.* 1971;28:150–161.

Chandraratna PA, Lopez JM, Cohen LS. Echocardiographic observations on the mechanism of production of the second heart sound. *Circulation.* 1975; 51:292–296. *S2 is caused by deceleration of columns of blood resulting from semilunar valve closure.*

ANSWER: B

AORTIC STENOSIS AND REGURGITATION CAN HAVE VALVULAR, SUPRAVALVULAR OR SUBVALVULAR CAUSES

Fixed nondynamic subvalvular aortic stenosis is rare. A discrete sub-aortic membrane is difficult to visualize on transthoracic echocardiography. Some patients have suboptimal images and a thin subaortic membrane may be completely missed. A fixed left ventricular outflow obstruction may be misdiagnosed as a dynamic subaortic gradient, such as is seen in hypertrophic cardiomyopathy.

FIGURE 3.8

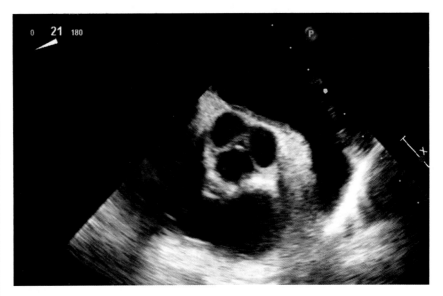

Supravalvular cause of aortic regurgitation: Trileaflet aortic valve with a central *regurgitant* orifice due to a dilated proximal ascending aorta (not evident in this view).

FIGURE 3.9

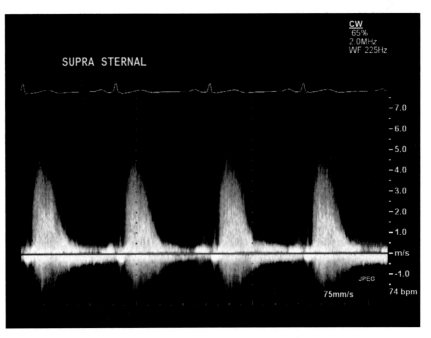

The right parasternal and suprasternal views align the Doppler beam with the aortic stenosis jet and may yield the highest flow velocities.

REFERENCES:

 Kelly DT, Wulfsberg E, Rowe RD. Discrete subaortic stenosis. *Circulation.* 1972;46:309–322. *Ejection clicks are rare. Peripheral pulses are normal. A precordial systolic thrill over the base of the heart is transmitted to the suprasternal notch. The murmur does not differ from the murmur of valvular aortic stenosis. Atrial S4 gallops and/or a single second heart sound indicate severe outflow obstruction.*

Edwards JE. Pathology of left ventricular outflow obstruction. *Circulation.* 1965; 31:586–599.

Katz NM, Buckley MJ, Liberthson RR. Discrete membranous subaortic stenosis: report of 31 patients, review of the literature, and delineation of management. Circulation. 1977;56:1034–1038.

Aboulhosn J, Child JS. Left ventricular outflow obstruction: subaortic stenosis, bicuspid aortic valve, supravalvar aortic stenosis, and coarctation of the aorta. *Circulation.* 2006;114:2412–2422. *Excellent review.*

Choi JY, Sullivan ID. Fixed subaortic stenosis: anatomical spectrum and nature of progression. Br Heart J. 1991;65:280–286. *Four types of fixed subaortic stenosis were identified: short segment (81%), long segment (12%), posterior displacement of the infundibular septum with additional discrete narrowing of the left ventricular outflow tract (5%), and redundant tissue arising from the membranous septum (2%).*

Maron BJ, Redwood DR, Roberts WC, et al. Tunnel subaortic stenosis: left ventricular outflow tract obstruction produced by fibromuscular tubular narrowing. *Circulation.* 1976;54:404–416.

Williams JC, Barratt-Boyes BG, Lowe JB. Supravalvular aortic stenosis. *Circulation.* 1961;24:1311–1318.

De Rubens Figueroa J, Rodríguez LM, Hach JL, et al. Cardiovascular spectrum in Williams-Beuren syndrome: the Mexican experience in 40 patients. *Tex Heart Inst J.* 2008;35:279–285.

Vince DJ. The role of rubella in the etiology of supravalvular aortic stenosis. *Can Med Assoc J.* 1970;103:1157–1160.

Varghese PJ, Izukawa T, Rowe RD. Supravalvular aortic stenosis as part of rubella syndrome, with discussion of pathogenesis. *Br Heart J.* 1969;31:59–62.

Ensing GJ, Schmidt MA, Hagler DJ, et al. Spectrum of findings in a family with nonsyndromic autosomal dominant supravalvular aortic stenosis: a Doppler echocardiographic study. *J Am Coll Cardiol.* 1989;13:413–419.

Espinola-Zavaleta N, Muñoz-Castellanos L, Kuri-Nivon M, et al. Aortic obstruction: anatomy and echocardiography. *Cardiovasc Ultrasound.* 2006;4:36.

CONTINUITY EQUATION TO CALCULATE AORTIC VALVE AREA

66 *In systole, flow is the same below the valve, across the* **99**
valve, and past the valve.

Flow is equal to velocity times the area. With flow remaining the same, any change in the area results in a proportional change in velocity.

Stroke volume = stroke volume.

Fat and short cylinder (A × v) = Thin and long cylinder (a × V)

To solve for aortic stenosis orifice area (a): Use (A × v) divided by V

Increasing flow with dobutamine to unmask nonsevere aortic stenosis:

1. Flow (v) gets disproportionately faster in the unchanged outflow (A).
2. V is proportionately slower in the case of a mobile aortic valve that opens further with the increased flow.
3. The calculated aortic valve area *increases* in cases of nonsevere stenosis.

The ratio between v and V is called the dimensionless index.

REFERENCES:

Burwash IG, Thomas DD, Sadahiro M, et al. Dependence of Gorlin formula and continuity equation valve areas on transvalvular volume flow rate in valvular aortic stenosis. *Circulation*. 1994;89:827–835.

deFilippi CR, Willet DL, Brickner ME, et al. Usefulness of dobutamine echocardiography in distinguishing severe from nonsevere valvular aortic stenosis in patients with depressed left ventricular function and low transvalvular gradients. *Am J Cardiol*. 1995; 75:191–194.

Schwammenthal E, Vered Z, Moshkowitz Y, et al. Dobutamine echocardiography in patients with aortic stenosis and left ventricular dysfunction: Predicting outcome as a function of management strategy. *Chest*. 2001;119:1766–1777.

Monin JL, Quere JP, Monchi M, et al. Low-gradient aortic stenosis: operative risk stratification and predictors for long-term outcome: a multicenter study using dobutamine stress hemodynamics. *Circulation*. 2003;108:319–324.

FIGURE 3.10

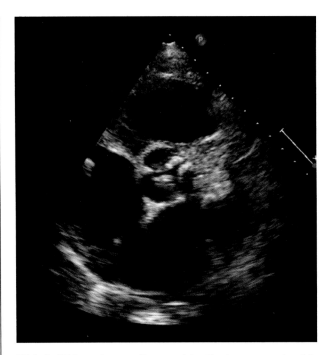

Pitfall: This echocardiographically innocent looking, slit-like appearance of the aortic valve is actually distorted by ultrasound artifacts; and can appear misleadingly small. Planimetry area should be compared to, and reconciled with: the Doppler findings (gradients and continuity area), and with the clinical findings.

FIGURE 3.11

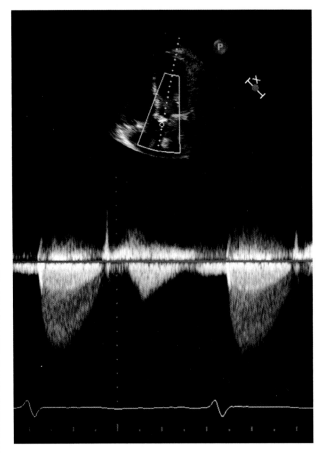

Dimensionless index.

FIGURE 3.12

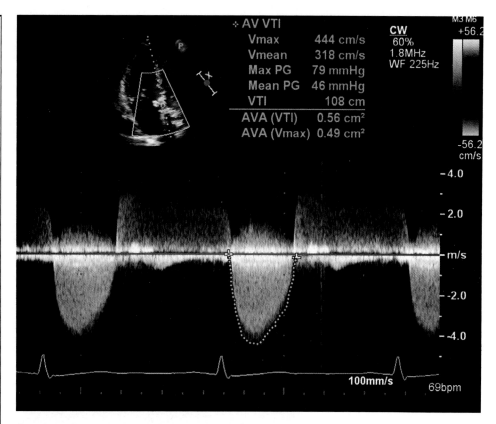

Aortic valve area is equal to the outflow area multiplied by the dimensionless index (v/V).

FIGURE 3.13

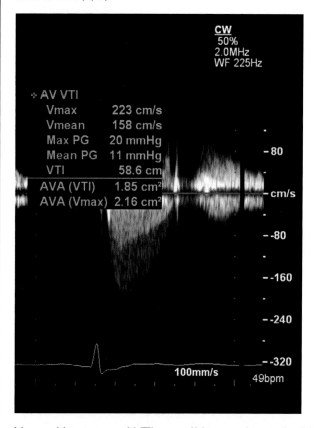

Vmax, Vmean, and VTI can all be used as velocities in the continuity equation. Pitfall: Do not compare apples with oranges – the velocities of v/V have to be of the same type.

FIGURE 3.14

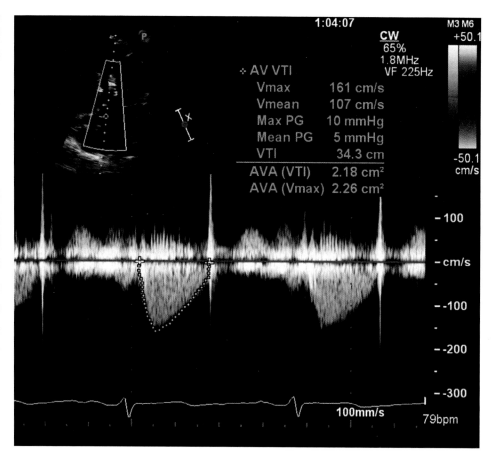

Pitfall: Gradients ($4V^2$) are more significantly affected by flow than velocities. They are chronically increased by aortic regurgitation, and decreased by left ventricular dysfunction. They are acutely increased by anxiety/tachycardia, and decreased by sedation. Continuity aortic valve area calculations use velocities (not gradients).

QR 3.3: Calcified aortic valve. Calcified mitral annulus. Left ventricular hypertrophy.

QR 3.4: Patchy aortic valve calcifications.

QR 3.5: Calcified aortic valve. Subcostal view.

REFERENCES:

Skjaerpe T, Hegrenaes L, Hatle L. Noninvasive estimation of valve area in patients with aortic stenosis by Doppler ultrasound and two-dimensional echocardiography. *Circulation*. 1985;72:810–818.

Hegrenaes L, Hatle L. Aortic stenosis in adults: non-invasive estimation of pressure differences by continuous wave Doppler echocardiography. *Br Heart J*. 1985;54:396–404.

Currie PJ, Seward JB, Reeder GS, et al. Continuous-wave Doppler echocardiographic assessment of severity of calcific aortic stenosis: a simultaneous Doppler-catheter correlative study in 100 adult patients. *Circulation*. 1985;71:1162–1169.

Zoghbi WA, Farmer KL, Soto JG, et al. Accurate noninvasive quantification of stenotic aortic valve area by Doppler echocardiography. *Circulation*. 1986;73:452–459.

de la Morena G, Saura D, Oliva MJ, et al. Real-time three-dimensional transoesophageal echocardiography in the assessment of aortic valve stenosis. *Eur J Echocardiogr*. 2010;11:9–13. *Aortic valve planimetry was possible in 95% of patients by using three-dimensional transesophageal echocardiography.*

Chang SA, Kim HK, Sohn DW. Impact of afterload on the assessment of severity of aortic stenosis. *J Cardiovasc Ultrasound*. 2012;20:79–84.

Dumesnil JG, Pibarot P, Carabello B. Paradoxical low flow and/or low gradient severe aortic stenosis despite preserved left ventricular ejection fraction: implications for diagnosis and treatment. *Eur Heart J*. 2010;31:281–289.

AORTIC STENOSIS VALVE AREA CALCULATION
IN THE CATH LAB

“   *In order to calculate aortic valve area, your IQ has to be at*   **”**
least as high as your patient's EF.

The valve area can be calculated in the cath lab by the simple Hakki formula: Cardiac output divided by the square root of the gradient across the aortic valve.

REFERENCE: Hakki AH, Iskandrian AS, Bemis CE, et al. A simplified valve formula for the calculation of stenotic cardiac valve areas. *Circulation.* 1981;63:1050–1055. *A simplified version of the original Gorlin formula using the cardiac output and the pressure difference across the valve can be used to measure the severity of aortic stenosis. Peak pressure difference across the valve can be used instead of the mean pressure difference.*

Pitfall of *echocardiographic* cardiac output calculation: The left ventricular outflow diameter can be overestimated or underestimated, giving a wrong stroke volume. Pitfall of pressure recovery is discussed in the two references below.

REFERENCES: Chambers J. Is pressure recovery an important cause of "Doppler aortic stenosis" with no gradient at cardiac catheterisation? *Heart.* 1996;76:381–383.

Baumgartner H, Khan S, De Robertis M, et al. Discrepancies between Doppler and catheter gradients in aortic prosthetic valves in vitro: a manifestation of localized gradients and pressure recovery. *Circulation.* 1990;82:1467–1475.

STROKE VOLUME

> *Echocardiographic stroke volume = cylinder base ×*
> *stroke distance.*

Stroke volume can be calculated by constructing an echocardiographic cylinder. The volume of a cylinder is the length of an area. Some people like the analogy of sand that is flattened out in a barrel.

Example: The area of the left ventricular outflow tract × the velocity time integral obtained in that spot = stroke volume.

Area: $\pi \times r^2 = .785 \times d^2$

Where does .785 come from?

$r = d/2$

$r^2 = d^2/4$

$\pi \times r^2 = \pi \times d^2/4 = \pi/4 \times d^2 = 3.14/4 \times d^2 = .785 \times d^2$

Length: The velocity time integral is the stroke distance. A change in the area results in a proportional change of the stroke distance.

• BAD NEWS: Two-dimensional echocardiography is a tomographic technique comparable with slicing a loaf of bread with a knife. The diameter can be overestimated or underestimated. A tangential slice will exaggerate the diameter. The diameter has to be measured at the *largest part* of a circle, or it will be underestimated.

Pitfalls in shunts, and in valvular regurgitation coexisting with valvular stenosis: Systemic and venous stroke volume will not match if there is a shunt. Stroke volumes will not match at different valves if some fraction of the forward stroke volume in a particular valve regurgitates backward during the same cardiac cycle.

STROKE VOLUME CALCULATIONS

QUESTION:

Doppler echocardiography can provide the stroke volume by measuring flow velocity at a measured flow area. Which resulting calculation is LEAST accurate?

A. Shunt calculation.

B. Stenotic orifice calculation.

C. Regurgitant orifice calculation.

D. Resistance calculation.

E. Cardiac output calculation.

Cardiac output is determined by simply multiplying the stroke volume by the heart rate. The inaccuracy of echocardiographic determination of pulmonary vascular resistance is not a calculation problem. Pulmonary vascular resistance is calculated as the ratio of transpulmonary gradient to transpulmonary flow. The flow area is the problem in this calculation. A dimensionless index that does not require flow area seems preferable, and may be useful for screening of elevated pulmonary vascular resistance without giving the actual number. This index measures the ratio between tricuspid regurgitation velocity and ventricular outflow stroke distance.

Shunt calculation is the least accurate because it requires two different flow areas. Each area comes with potential measurement errors. Stenotic and regurgitant orifice calculations are sufficiently accurate for routine clinical use.

FIGURE 3.15

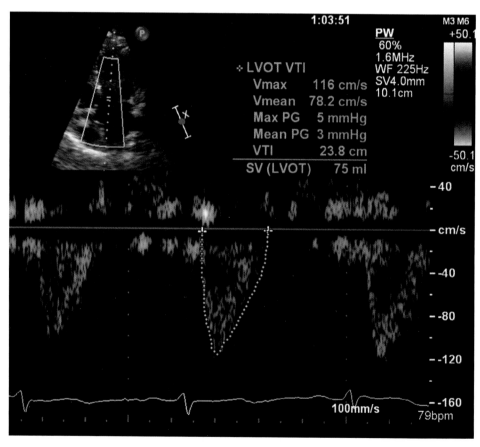

Stroke volume calculation.

REFERENCES:

 Enriquez-Sarano M, Bailey KR, Seward JB, et al. Quantitative Doppler assessment of valvular regurgitation. *Circulation*. 1993;87:841–848.

 Dumesnil JG, Shoucri RM. Effect of the geometry of the left ventricle on the calculation of ejection fraction. *Circulation*. 1982;65:91–98. *Ejection fraction is determined not only by the extent of myocardial shortening, but also by the relationship of ventricular wall thickness to ventricular cavity size.*

ANSWER: A

CARDIAC OUTPUT

QUESTION:

Which statement is FALSE?

A. Fick cardiac output is suited for atrial fibrillation.

B. Thermodilution cardiac output is made inaccurate by tricuspid regurgitation.

C. Pulmonary artery saturation below 65% indicates decreased cardiac output.

D. Pulmonary artery saturation above 80% indicates decreased cardiac output.

The *Fick* method uses the a-vO$_2$ difference. It works in atrial fibrillation because "steady state" is used. It is most accurate in low cardiac output states where there is a wide a-vO$_2$ difference. Oxygen extraction is greater with decreased cardiac output. This results in a low pulmonary artery saturation.

Thermodilution measures the "area under the curve" after a short set of cardiac cycles. The calculation is affected by significant tricuspid regurgitation, and possibly by the variable cardiac cycle length in atrial fibrillation.

REFERENCES:

Detry JM, Rousseau M, Vandenbroucke G, et al. Increased arteriovenous oxygen difference after physical training in coronary heart disease. *Circulation*. 1971;44:109–118.

Fares WH, Blanchard SK, Stouffer GA, et al. Thermodilution and Fick cardiac outputs differ: impact on pulmonary hypertension evaluation. *Can Respir J*. 2012;19:261–266.

Gonzalez J, Delafosse C, Fartoukh M, et al. Comparison of bedside measurement of cardiac output with the thermodilution method and the Fick method in mechanically ventilated patients. *Crit Care*. 2003;7:171–178.

ANSWER: D

LOW GRADIENT AORTIC STENOSIS

❝   *Short and fat = thin and long.*   **❞**

The velocity of blood flow across a stenotic aortic valve orifice increases with the degree of obstruction. Velocity is converted to gradient by squaring it and multiplying by four. A high gradient usually means severe stenosis. Low gradient with *decreased stroke volume* requires calculation of the stenotic orifice area. Aortic valve area is needed because gradients are influenced by loading conditions. The *magnitude of increase* in velocity is affected by the flow across the valve.

QR 3.6: Dimensionless index.

QR 3.7a: Aortic leaflet thickening. Decreased systolic excursion.

QR 3.7b: Aortic leaflet thickening. Decreased systolic excursion.

REFERENCES:

Pereira JJ, Lauer MS, Bashir M, et al. Survival after aortic valve replacement for severe aortic stenosis with low transvalvular gradients and severe left ventricular dysfunction. *J Am Coll Cardiol.* 2002;39:1356–1363.

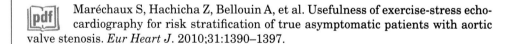

Maréchaux S, Hachicha Z, Bellouin A, et al. Usefulness of exercise-stress echocardiography for risk stratification of true asymptomatic patients with aortic valve stenosis. *Eur Heart J.* 2010;31:1390–1397.

Hachicha Z, Dumesnil JG, Bogaty P, et al. Paradoxical low-flow, low-gradient severe aortic stenosis despite preserved ejection fraction is associated with higher afterload and reduced survival. *Circulation.* 2007;115:2856–2864. *Patients with severe aortic stenosis may have low transvalvular flow and low gradients despite a normal LV ejection fraction. This pattern is in fact consistent with a more advanced stage of the disease and has a poorer prognosis. This condition may be misdiagnosed, leading to an inappropriate delay of aortic valve replacement surgery.*

BICUSPID AORTIC VALVE

QUESTION: **Which statement is true about bicuspid aortic valves?**

A. Auscultation has no role in the diagnosis.

B. Doming always indicates rheumatic etiology.

C. There are no associated abnormalities in the aorta.

D. None of the above.

Doming is present in congenitally bicuspid (nonrheumatic) aortic valves because of commissural fusion. Coarctation of the aorta is associated with bicuspid aortic valves. A bicuspid aortic valve should be suspected on auscultation when there is an ejection click.

FIGURE 3.16

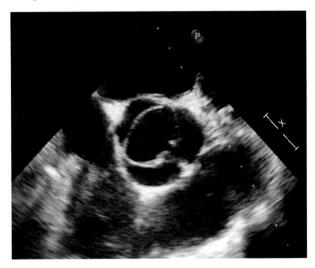

Bicuspid aortic valve. "Fish mouth" orifice in systole. Raphe at 5 o'clock.

FIGURE 3.17

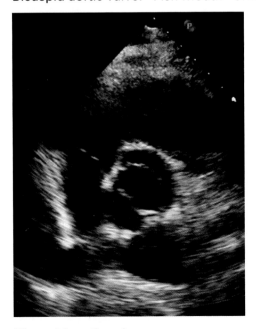

Bicuspid aortic valve.

QR 3.8a: Bicuspid aortic valve.

QR 3.8b: Bicuspid aortic valve.

QR 3.9: Eccentric aortic regurgitation with a doming bicuspid aortic valve.

QR 3.10: Artifact due to the raphe of a bicuspid aortic valve.

QR 3.11: Trivial eccentric aortic regurgitation.

REFERENCES

 Ward C. Clinical significance of the bicuspid aortic valve. *Heart.* 2000;83:81–85.

 Mordi I, Tzemos N. Bicuspid aortic valve disease: a comprehensive review. *Cardiol Res Pract.* 2012;2012:196037.

Michelena HI, Desjardins VA, Avierinos JF, et al. Natural history of asymptomatic patients with normally functioning or minimally dysfunctional bicuspid aortic valve in the community. *Circulation.* 2008;117:2776–2784.

Abdulkareem N, Smelt J, Jahangiri M. Bicuspid aortic valve aortopathy: genetics, pathophysiology and medical therapy. *Interact Cardiovasc Thorac Surg.* 2013;17:554–559.

Cho HJ, Jung JI, Kim HW, et al. Intracardiac eustachian valve cyst in an adult detected with other cardiac anomalies: usefulness of multidetector CT in diagnosis. *Korean J Radiol.* 2012;13:500–504.

ANSWER: D

AUSCULTATION OF THE BICUSPID AORTIC VALVE

" *Location, location, location.* "

A patient is referred for an echocardiogram to confirm the clinical suspicion of a bicuspid aortic valve. The transthoracic images of the aortic valve are suboptimal. Which of the following statements by the clinician should make the echocardiographer consider performing a confirmatory TEE?

A. The first heart sound was split at the lower left sternal border.

B. The first heart sound was similarly split at the apex and at the base.

C. The first heart sound was split at the apex only when using light pressure with the bell of the stethoscope.

The auscultatory hallmark of a bicuspid aortic valve is the early systolic ejection click. This ejection click must be distinguished at the bedside from a normally split first heart sound and from an atrial gallop (S4). The ejection click is a short, sharp sound that is easily heard both at the aortic area on the right side of the sternum and equally well (or better) at the apex.

The normal first heart sound has *no business* being split at the upper right sternal border. Normal splitting of the first heart sound is typically heard in a limited area at the lower left sternal border where the tricuspid closure component (T1) is heard, contributing to the splitting of M1 (mitral closure component) and T1.

A left atrial gallop is heard at the apex. It is usually a difficult-to-hear low frequency "thud." The bell of the stethoscope is pressed lightly against the skin with just enough pressure to create a seal and eliminate entry of distracting ambient noise via the bell. Further pressure may actually *filter out* the gallop by stretching the skin and "creating a diaphragm." Varying the pressure of the bell to intermittently muffle the gallop during auscultation can be used to confirm its presence by making it "come and go."

• CAUTION: Patients with right bundle branch block on the electrocardiogram frequently have a widely split first heart sound at the left lower sternal border. This may get confused with an atrial gallop.

REFERENCE: Vancheri F, Gibson D. Relation of third and fourth heart sounds to blood velocity during left ventricular filling. *Br Heart J*. 1989;61:144–148.

ANSWER: B

CHRONIC SEVERE AORTIC REGURGITATION

" *Di-crotic and bis-feriens mean "twice-striking" in* **"**
Greek and Latin respectively.

QUESTION: **Which pulse abnormality in chronic severe aortic regurgitation best illustrates the *dynamic nature* of the characteristically wide pulse pressure?**

A. Corrigan pulse: prominent pulsations of the carotid arteries.

B. Bisferiens pulse: double systolic arterial impulse, the so-called twice-beating heart.

C. De Musset sign: head nodding with each heartbeat.

D. Duroziez sign: systolic and diastolic femoral artery bruit.

E. Hill sign: accentuated leg systolic pressure with >40 mmHg difference from the brachial artery systolic pressure.

F. Müller sign: pulsation of the uvula with each heartbeat.

G. Palmar click: palpable systolic flushing of the palms.

H. Quincke pulse: cyclic reddening and blanching of the nail capillaries.

I. Traube sign: loud "pistol shot" sound heard over the femoral artery.

J. Water hammer pulse: brisk femoral pulsation similar to that felt with a water hammer—a Victorian toy. The water hammer was a glass tube filled partly with water or mercury in a vacuum. The water or mercury produced a slapping impact when the glass tube was turned over.

Hill sign variation: the forearm of the patient is encircled by the examiner and lifted up. When the forearm is lifted in the patient with chronic severe aortic regurgitation, the examiner will feel the patient's pulse. The maneuver increases the already wide pulse pressure by dropping the diastolic pressure even further. The combination of echocardiography with the physical examination cannot be overstated in aortic regurgitation.

The murmur of aortic regurgitation is fairly easy to convey to beginning listeners. The blowing decrescendo quality of the murmur is so unique and characteristic that an enthusiastic listener can acquire this skill by learning proper technique. Color flow Doppler is more sensitive than the stethoscope for the detection of aortic regurgitation.

Hence, the presence of any degree of aortic regurgitation on color flow Doppler should be considered an opportunity to go back and listen for the murmur.

Patients with aortic dissection can present with acute myocardial infarction because the dissection extends to the ostium of the right coronary artery, closing it off, and the patient presents with acute inferior myocardial infarction. The combination of acute inferior infarction with a new diastolic decrescendo murmur provides a *potentially lifesaving* clinical clue that the patient may actually have dissection as the cause of their acute myocardial infarction. Thrombolytic therapy and catheter intervention in this patient is not the proper course of therapy—emergency surgery is required.

It is useful to combine the echocardiographic features of aortic regurgitation with auscultatory hallmarks of aortic regurgitation. Echocardiography may explain some of the physical findings. For example, the echocardiographic finding of mitral valve preclosure corresponds to the decrease in intensity of the first heart sound. Diastolic flow reversal in the descending aorta can be seen on echo in severe aortic regurgitation. It can be indirectly demonstrated on physical examination by placing a stethoscope over the femoral artery and listening for a "pistol shot" sound.

FIGURE 3.18

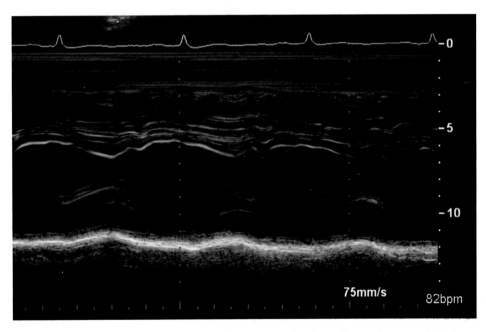

Diastolic "dip" of the interventricular septum in chronic aortic regurgitation.

FIGURE 3.19

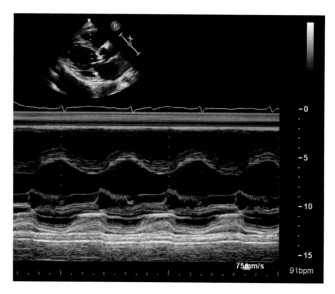

Diastolic flutter of the anterior mitral leaflet due to aortic regurgitation. The presence of this finding does not correlate with severity of aortic regurgitation. It is caused by the jet of aortic regurgitation.

FIGURE 3.20

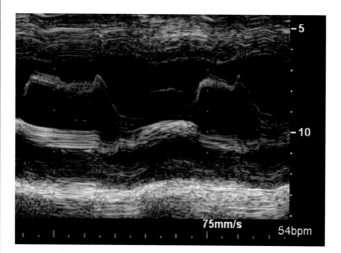

Diastolic flutter of the anterior mitral leaflet due to aortic regurgitation. Unrelated calcification of the posterior mitral annulus.

QR 3.12: Diastolic mitral regurgitation (red color flow) is typically found in *acute* **severe aortic regurgitation (where the left ventricular diastolic pressure rises above the left atrial pressure at end diastole).** The dilated left ventricular cavity in this case indicates that the aortic regurgitation is chronic.

QR 3.13: Severe aortic regurgitation with loss of leaflet coaptation. Decreased mitral leaflet opening. Severe left ventricular dysfunction.

FIGURE 3.21

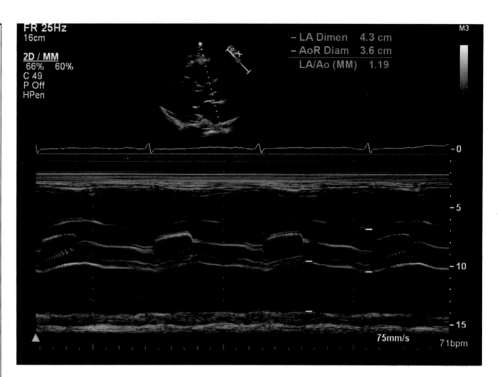

Normal *systolic* fluttering of the aortic leaflets.

REFERENCES:

O'Rourke MF. The arterial pulse in health and disease. *Am Heart J.* 1971;82:687–702.

Sapira JD. Quincke, de Musset, Duroziez, and Hill: some aortic regurgitations. *South Med J.* 1981;74:459–467.

Ewy GA, Rios JC, Marcus FI. The dicrotic arterial pulse. *Circulation.* 1969; 39:655–661. *The dicrotic pulse is felt as a faint rebound immediately after the second heart sound. It is different from the bisferiens pulse (sometimes found in aortic regurgitation) where both palpable peaks are felt well before the second heart sound.*

Orchard RC, Craige E. Dicrotic pulse after open heart surgery. *Circulation.* 1980;62:1107–1114. *A dicrotic pulse may be found after aortic valve replacement in aortic regurgitation patients with severely dilated left ventricles and decreased systolic function.*

Smith D, Craige E. Mechanism of the dicrotic pulse. *Br Heart J.* 1986;56: 531–534.

Lange RL, Hecht HH. Genesis of pistol-shot and Korotkoff sounds. *Circulation.* 1958;18:975–978.

Abdulla AM, Frank MJ, Erdin RA Jr, et al. Clinical significance and hemodynamic correlates of the third heart sound gallop in aortic regurgitation. A guide to optimal timing of cardiac catheterization. *Circulation.* 1981;64:464–471. *The finding of a ventricular S3 gallop in patients with chronic aortic regurgitation indicates left ventricular dysfunction.*

ANSWER: E

ACUTE SEVERE AORTIC REGURGITATION

A 30-year-old patient has color flow Doppler evidence of aortic regurgitation (AR).

Which of the following Doppler signs is the most useful indicator that the severe aortic regurgitation is acute?

A. Large color flow jet.

B. Aortic leaflet morphology on two-dimensional echo.

C. Diastolic flow reversal.

D. Diastolic mitral regurgitation.

E. Mitral valve preclosure.

Acute severe AR in a young patient may be due to leaflet destruction from endocarditis.

• CAUTION: The appearance of a flail leaflet in the left ventricular outflow may simulate a vegetation when there is no endocarditis.

Disruption of leaflet coaptation may also be due to aortic dissection, or due to trauma without dissection. Diastolic flow reversal in the descending thoracic aorta is a specific sign of severe aortic regurgitation. It is influenced by heart rate. Age is relevant to the interpretation. Young patients have more prominent diastolic recoil than older patients. The reversal has to be holodiastolic. The end-diastolic velocity will be 20 cm/sec or greater in severe regurgitation.

Diastolic mitral regurgitation is useful but rare in acute AR. It may be accompanied by mitral valve preclosure. It is influenced by the PR interval and may occur intermittently in complete heart block. It may be missed because the onset is subtle. There may be mid-diastolic opening of the aortic valve and/or premature closure of the mitral valve.

As the rapidly rising left ventricular diastolic pressure reaches the falling aortic root pressure, the aortic cusps may simply float into the open position. Late-diastolic elastic recoil of the acutely over-distended left ventricular myocardium might contribute to reopening of the aortic valve. The force of atrial contraction, increasing the end-diastolic left ventricular pressure, might cause the aortic valve to open. This could occur even if the mitral valve had closed prematurely, by forceful downward displacement of the upward-tensed (but still closed) mitral leaflets.

The presence of a markedly compliant precapillary arteriolar bed, manifest by a very low peripheral vascular resistance, would complement any of these explanations by providing unimpeded diastolic runoff into a very low pressure distal compartment. Diastolic shuddering of the anterior mitral leaflet is *not* related to severity or acuteness of AR.

Bedside examination **pearls** in acute severe AR: The mitral component of the first heart sound is decreased or completely inaudible when there is diastolic mitral regurgitation and mitral valve preclosure. The tricuspid component should still be audible at the left lower sternal border. There may be an S3 gallop, which is rarely found in compensated chronic severe AR. The prominent physical findings found in chronic severe AR can be conspicuously absent.

FIGURE 3.22

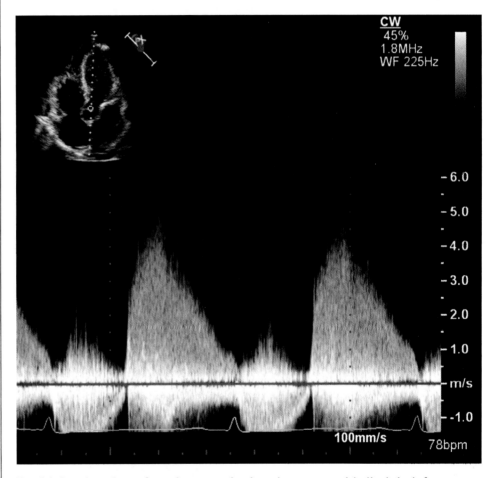

Rapid deceleration of aortic regurgitation due to a rapid climb in left ventricular end-diastolic pressure.

QR 3.14a: Diastolic flow reversal in the descending aorta.

QR 3.14b: Diastolic flow reversal in the descending aorta.

FIGURE 3.23

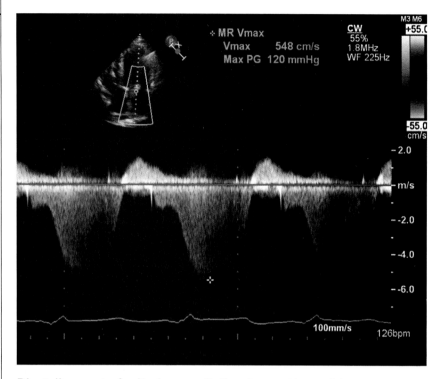

Diastolic onset of mitral regurgitation in a patient with acute severe aortic regurgitation.

FIGURE 3.24

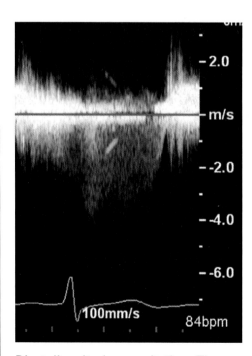

Diastolic mitral regurgitation. The regurgitant flow begins before the QRS.

FIGURE 3.25

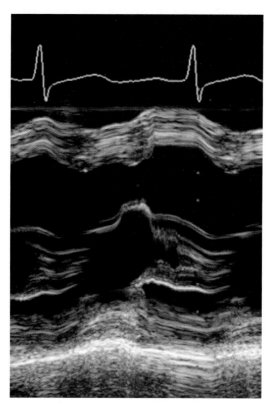

M-mode of mitral valve preclosure.

FIGURE 3.26

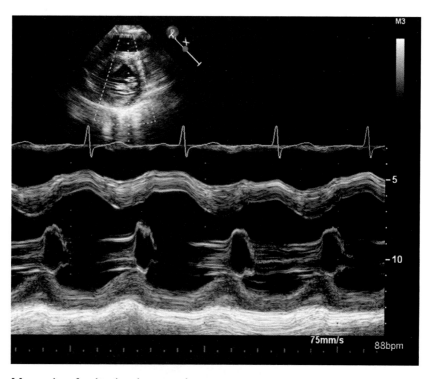

M-mode of mitral valve preclosure.

QR 3.15: Diastolic mitral regurgitation on color M-mode—red color flow before the QRS.

QR 3.16a: Continuous systolic and diastolic aortic regurgitation in a patient with a ventricular assist device, and no forward flow through the aortic valve in systole.

QR 3.16b: Continuous systolic and diastolic aortic regurgitation in a patient with a ventricular assist device, and no forward flow through the aortic valve in systole.

QR 3.17: Acute severe aortic regurgitation due to endocarditis.

REFERENCES:

 Samstad SO, Hegrenaes L, Skjaerpe T, et al. Half time of the diastolic aortoventricular pressure difference by continuous wave Doppler ultrasound: a measure of the severity of aortic regurgitation? *Br Heart J*. 1989;61:336–343.

Oh JK,, Hatle LK, Sinak LJ, et al. Characteristic Doppler echocardiographic pattern of mitral inflow velocity in severe aortic regurgitation. *J Am Coll Cardiol*. 1989;14:1712–1717.

 Weaver WF, Wilson CS, Rourke T, et al. Mid-diastolic aortic valve opening in severe acute aortic regurgitation. *Circulation*. 1977;55:145–148.

Nakao S, Nagatomo T, Kiyonaga K, et al. Influences of localized aortic valve damage on coronary artery blood flow in acute aortic regurgitation: an experimental study. *Circulation*. 1987;76:201–207. *Coronary blood flow is significantly decreased when the corresponding aortic cusp is damaged.*

Lakier JB, Fritz VU, Pocock WA, et al. Mitral components of the first heart sound. *Br Heart J*. 1972;34:160–166.

Sainani GS, Szatkowski J. Rupture of normal aortic valve after physical strain. *Br Heart J*. 1969;31:653–655. *A patient had a "seagull" or "cooing-dove" type of diastolic murmur, which was so loud that it was audible over the shoulders, arms, abdomen, low back, and neck region.*

[pdf] Estevez CM, Dillon JC, Walker PD, et al. Echocardiographic manifestations of aortic cusp rupture in a myxomatous aortic valve. *Chest.* 1976;69:685–687. *Echocardiographic features associated with valvular vegetations are not specific for endocarditis. Aortic cusp rupture revealed chaotic systolic motion of one of the aortic cusps, diastolic aortic valvular fluttering, and abnormal diastolic echoes in the left ventricular outflow tract.*

[pdf] Becker AE, Düren DR. Spontaneous rupture of bicuspid aortic valve. An unusual cause of aortic insufficiency. *Chest.* 1977;72:361–362. *The conjoined cusp of an unusual bicuspid valve had prolapsed, due to rupture of a fibrous strand which previously had anchored the free rim of the cusp to the inner wall of the aorta. Spontaneous rupture of the cord caused the sudden aggravation of aortic regurgitation. There were no signs of endocarditis.*

ANSWER: C

SNAPS, PLOPS, KNOCKS, AND GALLOPS

QUESTION: **Complete the phrases below using the corresponding "buzz" words above.**

A. Mitral stenosis opening.....

B. Pericardial.....

C. Tumor....

D. Ventricular...

The colorful names above are used to indicate an abnormality of the heart. They are all *diastolic* heart sounds. The opening snap is discussed in detail in the mitral stenosis section. Tumor plop refers to the extremely rare instance where a left atrial myxoma is heard to stop short in early diastole. Coincidentally, the opening snap is heard at about the same time. Both the snap and the plop may also be loud enough to be palpable during the precordial examination.

Prior to the availability of echocardiography, it was sometimes difficult to distinguish left atrial myxoma from mitral stenosis on auscultation. The pericardial knock is a rare early diastolic heart sound. It has some unique auscultatory features and associated physical findings. It gets louder on squatting. There is a dramatic jugular venous 'y' descent (seen at about the same time that the knock is heard—after S2). This should suggest the diagnosis of pericardial constriction. Echocardiographic evaluation should then be expanded to look for expiratory reversal of hepatic vein flow, respiratory discordance of mitral and tricuspid early inflow velocities, and a respiratory "bounce" of the interventricular septum. There may also be prominent but nonspecific biatrial enlargement.

The triple heart sounds that simulate the gallop of a horse:

Ten..Neh....See (S4..S1....S2) or Ken...Tuh...Keee (S1...S2...S3)

This is an acquired skill that takes time to master, but the reward at the bedside is well worth the effort!

REFERENCES:

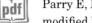 Pitt A, Pitt B, Schaefer J, et al. Myxoma of the left atrium. Hemodynamic and phonocardiographic consequences of sudden tumor movement. *Circulation*. 1967;36:408–416.

Lange RL, Botticelli JT, Tsagaris TJ, et al. Diagnostic signs in compressive cardiac disorders. Constrictive pericarditis, pericardial effusion, and tamponade. *Circulation*. 1966;33:763–777.

Gibson TC, Grossman W, McLaurin LP, et al. An echocardiographic study of the interventricular septum in constrictive pericarditis. *Br Heart J*. 1976;38:738–743. *Echocardiographic timing of the pericardial knock is illustrated in Figures 1 and 2.*

Candell-Riera J, García del Castillo H, Permanyer-Miralda G, et al. Echocardiographic features of the interventricular septum in chronic constrictive pericarditis. *Circulation*. 1978;57:1154–1158. *Echocardiographic timing of the "M" or "W" jugular venous pulse contour of constrictive pericarditis is illustrated. The trough of the 'y' descent coincides with the pericardial knock.*

Parry E, Mounsey P. Gallop sounds in hypertension and myocardial ischaemia modified by respiration and other manoeuvres. *Br Heart J*. 1961;23:393–404.

MITRAL STENOSIS

66 *Echocardiography has supplanted the physical examination* 99
for the diagnosis and determination of severity of mitral stenosis.
The physical examination continues to be used for routine
follow-up evaluation.

QUESTION: **A 40-year-old woman with history of rheumatic fever and recent onset of dyspnea has an echocardiogram performed that shows a "hockey stick" mitral leaflet. Which statement is FALSE?**

A. The second heart sound may now be increased.

B. The first heart sound may now be decreased.

C. The mitral valve now opens earlier than on a previous study.

D. The only possible cause is rheumatic fever.

Mitral stenosis is quickly recognized in the initial set of parasternal echocardiographic images. There is doming and thickening of the anterior mitral leaflet with a "hockey stick" appearance due to the fact that the anterior mitral leaflet was fused by inflammation to the posterior mitral leaflet decades ago during the acute inflammatory bout of rheumatic fever. Classic question to a medical student during teaching rounds: What are the three etiologies of mitral stenosis?

Answer (which is actually wrong): Rheumatic fever, rheumatic fever, and rheumatic fever.

Better answer (only known to readers of this book):

1. Rheumatic fever
2. Parachute mitral valve: Rare congenital fusion of the papillary muscles into a single papillary muscle trunk. The chordal attachment to a single papillary muscle results in variable degrees of mitral stenosis.

Two other rare congenital abnormalities in the left atrium may create the respiratory manifestations of mitral stenosis: There may be a supramitral membrane or cor triatriatum.

Echocardiographic and auscultatory consequences of chronic severe mitral stenosis:

1. Mitral valve calcification and thickening (may decrease the previously loud M1).
2. Pulmonary hypertension (loud P2 on auscultation).
3. Tricuspid regurgitation (may decrease the loudness of T1).
4. Left atrial thrombus.

FIGURE 3.27

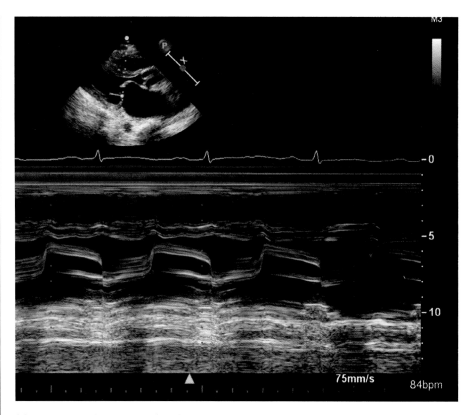

Mitral stenosis with a "hockey stick" anterior mitral leaflet on two dimensional image (shown on the upper part of the image). M-mode beam passing through the anterior and posterior mitral leaflets shows the classic plateau of the anterior mitral leaflet EF slope. There is also a second, more subtle finding. The posterior mitral leaflet is being pulled anteriorly by the bigger anterior leaflet. This is due to the commissural fusion caused by inflammation during the initial episode of rheumatic fever.

FIGURE 3.28

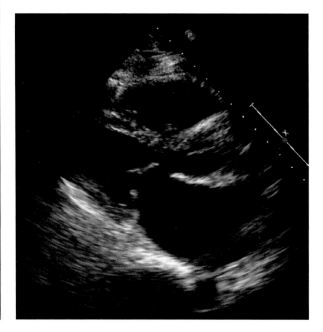

Mitral stenosis. Minimal leaflet thickening.

FIGURE 3.29

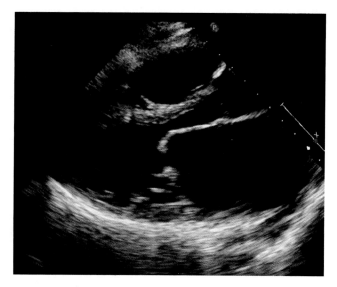

Mitral stenosis. Moderate thickening of the mitral leaflet commisures.

FIGURE 3.30

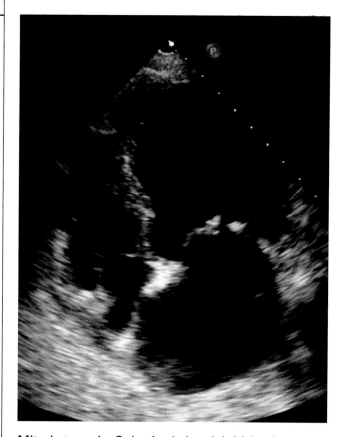

Mitral stenosis. Submitral chordal thickening.

FIGURE 3.31

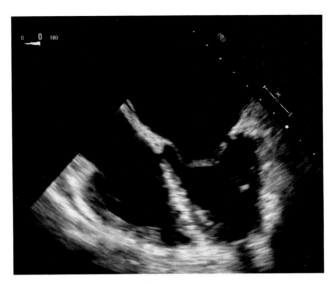

TEE in mitral stenosis. Severely dilated left atrium. Doming of the anterior mitral leaflet. Anterior diastolic motion of the posterior mitral leaflet. Note: TEE is rarely needed to determine the severity of mitral stenosis. It is typically used to look for thrombus in the left atrial appendage, and to help quantitate any coexisting mitral regurgitation.

FIGURE 3.32

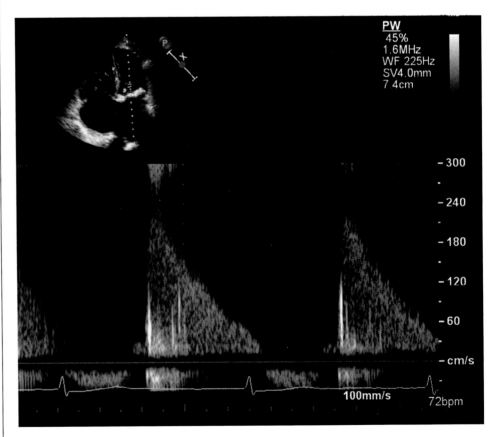

"Eyeball" deceleration time is easily determined to be under 600 msec in this patient, hence mitral stenosis is not severe (760/600 > 1). Pressure half time is equal to .29 × deceleration time. (.29 × 760 = 220.4)

QR 3.18a: Color flow can be used to calculate mitral stenosis orifice area.

QR 3.18b: Color flow can be used to calculate mitral stenosis orifice area.

QR 3.18c: Color flow can be used to calculate mitral stenosis orifice area.

FIGURE 3.33

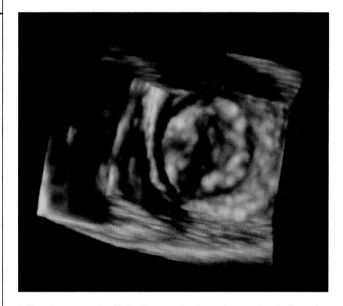

Mitral stenosis "bird's eye" view from the left atrium.

FIGURE 3.34

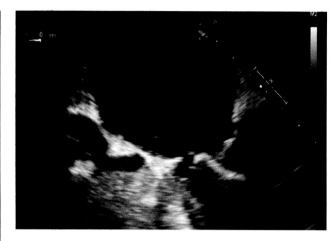

Mitral stenosis. TEE-guided balloon valvuloplasty.

QR 3.19a: Anterior mitral leaflet doming in mitral stenosis.

QR 3.19b: Anterior mitral leaflet doming in mitral stenosis.

QR 3.19c: Anterior mitral leaflet doming in mitral stenosis.

QR 3.19d: Anterior mitral leaflet doming in mitral stenosis.

QR 3.20: Massively dilated left atrium in a patient with mitral stenosis.

QR 3.21a: Cor triatriatum was sometimes clinically confused with mitral stenosis prior to the advent of echocardiography.

QR 3.21b: Cor triatriatum was sometimes clinically confused with mitral stenosis prior to the advent of echocardiography.

REFERENCES:

Remenyi B, Gentles TL. Congenital mitral valve lesions: correlation between morphology and imaging. *Ann Pediatr Cardiol*. 2012;5:3–12.

Abascal VM, Wilkins GT, Choong CY, et al. Echocardiographic evaluation of mitral valve structure and function in patients followed for at least 6 months after percutaneous balloon mitral valvuloplasty. *J Am Coll Cardiol*. 1988;12:606–615. *Echocardiographic scores of valvular morphology were obtained by assigning scores of 0 to 4 (with increasing abnormality) to each of four morphologic characteristics of the valve: leaflet mobility, thickening, calcification, and subvalvular thickening (but not calcification).*

ANSWER: D

THE OPENING SNAP OF MITRAL STENOSIS

" *Use of echocardiography to sort out the auscultatory findings* **"**
(or lack thereof).

The loud first heart sound of mitral stenosis, followed by the second heart sound (made louder if there is pulmonary hypertension), and then followed by the (usually) loud opening snap combine to give *an unmistakable* loud *triple rhythm* on auscultation. Echocardiography can be useful for determining the reason why the opening snap is conspicuously difficult to hear in some mitral stenosis patients.

A heavily calcified, immobile stenotic mitral valve is no longer PLIABLE, and both the loud first heart sound and the loud opening snap decrease in intensity, or actually become inaudible on auscultation. Moderate-to-severe mitral regurgitation (perhaps due to prior mitral valvuloplasty) may mask or attenuate the first heart sound. The opening snap may come earlier because of the elevated left atrial pressure and may "blend in" with the second heart sound on auscultation.

The opening snap may be misinterpreted as a widely split second heart sound. Raising the legs during auscultation (to increase venous return) may help sort this out:

The second heart sound splits *more* with *increased* venous return, because pulmonic valve closure gets delayed. The interval between an audibly single second heart sound and the opening snap does the opposite. Increased venous return elevates left atrial pressure and the mitral valve "snaps open" earlier, hence closer, to the second heart sound. It may also help to pay attention to the respiratory cycle. A widely split second heart sound may still perceptibly change with respiration.

Finally, if there is *no* bundle branch block on the ECG, why should the "second heart sound" be so widely split?

• ECG PEARL: Think of severe mitral stenosis when there is *left* atrial enlargement with *right* ventricular hypertrophy on the ECG.

REFERENCES:

 Julian D, Davies LG. Heart sounds and intracardiac pressures in mitral steno- sis. *Br Heart J.* 1957;19:486–494. *The time of occurrence of the opening snap, expressed as the A-OS interval (from the onset of the first component of aortic valve closure to the opening snap) showed a fair correlation with the left atrial pressure. This relationship was also dependent on the level of pressure in the left ventricle at the time of aortic valve closure. High aortic pressures make the opening snap later, and low aortic pressures make it earlier.*

Mounsey P. The opening snap of mitral stenosis. *Br Heart J.* 1953;15:135–142. *Auscultatory features and differential diagnosis of the opening snap.*

DIASTOLIC RUMBLE OF MITRAL STENOSIS

"   *rrrrrrrFoot........... Tah! Tah!*   **"**

The diastolic rumble is notoriously difficult to hear and to recognize on auscultation. The bell of the stethoscope (yes, you NEED the bell) is held lightly at the point of apical impulse with just enough pressure on the skin to create a seal that blocks out ambient noise.

The low-frequency nature of this diastolic flow murmur through the stenotic mitral valve orifice has been compared with "distant thunder," or a "rolling bowling ball." Our favorite description of a diastolic rumble is: "the distant sound of a horse-drawn carriage on a rickety wooden bridge."

Duroziez (the femoral pulse guy) used a variation of *"rrrrrrrFoot"* (the increasing loudness in the growl of a dog) as a phonic illustration of the presystolic accentuation caused by atrial contraction. The "Foot" includes the loud first heart sound, and is followed by the second heart sound *(tah)* and the opening snap *(tah)*.

The presystolic component of the diastolic rumble "fluffs-out" the first heart sound by blending into it. The unique combination of acoustic phenomena in mitral stenosis allows the experienced examiner to readily make the diagnosis of mitral stenosis on auscultation. Unfortunately, the only way to become "experienced" today is to listen to multiple *recordings* of different patients with mitral stenosis.

Fortunately, the authors below searched YouTube and made the recommendations that follow the reference:

REFERENCES:

Camm CF, Sunderland N, Camm AJ. A quality assessment of cardiac auscultation material on YouTube. *Clin Cardiol*. 2013;36:77–81.

http://www.youtube.com/watch?v=OQ9xrxDg3uc. Accessed November 30, 2013.
"Encompassed a range of murmurs with good audio quality and video animation."

http://www.youtube.com/watch?v=V5kSBrSA-sA. Accessed November 30, 2013.
"A video series containing lectures on heart murmurs, which was particularly comprehensive but contained fewer auscultation examples."

http://www.youtube.com/watch?v=xS3jX1FYG-M. Accessed November 30, 2013.
"A broad range of high-quality heart sounds and murmurs but lacked educational content to supplement this."

AORTIC REGURGITATION AND MITRAL STENOSIS

Aortic regurgitation (easily seen on echocardiography) causes confusion on auscultation in patients with coexisting mitral stenosis. Aortic regurgitation may decrease the intensity of the first heart sound (and of the opening snap) by limiting the excursion of the anterior mitral leaflet (confirmable by echocardiography).

Before echocardiography was available, the diastolic rumble of mitral stenosis was sometimes confused with the rumbling mid- to late-diastolic murmur of severe aortic regurgitation (described by Austin Flint). Severe aortic regurgitation can create *functional* mitral stenosis. The aortic regurgitation jet prevents the mitral valve from opening fully in diastole (confirmable by echocardiography).

REFERENCES:

Fortuin NJ, Craige E. On the mechanism of the Austin Flint murmur. *Circulation*. 1972;45:558–570. *This is a two-component murmur with both mid-diastolic and pre-systolic timing.*

Segal JP, Harvey WP, Corrado MA. The Austin Flint murmur: its differentiation from the murmur of rheumatic mitral stenosis. *Circulation*. 1958;18:1025–33.

Flachskampf FA, Weyman AE, Gillam L, et al. Aortic regurgitation shortens Doppler pressure half-time in mitral stenosis: clinical evidence, in vitro simulation and theoretic analysis. *J Am Coll Cardiol*. 1990;16:396–404. *Aortic regurgitation shortens directly-measured pressure half-time proportional to the regurgitant fraction – leading to mitral valve area overestimation. However, an increase in left ventricular compliance could offset this effect.*

Karp K, Teien D, Bjerle P, et al. Reassessment of valve area determinations in mitral stenosis by the pressure half-time method: impact of left ventricular stiffness and peak diastolic pressure difference. *J Am Coll Cardiol*. 1989;13:594–9. *Pressure half-time is shortened and valve area is overestimated if left ventricular stiffness is increased. This is often the case in patients with mitral stenosis associated with coronary heart disease, or with aortic stenosis.*

Fleming PR. The mechanism of the pulsus bisferiens. *Br Heart J*. 1957;19:519–24. *Patients with combined aortic stenosis and aortic regurgitation may have a pulse with two systolic upstrokes – the bisferiens pulse. Bedside examination technique: Raise the patient's wrist to shoulder level before palpating their radial pulse.*

Ikram H, Nixon PG, Fox JA. The haemodynamic implications of the bisferiens pulse. *Br Heart J*. 1964;26:452–9. *Extensive illustrations of the carotid pulse contour in aortic valve disease.*

Carlisle RP, Hecht HH, Lange RL. Observations on vascular sounds: the pistol-shot sound and the Korotkoff sound. *Circulation*. 1956;13:873–83. *Includes an explanation for the "zero diastolic" cuff readings in some patients with aortic regurgitation.*

Lange RL, Hecht HH. Genesis of pistol-shot and Korotkoff sounds. *Circulation*. 1958;18:975–8. *A "water-hammer" requires a compression wave at a velocity that approaches the speed of sound in liquid.*

NOT MITRAL STENOSIS

> **❝** *An elevated wedge pressure and a significantly lower left* **❞**
> *ventricular diastolic pressure during cardiac catheterization*
> *are not sufficient for the diagnosis of mitral stenosis.*

The wedge pressure is equivalent to mean left atrial pressure. Using the wedge to establish the mitral valve gradient is not reliable. The wedge pressure needs to be looked at for all the individual deflections, as they relate to the corresponding simultaneous diastolic mitral Doppler inflow patterns.

REFERENCES:

Nishimura RA, Rihal CS, Tajik AJ, et al. Accurate measurement of the transmitral gradient in patients with mitral stenosis: a simultaneous catheterization and Doppler echocardiographic study. *J Am Coll Cardiol*. 1994;24:152–158. *The Doppler-derived gradient is more accurate than pulmonary capillary wedge pressure for determination of the mean mitral valve gradient.*

Bramwell C. Signs simulating those of mitral stenosis. *Br Heart J*. 1943;5:24–26. *Auscultatory findings in army recruits and athletes. Blood flow through the mitral valve changes with body position. Blood is flowing almost directly against gravity with the patient on their back. The blood flows horizontally through the valve with the patient in the left lateral decubitus position. The observations in this study are relevant to positioning of the patient during the echocardiographic examination.*

MITRAL VALVE PROLAPSE—HEMODYNAMIC IMPORTANCE

In evaluating mitral valve regurgitation, the following sequence of echocardiographic findings can be discovered. Each finding has clinical implications. Together, the findings can tell a story.

The M-mode pattern of mitral valve prolapse is unmistakable but does not provide the hemodynamic importance. An additional finding of *flail chordae* on two-dimensional transthoracic, or if necessary transesophageal, echo usually indicates the need for surgical intervention. Mitral annular calcium, left atrial enlargement, and atrial fibrillation suggest chronicity. Doppler techniques evaluate severity.

QR 3.22a: Mid-to-late systolic mitral regurgitation in mitral valve prolapse.

QR 3.22b: Mid-to-late systolic mitral regurgitation in mitral valve prolapse.

FIGURE 3.35

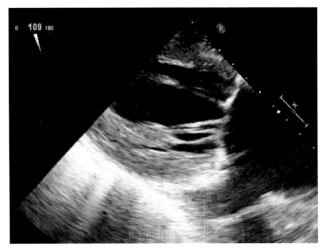

Transgastric TEE image of the mitral valve. Mild chordal thickening. No prolapse. Note: In this view the inferior wall is at the top.

QR 3.23: Color flow of mitral regurgitation must be distinguished from pulmonary vein inflow.

REFERENCE:

Devereux RB, Perloff JK, Reichek N, et al. Mitral valve prolapse. *Circulation.* 1976;54:3–14. *Excellent review. Postural changes affect the classic auscultatory signs (see Figure 6 in the article).*

MITRAL VALVE PROLAPSE DUE TO CORONARY ARTERY DISEASE

Posterior mitral leaflet prolapse may be the result of prior *inferior* myocardial infarction. The inferior wall motion abnormality may be subtle on echo. Looking for Q waves in leads II, III, and aVF on the ECG may be more useful. The findings of mitral annular calcium and left atrial enlargement on echo suggest chronicity.

FIGURE 3.36

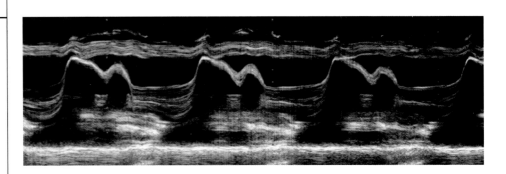

FIGURE 3.37

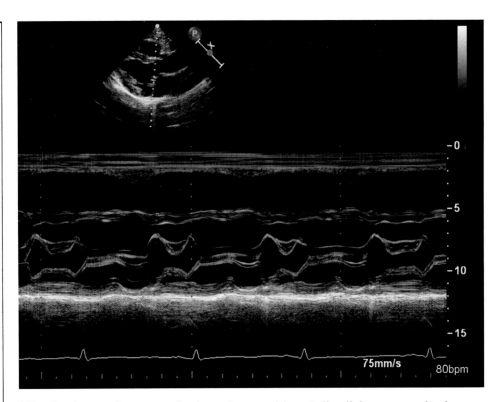

Mitral valve prolapse can be heard as a mid-systolic click on auscultation. "Luh" at the time of mitral valve closure. "Kit" in mid-systole as the valve buckles. "Up" at the time of mitral valve opening and aortic valve closure (S2). It sounds like: "look it up."

FIGURE 3.38

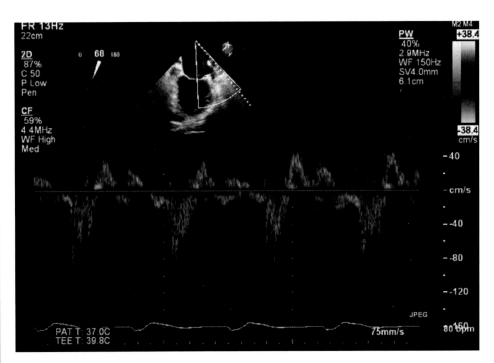

Late systolic flow reversal in the left pulmonary vein, indicating severe mitral regurgitation.

FIGURE 3.39

Timing of pulmonary vein flow reversal in severe mitral regurgitation.

 QR 3.24a: Posterior mitral leaflet prolapse.

 QR 3.24b: Posterior mitral leaflet prolapse.

 QR 3.24c: Posterior mitral leaflet prolapse.

 QR 3.24d: Posterior mitral leaflet prolapse.

 QR 3.24e: Posterior mitral leaflet prolapse.

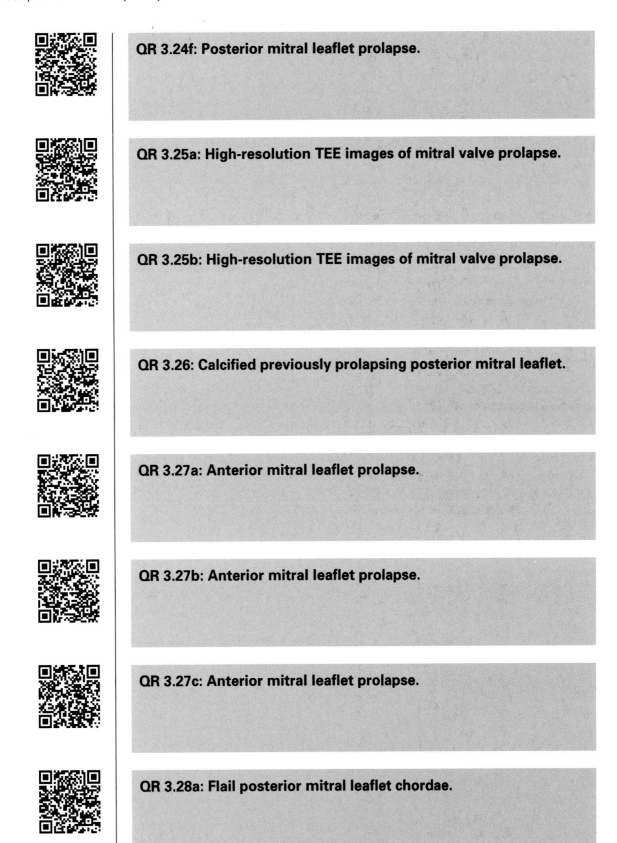

QR 3.24f: Posterior mitral leaflet prolapse.

QR 3.25a: High-resolution TEE images of mitral valve prolapse.

QR 3.25b: High-resolution TEE images of mitral valve prolapse.

QR 3.26: Calcified previously prolapsing posterior mitral leaflet.

QR 3.27a: Anterior mitral leaflet prolapse.

QR 3.27b: Anterior mitral leaflet prolapse.

QR 3.27c: Anterior mitral leaflet prolapse.

QR 3.28a: Flail posterior mitral leaflet chordae.

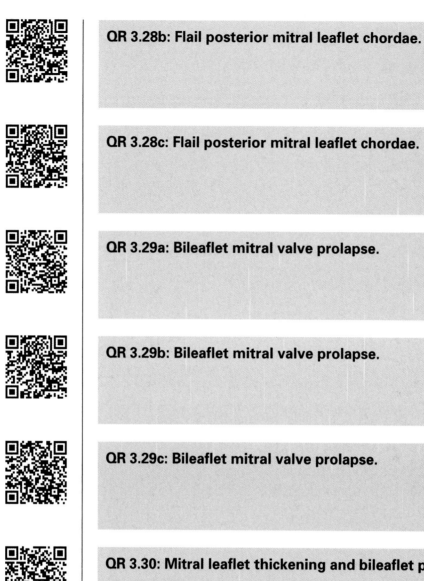

QR 3.28b: Flail posterior mitral leaflet chordae.

QR 3.28c: Flail posterior mitral leaflet chordae.

QR 3.29a: Bileaflet mitral valve prolapse.

QR 3.29b: Bileaflet mitral valve prolapse.

QR 3.29c: Bileaflet mitral valve prolapse.

QR 3.30: Mitral leaflet thickening and bileaflet prolapse.

QR 3.31a: Borderline posterior mitral leaflet prolapse.

QR 3.31b: Borderline posterior mitral leaflet prolapse.

REFERENCES:

 Voci P, Bilotta F, Caretta Q, et al. Papillary muscle perfusion pattern. A hypothesis for ischemic papillary muscle dysfunction. *Circulation*. 1995;91:1714–1718. *The posteromedial papillary muscle receives blood, in most cases, from a single supply from the posterior descending branch of a dominant right coronary artery. Rupture of the anterolateral papillary muscle is less common (25% of papillary muscle rupture cases). The reason for this is a dual blood supply from the first obtuse marginal artery, originating from the left circumflex artery, and from the first diagonal branch, originating from the left anterior descending artery.*

 Levine RA, Triulzi MO, Harrigan P, et al. The relationship of mitral annular shape to the diagnosis of mitral valve prolapse. *Circulation*. 1987;75: 756–767.

Nishimura RA, MCGoon MD, Shub C, et al. Echocardiographically documented mitral valve prolapse: long-term follow-up of 237 patients. *N Engl J Med*. 1985;313:1305–1309. *Most patients with echocardiographic evidence of mitral valve prolapse have a benign course, but subsets at high risk for the development of progressive mitral regurgitation, sudden death, cerebral embolic events, or infective endocarditis can be identified by echocardiography.*

 Avierinos JF, Gersh BJ, Melton LJ III, et al. Natural history of asymptomatic mitral valve prolapse in the community. *Circulation*. 2002;106:1355–1361.

MITRAL ANNULAR CALCIUM

QUESTION:

Which of the following disorders have been associated with mitral annular calcification?

A. Cardiac conduction disorders.

B. Atrial fibrillation.

C. Atherosclerosis of the aorta.

D. Stroke.

E. All of the above with even more disorders below.

Mitral annular calcification (MAC) is a common finding in the elderly. It is also found in younger patients with endstage renal disease. MAC may predispose the mitral valve to infection with endocarditis in this population of patients.

MAC typically involves the posterior mitral leaflet annulus where it joins the left ventricular wall. A rare caseous variant may be manifested on the echocardiogram as calcification with an echolucent center. The appearance may suggest endocarditis with an abscess, and the mitral valve has to be carefully scrutinized for vegetations or leaflet perforation.

The extent of calcification does not correlate with the degree of mitral valve obstruction. Planimetry of the mitral area may not be possible when there are excessive artifacts from the calcium. Doppler is required (to determine whether suspected valvular stenosis is really present) when leaflet mobility is unclear on two-dimensional echo images.

There are *pitfalls* in the echocardiographic interpretation of associated findings:

- Pressure half time may be misleading (but the isovolumic relaxation time should not be prolonged in valvular stenosis).
- The presence of MAC affects the velocity of adjacent myocardium. Consequently, tissue Doppler interpretation may also be misleading.
- The left atrium may be enlarged due to age, diastolic dysfunction, or associated mitral regurgitation.

QR 3.32a: Mitral annular calcium.

QR 3.32b: Mitral annular calcium.

FIGURE 3.40

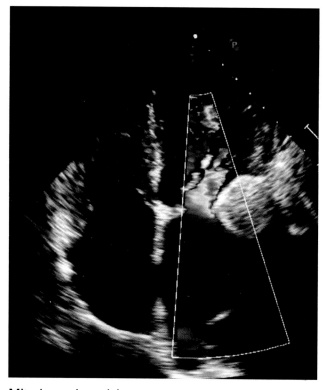

Mitral annular calcium.

QR 3.32c: Mitral annular calcium.

QR 3.32d: Mitral annular calcium.

QR 3.33: Mitral valve prolapse with consequent mitral annular calcification and possible superimposed vegetation. Caution: An echocardiographic diagnosis of a superimposed vegetation will likely result in mitral valve replacement instead of an attempt to repair the valve.

QR 3.34: Calcified papillary muscle tip.

QR 3.35: Calcified papillary muscle tips. Pacemaker wire in the right ventricle.

REFERENCES:

Pomerance A. Pathological and clinical study of calcification of the mitral valve ring. *J Clin Pathol.* 1970;23:354–361.

Carpentier AF, Pellerin M, Fuzellier JF, et al. Extensive calcification of the mitral valve annulus: pathology and surgical management. *J Thorac Cardiovasc Surg.* 1996;111:718–729; discussion 729–730. *Extensive, expert surgical paper. Complete annulus decalcification and valve repair can be done safely in patients with mitral valve regurgitation even when the calcification process deeply involves the myocardium.*

ANSWER: E

MITRAL REGURGITATION—CONTINUOUS WAVE DOPPLER

QUESTION:

Which of the following aspects of the mitral regurgitation continuous Doppler flow jet is NOT clinically useful?

A. Flow acceleration.

B. Flow deceleration.

C. Peak velocity.

D. Time of onset in relation to the QRS.

E. Envelope contour.

The time it takes for mitral regurgitant flow to *accelerate* from 1 to 3 m per second is used to determine left ventricular dP/dt. It can provide instant feedback about immediate worsening or improvement in global systolic left ventricular function. This is one of the parameters used for echocardiographic guidance of pacemaker optimization in patients with left ventricular dysfunction.

Flow deceleration is affected by an abnormally rapid rise in left atrial pressure in patients with acute severe mitral regurgitation. It serves as a "red flag" in patients with impinging eccentric color flow jets. Color flow Doppler can significantly underestimate severity of valvular regurgitation when there is loss of leaflet coaptation and/or when the color flow jet is eccentric.

The peak velocity of the mitral regurgitation jet is normally 5 m per second and does not change in clinically useful fashion with changing left atrial pressure. It may therefore come as a surprise that although it should work in theory, using the mitral regurgitation velocity with the Bernoulli equation does not help clinically in the determination of left atrial pressure.

The time of onset in relation to the QRS can identify the rare patient with diastolic mitral regurgitation due to acute severe aortic regurgitation. It is quite common to find delayed onset of mitral regurgitation in patients with mitral valve prolapse. A "lobster claw" contour can be found in apical hypertrophic cardiomyopathy. It can be confused with mitral regurgitation with an incomplete envelope. The "hypertrophic claw" is recorded in the left ventricular cavity not in the left atrium.

QR 3.36a: Apical left ventricular hypertrophy.

FIGURE 3.41

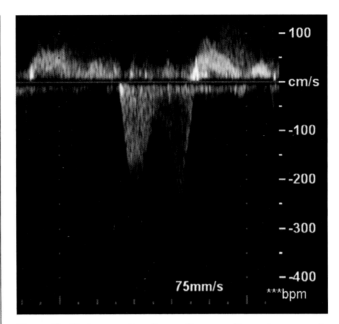

Systolic "lobster claw" continuous Doppler waveform in hypertrophic cardiomyopathy.

QR 3.36b: Apical left ventricular hypertrophy.

QR 3.36c: Apical left ventricular hypertrophy.

QR 3.37: Spade shape of color flow Doppler in apical left ventricular hypertrophy.

REFERENCES:

Bargiggia GS, Bertucci C, Recusani F, et al. A new method for estimating left ventricular dP/dt by continuous wave Doppler-echocardiography. Validation studies at cardiac catheterization. *Circulation*. 1989;80:1287–1292.

Chen C, Rodriguez L, Guerrero JL, et al. Noninvasive estimation of the instantaneous first derivative of left ventricular pressure using continuous-wave Doppler echocardiography. *Circulation*. 1991;83:2101–2110.

ANSWER: Some aspects of answer C are surprisingly not clinically useful.

MITRAL REGURGITATION AND THE RADIUS OF COLOR FLOW DOPPLER CONVERGENCE

" *Three easy PISAs.* **"**

Which of the following three color flow parameters is unrelated to the remaining two?

A. PISA.

B. Vena contracta.

C. Regurgitant jet area.

PISA

Proximal isovelocity surface area depicts the convergence of blood flow into a regurgitant orifice. "Eyeball" determination that mitral regurgitation is severe can be done by looking at the PISA radius. The purpose is to estimate the effective regurgitant orifice area, *e*ffectionately known as the ERO. Severe mitral regurgitation has an ERO >0.38 cm^2.

PISA and the math behind the following three radius measurements are painstakingly and laboriously explained in the references. Mitral regurgitation velocity has to be around 5 m/sec for the math to be correct.

Rule 1: ERO = $r^2/2$ (when aliasing velocity is set to 40 cm/sec)

Rule 2 is the quick "eyeball" method: Regurgitation is severe if PISA radius is 1 cm or greater

(aliasing velocity has to be set to 30 cm/sec)

Rule 3 works for any aliasing velocity: Regurgitation is severe if $1.9 \times r^2 \times$ aliasing velocity = 60 or greater.

Vena Contracta

Vena contracta is straightforward: Regurgitation is severe if the two-dimensional diameter is 7 mm or greater. The vena contracta shows some part of the actual regurgitant orifice. It is the "waist" between the PISA and the regurgitant jet in the left atrium. Vena contracta was initially validated by comparing it with the simultaneous PISA. When present on the echo, it is used clinically to validate the PISA measurements above. Three-dimensional reconstruction of the vena contracta is laborious, but can show the entire regurgitant orifice, the holy grail of the three rules above.

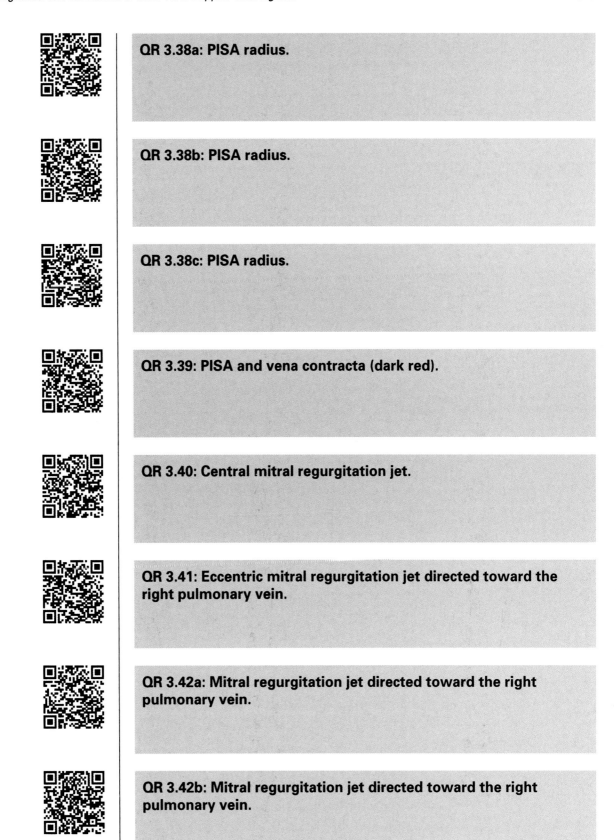

QR 3.38a: PISA radius.

QR 3.38b: PISA radius.

QR 3.38c: PISA radius.

QR 3.39: PISA and vena contracta (dark red).

QR 3.40: Central mitral regurgitation jet.

QR 3.41: Eccentric mitral regurgitation jet directed toward the right pulmonary vein.

QR 3.42a: Mitral regurgitation jet directed toward the right pulmonary vein.

QR 3.42b: Mitral regurgitation jet directed toward the right pulmonary vein.

QR 3.43: Normal pulmonary vein inflow should not be confused with mitral regurgitation.

REFERENCES:

 Irvine T, Li XK, Sahn DJ, et al. Assessment of mitral regurgitation. *Heart.* 2002;88(Suppl 4):iv11–iv19.

 Hall SA, Brickner ME, Willett DL, et al. Assessment of mitral regurgitation severity by Doppler color flow mapping of the vena contracta. *Circulation.* 1997;95:636–642.

Enriquez-Sarano M, Seward JB, Bailey KR, et al. Effective regurgitant orifice area: a noninvasive Doppler development of an old hemodynamic concept. *J Am Coll Cardiol.* 1994;23:443–451.

Enriquez-Sarano M, Avierinos JF, Messika-Zeitoun D, et al. Quantitative determinants of the outcome of asymptomatic mitral regurgitation. *N Engl J Med.* 2005;352:875–883. *Quantitative grading of mitral regurgitation is a powerful predictor of the clinical outcome of asymptomatic mitral regurgitation.*

Castello R, Pearson AC, Lenzen P, et al. Effect of mitral regurgitation on pulmonary venous velocities derived from transesophageal echocardiography color-guided pulsed Doppler imaging. *J Am Coll Cardiol.* 1991;17:1499–1506. *The sensitivity of reversed systolic flow for severe mitral regurgitation was 90% (9 of 10), the specificity was 100% (65 of 65), the positive predictive value was 100% (9 of 9), the negative predictive value was 98% (65 of 66) and the predictive accuracy was 99% (74 of 75).*

ANSWER: Always pick the longest answer.

TRICUSPID REGURGITATION APHORISMS

"   *Color flow Doppler reliably detects all degrees of tricuspid*   **"**
regurgitation—except perhaps when you need it most—when
it is wide open.

The size of the color flow jet is the starting point for determining severity.

Other measures and findings include:

• Doppler characteristics such as signal strength and signal duration.
• Contour by continuous wave may show early systolic deceleration and late systolic cutoff.
• PISA and vena contracta indicate regurgitant volume.
• Increased right atrial and right ventricular size should be noted.

The shape of the interventricular septum helps to differentiate between severe right ventricular *pressure* overload and severe right ventricular *volume* overload. Loss of leaflet coaptation can be demonstrated with two-dimensional echo. Leaflet thickening and retraction are found in *carcinoid* tricuspid valve disease. Chordal rupture can occur with trauma.

Leaflet destruction may be seen with endocarditis. Pacemaker wires and catheters across the tricuspid valve cause variable degrees of regurgitation. Bedside examination after the echocardiographic diagnosis is useful for follow-up decisions.

The neck vein findings may be influenced by pericardial compliance. An increase in the loudness of the tricuspid regurgitation murmur during inspiration is a classic finding. The Doppler tricuspid regurgitation signal also increases during respiration.

The following *bedside technique* may be useful to evaluate a murmur for respiratory variation:

Inspiration may be too distracting to comment on the change in loudness of the tricuspid regurgitation murmur. During held deep expiration, left-sided murmurs should become MORE audible because there is less interposed air between the stethoscope and the heart.

During held deep expiration, tricuspid regurgitation becomes LESS audible.

FIGURE 3.42

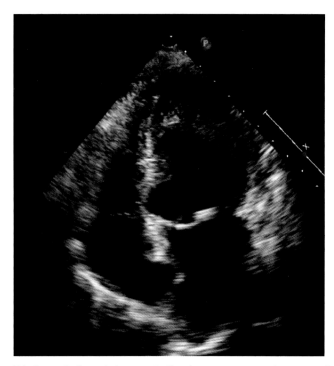

Right to left atrial septal displacement can be seen in recent onset tricuspid regurgitation with a noncompliant right atrium.

QR 3.44: The tricuspid regurgitation v wave cutoff sign indicates elevated end-systolic right atrial pressure.

QR 3.45a: Severe tricuspid regurgitation and/or severe pulmonary hypertension can cause systolic flow reversal in the hepatic veins.

QR 3.45b: Severe tricuspid regurgitation and/or severe pulmonary hypertension can cause systolic flow reversal in the hepatic veins.

QR 3.45c: Severe tricuspid regurgitation and/or severe pulmonary hypertension can cause systolic flow reversal in the hepatic veins.

QR 3.45d: Severe tricuspid regurgitation and/or severe pulmonary hypertension can cause systolic flow reversal in the hepatic veins.

QR 3.45e: Severe tricuspid regurgitation and/or severe pulmonary hypertension can cause systolic flow reversal in the hepatic veins.

QR 3.45f: Severe tricuspid regurgitation and/or severe pulmonary hypertension can cause systolic flow reversal in the hepatic veins.

QR 3.46: Phasic respiratory hepatic vein flow changes (unaffected by the first premature ventricular contraction).

QR 3.47: Pulsatile to-and-fro hepatic vein flow. Pulmonary hypertension and sinus tachycardia.

QR 3.48a: Severe tricuspid regurgitation. Color flow of systolic hepatic vein flow reversal (red). A color M-mode beam can be used to time the reversal with the ECG.

QR 3.48b: Severe tricuspid regurgitation. Color flow of systolic hepatic vein flow reversal (red). A color M-mode beam can be used to time the reversal with the ECG.

QR 3.48c: Severe tricuspid regurgitation. Color flow of systolic hepatic vein flow reversal (red). A color M-mode beam can be used to time the reversal with the ECG.

QR 3.48d: Severe tricuspid regurgitation. Color flow of systolic hepatic vein flow reversal (red). A color M-mode beam can be used to time the reversal with the ECG.

QR 3.48e: Severe tricuspid regurgitation. Color flow of systolic hepatic vein flow reversal (red). A color M-mode beam can be used to time the reversal with the ECG.

QR 3.48f: Severe tricuspid regurgitation. Color flow of systolic hepatic vein flow reversal (red). A color M-mode beam can be used to time the reversal with the ECG.

QR 3.48g: Severe tricuspid regurgitation. Color flow of systolic hepatic vein flow reversal (red). A color M-mode beam can be used to time the reversal with the ECG.

QR 3.48h: Severe tricuspid regurgitation. Color flow of systolic hepatic vein flow reversal (red). A color M-mode beam can be used to time the reversal with the ECG.

QR 3.49a: Severe tricuspid regurgitation demonstrated by reversal of saline contrast into the hepatic veins after injection into an arm vein.

QR 3.49b: Severe tricuspid regurgitation demonstrated by reversal of saline contrast into the hepatic veins after injection into an arm vein.

QR 3.50: Dilated inferior vena cava due to elevated right atrial pressure.

QR 3.51a: Normal inferior vena cava oscillation in a patient with normal right atrial pressure.

QR 3.51b: Normal inferior vena cava oscillation in a patient with normal right atrial pressure.

QR 3.52: Normal brief hepatic vein flow reversal following the atrial contraction.

QR 3.53: Visual exercise. Try to time the red hepatic vein flow reversal with the adjacent tricuspid annulus motion. This is as challenging as inspection of jugular vein flow in search of the atrial contraction wave. You can cheat and use color flow M-mode with an ECG to hone your visual timing skills.

QR 3.54: Normal inspiratory increase in hepatic vein flow toward the heart (blue color flow).

QR 3.55: Chronic severe tricuspid regurgitation. The pacemaker wire restricts tricuspid leaflet closure.

QR 3.56: Severe tricuspid regurgitation.

QR 3.57a: Severe tricuspid regurgitation with loss of leaflet coaptation.

QR 3.57b: Severe tricuspid regurgitation with loss of leaflet coaptation.

QR 3.57c: Severe tricuspid regurgitation with loss of leaflet coaptation.

QR 3.58: Tricuspid regurgitation from the mid-esophagus.

QR 3.59: Tricuspid regurgitation directed toward the eustachian valve.

REFERENCES:

Nath J, Foster E, Heidenreich PA. Impact of tricuspid regurgitation on long-term survival. *J Am Coll Cardiol.* 2004;43:405–409. *Increasing severity is associated with worse survival in men (veteran hospital study) regardless of left ventricular ejection fraction, or pulmonary artery pressure. Severe tricuspid regurgitation is associated with a poor prognosis, independent of age, biventricular systolic function, right ventricular size, or dilation of the inferior vena cava.*

Sepulveda G, Lukas DS. The diagnosis of tricuspid insufficiency; clinical features in 60 cases with associated mitral valve disease. *Circulation.* 1955;11: 552–563.

Morgan JR, Forker AD. Isolated tricuspid insufficiency. *Circulation.* 1971; 43:559–564. *A useful test is the Valsalva maneuver; the murmur of tricuspid insufficiency will return in about 1 second on release of Valsalva, whereas left heart murmurs will usually not return for 3 seconds or longer.*

Brickner PW, Scudder WT, Weinrib M. Pulsating varicose veins in functional tricuspid insufficiency. Case report and venous pressure tracing. *Circulation.* 1962;25:126–129. *As the degree of cardiac compensation improves, the physical signs of tricuspid insufficiency disappear.*

Verel D, Sandler G, Mazurkie SJ. Tricuspid incompetence in cor pulmonale. *Br Heart J.* 1962;24:441–444. *In patients with emphysema, cor pulmonale, or rheumatic heart disease, the site of maximal intensity of the tricuspid insufficiency murmur is commonly over the free edge of the liver.*

Muller O, Shillingford J. Tricuspid incompetence. *Br Heart J.* 1954;16:195–207. *Detailed description of the murmur.*

Hultgren HN. Venous pistol shot sounds. *Am J Cardiol.* 1962;10:667–672.

Hansing CE, Rowe GG. Tricuspid insufficiency. A study of hemodynamics and pathogenesis. *Circulation.* 1972;45:793–799. *Duroziez described a xiphoid systolic murmur, enlarged right atrium, distended neck veins with systolic pulsation, hepatic enlargement and pulsation, and peripheral cyanosis.*

Practical Tips from the Article Above

The characteristic murmur with its inspiratory accentuation may be missed even in cases with severe tricuspid insufficiency.

Jugular venous V waves are not always present and may be obscured by distended neck veins.

The hepatic pulsation is readily detected only with severe tricuspid insufficiency and may be confused with a transmitted pulse from the aorta or right ventricle.

The severity of tricuspid insufficiency is influenced by exercise, deep breathing, and cardiac function.

PULMONARY VALVE REGURGITATION ON ECHO

❝   *An audible murmur is relevant!*   **❞**

Pulmonary regurgitation is easily recorded during the initial parasternal echocardiographic views as a color flow jet. The jet is present in the majority of adult patients and does not indicate pulmonic valve pathology. This normal color flow pattern is usually interpreted and reported as a trace-to-mild pulmonic regurgitation.

Unfortunately, there is no gold standard for reference, so it is not possible to standardize criteria for severity. However, the normal diastolic regurgitation jet *should not be audible* on auscultation. Pulmonary regurgitation is influenced by respiration. The right atrial contraction slows down the regurgitation jet.

The peak *early* velocity of the pulmonary regurgitation jet is determined by the initial early diastolic gradient between the pulmonary artery and the right ventricle. The peak *late* velocity of the pulmonary regurgitation jet is determined by the end-diastolic gradient between the pulmonary artery and the right ventricle, and can be used to estimate the right ventricular end-diastolic pressure. The M-mode pattern has been used for pulmonary hypertension and for pulmonic valve stenosis.

QR 3.60a: Color flow of mild pulmonic valve regurgitating very close to the area where the proximal left main coronary artery can be visualized. Timing the color flow with color M-mode can be useful. Pulmonic regurgitation is limited to diastole. Coronary flow occurs both in systole and in diastole. Unusually prominent coronary artery color flow can be a clue to possible left main coronary artery stenosis. In this case, the flow represents pulmonic regurgitation. We asked singer Tom Jones how often patients with mild pulmonic regurgitation have multiple small jets on color flow Doppler. He said it is not unusual.

QR 3.60b: Color flow of mild pulmonic valve regurgitation originating very close to the area where the proximal left main coronary artery can be visualized.

QR 3.60c: Color flow of mild pulmonic valve regurgitation originating very close to the area where the proximal left main coronary artery can be visualized.

QR 3.61a: Color flow in the left main coronary artery.

QR 3.61b: Color flow in the left main coronary artery.

QR 3.61c: Color flow in the left main coronary artery.

REFERENCES:

 Simpson IA, De Belder MA, Kenny A, et al. How to quantitate valve regurgitation by echo Doppler techniques. British Society of Echocardiography. *Br Heart J*. 1995;73(5 Suppl 2):1–9.

 Bruce CJ, Connolly HM. Right-sided valve disease deserves a little more respect. *Circulation*. 2009;119:2726–2734.

Cohn KE, Hultgren HN. The Graham-Steell murmur re-evaluated. *N Engl J Med*. 1966;274:486–489.

 Masuyama T, Kodama K, Kitabatake A, et al. Continuous-wave Doppler echocardiographic detection of pulmonary regurgitation and its application to non-invasive estimation of pulmonary artery pressure. *Circulation*. 1986;74:484–492.

PROSTHETIC VALVES

66 *Sometimes it's not so good to walk around with a song in your heart.* **99**

QUESTION: **Which finding is NOT a feature of a bioprosthetic valve?**

A. Three bright immobile reflections with an attenuation artifact.

B. Horizontal stripes on the continuous wave Doppler signal (that may indicate valve failure).

C. Parallel "comet tail" reverberation artifacts on TEE of a mitral prosthesis.

D. Musical cooing "seagull" murmur (that may indicate valve failure).

The echocardiographic hallmark of a bioprosthetic valve is the presence of three struts. The vibrations produced by a tear in a bioprosthetic leaflet may create a "musical instrument" that is detectable on auscultation (and on Doppler examination).

Bedside Auscultation Challenge:

Mitral vs. Aortic *Mechanical* Prosthesis

Mechanical valves may have a faint opening click on auscultation (in addition to the loud closure CLICK). The challenge to the reader is to time the two different sounding clicks along with the native closure sound and determine if the patient has a mitral or aortic mechanical prosthesis.

	S1	S2

Mitral mechanical on auscultation: CLICK .... Dub click

Aortic mechanical on auscultation: Lub click............. CLICK

CLICK = loud closure click

Lub Dub = native remaining valve closure sounds

Faint click = prosthesis opening ejection click

.... = the dots represent systole (S1[Lub].......... S2[Dub])

Echocardiography will easily determine mitral versus aortic location of a prosthesis, but it may sometimes come up short in distinguishing a mechanical from a biological prosthesis. In such cases, aside from asking the patient (duh!), and using the stethoscope as discussed above, one can use fluoroscopy to image the prosthesis.

FIGURE 3.43

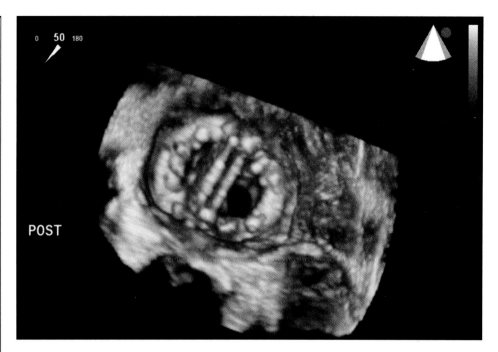

Mitral bileaflet prosthesis.

FIGURE 3.44

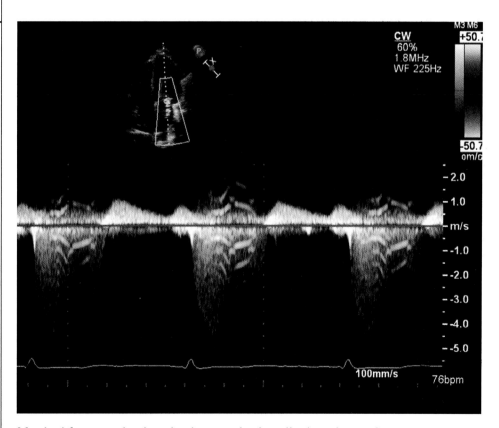

Musical frequencies in mitral regurgitation displayed as stripes.

FIGURE 3.45

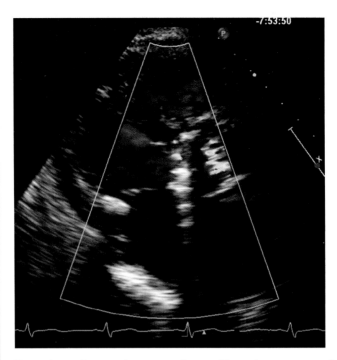

Reverberation and attenuation artifact due to a mechanical aortic prosthesis.

FIGURE 3.46

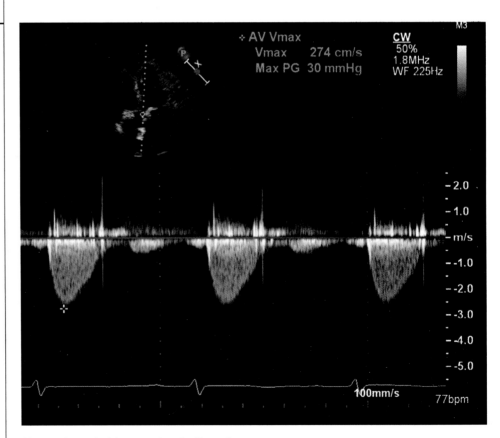

Normal aortic bioprosthesis Doppler.

FIGURE 3.47

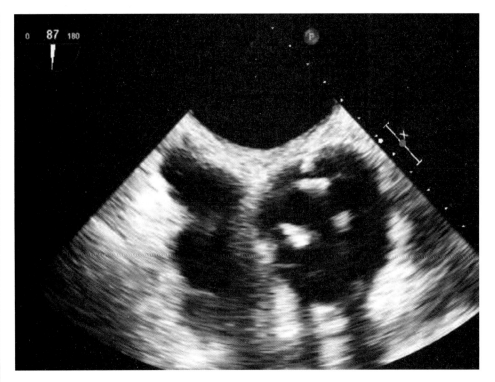

Aortic bioprosthesis struts on TEE.

FIGURE 3.48

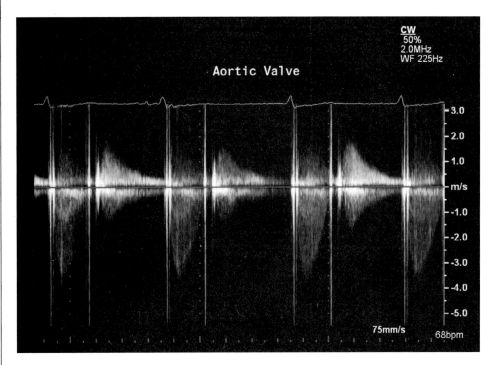

Aortic mechanical prosthesis opening and closing.

QR 3.62: Aortic prosthesis dehiscence.

QR 3.63: Abnormal bileaflet mechanical mitral prosthesis. The opening of the leaflet on the left is slightly delayed.

QR 3.64a: Aortic bioprosthesis struts on TEE.

QR 3.64b: Aortic bioprosthesis struts on TEE.

QR 3.65a: Mitral bioprosthesis.

QR 3.65b: Mitral bioprosthesis.

QR 3.66: Paravalvular mitral regurgitation. Mechanical mitral prosthesis.

QR 3.67a: Partial dehiscence of a prosthetic mitral ring.

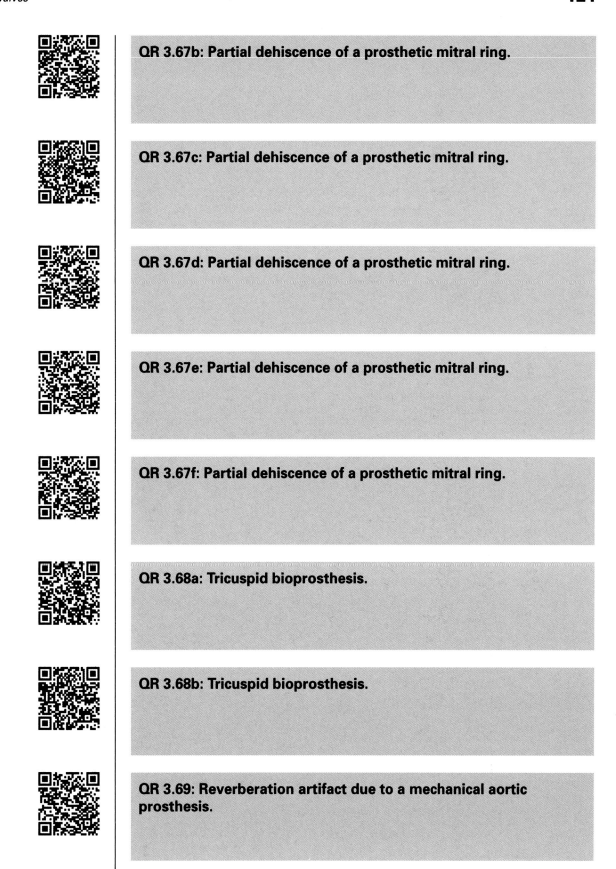

QR 3.67b: Partial dehiscence of a prosthetic mitral ring.

QR 3.67c: Partial dehiscence of a prosthetic mitral ring.

QR 3.67d: Partial dehiscence of a prosthetic mitral ring.

QR 3.67e: Partial dehiscence of a prosthetic mitral ring.

QR 3.67f: Partial dehiscence of a prosthetic mitral ring.

QR 3.68a: Tricuspid bioprosthesis.

QR 3.68b: Tricuspid bioprosthesis.

QR 3.69: Reverberation artifact due to a mechanical aortic prosthesis.

QR 3.70a: Mitral and aortic bioprosthesis.

QR 3.70b: Mitral and aortic bioprosthesis.

QR 3.71a: Fluoroscopic appearance of a mechanical mitral bileaflet prosthesis.

QR 3.71b: Fluoroscopic appearance of a mechanical mitral bileaflet prosthesis.

QR 3.72a: Fluoroscopic appearance of a ball-in-cage Starr-Edwards aortic prosthesis.

QR 3.72b: Fluoroscopic appearance of a ball-in-cage Starr-Edwards aortic prosthesis.

REFERENCES:

Burstow DJ, Nishimura RA, Bailey KR, et al. Continuous wave Doppler echocardiographic measurement of prosthetic valve gradients. A simultaneous Doppler-catheter correlative study. *Circulation.* 1989;80:504–514.

Chafizadeh ER, Zoghbi WA. Doppler echocardiographic assessment of the St. Jude Medical prosthetic valve in the aortic position using the continuity equation. *Circulation.* 1991;83:213–223.

ANSWER: C

PATIENT PROSTHESIS MISMATCH

QUESTION:

An echocardiogram *following* aortic valve replacement shows a peak systolic gradient of 64 mmHg. Which preoperative finding would have helped predict this undesirable postoperative outcome?

A. Age.

B. Gender.

C. Body habitus.

D. Etiology of native valve disease.

Patients with a small body mass index, and hence, a small size aorta may wind up with a small-diameter aortic prosthesis that has a significant gradient.

REFERENCES:

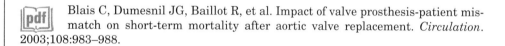 Mohty D, Malouf JF, Girard SE, et al. Impact of prosthesis-patient mismatch on long-term survival in patients with small St. Jude Medical mechanical prostheses in the aortic position. *Circulation.* 2006;113:420–426.

Blais C, Dumesnil JG, Baillot R, et al. Impact of valve prosthesis-patient mismatch on short-term mortality after aortic valve replacement. *Circulation.* 2003;108:983–988.

Rahimtoola SH. The problem of valve prosthesis-patient mismatch. *Circulation.* 1978;58:20–24.

ANSWER: Always pick C

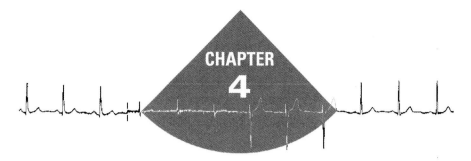

PREGNANCY

PREGNANCY AND ECHOCARDIOGRAPHY

QUESTION:

Echo may be ordered during pregnancy for the following reasons. In which case is echo LEAST likely to provide additional useful clinical insight?

A. New murmur.

B. New atrial S4 gallop.

C. Maternal congenital heart disease.

D. New onset of hypertension.

E. New dyspnea on exertion.

F. New arrhythmias.

Echocardiography is a safe and accepted tool for evaluation of cardiac disease during pregnancy. It is used in conjunction with the history, physical examination, and electrocardiogram. The cardiac evaluation seeks to determine the risk of continuing the pregnancy. Stenotic lesions increase risk, while regurgitant lesions typically do not. Marfan syndrome and severe pulmonary hypertension pose a prohibitive risk. Although a ventricular S3 gallop may be normal during late pregnancy, an atrial S4 gallop is not.

ANSWER: Hard to say. Answers A and E are discussed in the subsequent sections.

FLOW MURMUR OF PREGNANCY

The judicious use of echocardiography helps make the distinction between the common normal flow murmur of pregnancy and a pathological murmur.

Serial cardiac auscultation (rather than serial echocardiography) remains the diagnostic tool of choice during follow-up visits for the remaining course of the pregnancy. The nature of a flow murmur is

125

different than that of a pathological murmur. Flow murmurs can change with body position and with respiration. A flow murmur is usually *localized*—it is most likely to be heard at the upper left sternal border. Loud systolic murmurs (and most diastolic murmurs) are likely to be pathological rather than flow murmurs.

The best way to acquire confidence in murmur differentiation is to listen to many pathological murmurs. Mitral regurgitation and aortic stenosis are common pathological murmurs in routine adult practice. Mitral regurgitation murmurs can be blowing. Aortic stenosis murmurs can be harsh. Repeated auscultation of these murmurs will build the skill to identify the subtle auditory differences in the nature of a flow murmur.

The pitch of a flow murmur is typically more "gentle to the ears," and it too is best learned and recognized by listening to many examples. If one has the opportunity to care for many pregnant patients, one should listen to their flow murmurs during each and every visit.

Pre Pep Talk Question: How do you get to Carnegie Hall?

Answer: Practice, practice, practice.

Pep Talk:

To the reader who is skeptical about their skills in auscultation, we would like to offer the following words of encouragement: The human mind has the capacity to find (and subconsciously memorize) subtle unique auditory features of the murmurs of different patients.

We offer as proof for this—the fact that all of us have gotten a phone call from someone (perhaps a long-lost friend) and immediately identified the person after a word or two—*just by hearing their voice*. This can also happen with repetitive methodical auscultation. How frequently do YOU listen to the murmur of the high-risk patient during the course of their pregnancy?

THE MAMMARY SOUFFLE

This is a continuous arterial murmur of pregnancy.

It is due to enlarged tortuous branches of the internal mammary artery. It arises at the site of anastomosis between branches of aortic intercostal arteries and branches of the internal mammary artery, during the last month of pregnancy and during lactation. The murmur is obliterated by pressing down with the stethoscope, or by finger pressure next to the stethoscope.

QR 4.1: Prominent pulsatility of the aorta during late pregnancy due to the increased cardiac output state.

REFERENCES:

 Jahjah L, Vandenbossche JL. Continuous heart murmur in a 26-year-old woman. *Eur J Echocardiogr.* 2009;10:442–443.

 Tabatznik B, Randall TW, Hersch C. The mammary souffle of pregnancy and lactation. *Circulation.* 1960;22:1069–1073.

 Scott JT, Murphy EA. Mammary souffle of pregnancy: report of two cases simulating patent ductus arteriosus. *Circulation.* 1958;18:1038–1043.

DYSPNEA DURING PREGNANCY

QUESTION:

A patient becomes progressively more short of breath at the 30th week of pregnancy. Which echocardiographic finding is indicative of an increased maternal risk for an adverse cardiac event during this pregnancy? More than one answer may be correct.

A. Mitral pressure half time of 300 msec.

B. Tricuspid regurgitation maximum velocity of 5 m/s.

C. Bicuspid aortic valve with a systolic maximum velocity of 3 m/s.

D. Secundum atrial septal defect.

Progressive dyspnea on exertion is a common complaint in late pregnancy.

Echocardiography plays a pivotal role in the evaluation of this typically benign, but potentially ominous symptom. Obstructive left heart lesions such as mitral stenosis should be suspected on the physical examination and should prompt an echocardiographic evaluation.

Severe pulmonary hypertension is a *contraindication* to pregnancy. The decreased peripheral vascular resistance of pregnancy helps explain why atrial septal defects are usually well tolerated, and why the left-to-right shunt may not change for the worse as pregnancy progresses.

• BEDSIDE TIP: The flow murmur of an undiagnosed secundum atrial septal defect may get mistakenly *dismissed* on physical examination as an unusually loud flow murmur of pregnancy.

REFERENCES:

Penning S, Robinson KD, Major CA, et al. A comparison of echocardiography and pulmonary artery catheterization for evaluation of pulmonary artery pressures in pregnant patients with suspected pulmonary hypertension. *Am J Obstet Gynecol.* 2001;184:1568–1570. *Echocardiography overestimates pulmonary artery pressures compared with catheterization in pregnant patients. Patients with structural cardiac defects appear to have a significantly greater discrepancy in pulmonary artery pressures. One-third of pregnant patients with normal pulmonary artery pressures may be misclassified as having pulmonary artery hypertension. Plethora of the inferior vena cava on the echocardiogram is also unreliable due to the volume overload of pregnancy.*

 Janda S, Shahidi N, Gin K, et al. Diagnostic accuracy of echocardiography for pulmonary hypertension: a systematic review and meta-analysis. *Heart.* 2011;97:612–622.

 Thaman R, Varnava A, Hamid MS, et al. Pregnancy related complications in women with hypertrophic cardiomyopathy. *Heart.* 2003;89:752–756.

Shotan A, Ostrzega E, Mehra A, et al. Incidence of arrhythmias in normal pregnancy and relation to palpitations, dizziness, and syncope. *Am J Cardiol.* 1997;79:1061–1064. *This study confirms an increased incidence of arrhythmias during normal pregnancy. These arrhythmias consist mostly of APCs and VPCs. The number of simple and multifocal VPCs is higher in patients presenting with symptoms of palpitations, dizziness, or syncope. There is no correlation between the incidence of arrhythmias and symptoms. Only 10% of symptomatic episodes were accompanied by the presence of arrhythmias. On the other hand, other studies show that arrhythmias associated with structural heart disease on echocardiography are a cause for concern.*

 Natale A, Davidson T, Geiger MJ, et al. Implantable cardioverter-defibrillators and pregnancy: a safe combination? *Circulation.* 1997;96:2808–2812. *The mere presence of an ICD should not defer a woman from becoming pregnant unless echocardiography reveals underlying structural cardiac disease that is considered a contraindication.*

 Katz R, Karliner JS, Resnik R. Effects of a natural volume overload state (pregnancy) on left ventricular performance in normal human subjects. *Circulation.* 1978;58(3 Pt 1):434–441.

ANSWERS: A and B

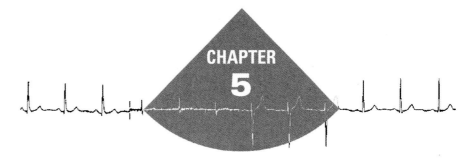

CHAPTER 5

MURMURS

VENOUS HUM

" *A Continuous Murmur with no Ductus.* "

Which statement is FALSE?

A. Venous hum is a continuous but innocent murmur.

B. It gets louder by turning the head away from the examiner.

C. It is louder in the recumbent position.

D. It can be made to disappear in a split second.

A continuous murmur is usually considered to be evidence of a patent ductus arteriosus (PDA) by the casual examiner. PDA is *rare* after the neonatal period. On physical examination of a young patient (usually in their early teens), it is quite *common* to discover the presence of another continuous murmur. This is an innocent murmur. It is called a venous hum. It need not prompt a referral for an echocardiogram.

The venous hum is heard during auscultation of the right side of the neck in the *sitting* position. It is due to torrential venous flow from the head vessels to the right heart in young patients with very compliant right cardiac chambers. It is (to put it simply) driven by gravity. It disappears in the recumbent position.

The loudness of this murmur increases on the right side of the neck when the patient's head is turned to the left (because the caliber of the right jugular vein is narrowed and blood flow becomes even more turbulent). This innocent continuous murmur may, in some cases, transmit and extend to the chest, making it prone to misinterpretation. When this innocent murmur is heard in the chest, the first inclination may be to diagnose a PDA.

The "cure" for this presumed PDA is very simple. Compressing the neck with the examiner's finger just *above* the stethoscope will make the murmur completely disappear (by stopping blood flow). The prominent bounding arterial pulse of PDA is "conspicuous by being absent" in the patient with an innocent venous hum.

The only other consideration is that a venous hum and a PDA are not mutually exclusive and BOTH may be present in the same patient. If the continuous murmur continues to be heard in the recumbent position, an echocardiogram *is* indicated.

ANSWER: C

AUSCULTATION PEARLS IN PATENT DUCTUS ARTERIOSUS

A small ductal shunt may prompt referral for echocardiography because of a nondiagnostic systolic murmur.

Signs and symptoms are usually proportionate to the size of the shunt from aorta to pulmonary artery. The murmur of a persistently patent ductus is usually detected in the first few weeks of life. It may only be systolic rather than the typical continuous murmur.

The typical murmur increases in intensity through systole becoming loudest at the time of aortic valve closure. It *continues* without interruption into diastole, decreasing in intensity but assuming a higher frequency. There may be "shaking dice" noises, or multiple clicks in systole. Increased flow through the mitral valve may result in an apical diastolic rumble.

As mentioned in the previous section, the ductus murmur can be distinguished from a venous hum by the location where it is heard loudest and by turning the head during auscultation. The hum disappears when the head is turned. The ductal murmur is loudest at the second left intercostal space. The venous hum may be loudest at the supraclavicular fossa, or on the right side of the sternum. Venous hums are also modified by respiration and by a change in body position.

Other causes of continuous murmurs include ruptured sinus of Valsalva aneurysm, coronary artery fistula, aortopulmonary window, and collateral flow murmurs in tetralogy with pulmonary atresia. Tetralogy of Fallot with pulmonary atresia should always be suspected in a cyanotic neonate with continuous murmurs heard over the back.

QR 5.1a: Patent ductus arteriosus.

QR 5.1b: Patent ductus arteriosus.

QR 5.2: Overriding aorta in tetralogy of Fallot.

QR 5.3: Repaired tetralogy of Fallot.

QR 5.4a: Right coronary artery manifested intermittently as two parallel "railroad track" reflections.

QR 5.4b: Right coronary artery manifested intermittently as two parallel "railroad track" reflections.

QR 5.4c: Right coronary artery manifested intermittently as two parallel "railroad track" reflections. The coronary arteries must be identified in tetralogy prior to repair. Inadvertent division of a coronary artery can occur during surgery of the right ventricular infundibulum.

REFERENCE: Gatzoulis MA, Soukias N, Ho SY, et al. Echocardiographic and morphological correlations in tetralogy of Fallot. *Eur Heart J.* 1999;20: 221–231.

SILENT BUT PATENT DUCTUS ARTERIOSUS

"   *A Ductus with no Murmur.*   **"**

A routine echocardiogram in a 40-year-old patient with systolic hypertension and a wide pulse pressure reveals the presence of diastolic and systolic flow reversal in the pulmonary artery. There are no murmurs on careful auscultation. The accepted intervention is:

A. Coil occlusion of the patent but "silent" ductus arteriosus.

B. Standard treatment of hypertension.

Color Doppler is the standard for diagnosis of PDA. Some patients with a small PDA may have color flow evidence of the ductus but no murmur. Careful auscultation in the left infraclavicular area *after* the echo may reveal a soft murmur. The murmur may be continuous, or just systolic. It may only be heard intermittently.

> **QR 5.5: Silent patent ductus arteriosus.** Neither the ductus nor the pulmonic regurgitation was heard on auscultation.

 Dammann JF Jr, Sell CG. Patent ductus arteriosus in the absence of a continuous murmur. *Circulation*. 1952;6:110–124.

 Evans DW, Heath D. Disappearance of the continuous murmur in a case of patent ductus arteriosus. *Br Heart J*. 1961;23:469–472.

ANSWER: B, but if you go to a barber (aka interventional cardiologist) you may walk out with a haircut (aka a coil occluder)

DUCTAL ARCH IN THE FETUS

In the fetus, the main pulmonary artery connects to the aorta with the ductus.

The appearance can be confused with the true arch. The ductal arch does *not* give rise to the innominate or right common carotid arteries. The left subclavian can create confusion because its normal takeoff from the aorta *can* be shown in the same plane as the ductal arch.

STILL'S INNOCENT CHILDHOOD MURMUR

Adapted from Still's original description:

It is found in children between the ages of two and six. *Twanging* sound, somewhat musical, like a tense string. The usual location is just below the level of the left nipple, halfway between the left margin of the sternum, and the vertical left nipple line. It is *not* heard in the axilla. Audibility is variable during auscultation, being scarcely noticeable with some heartbeats and being easily heard with others.

Useful observations by others:

Low to medium pitch.

Early to mid-systolic, but separated from the first heart sound.

Loudness may vary from examination to examination.

It may be altered by respiration and by body position.

Lifting the legs in the recumbent position may make it louder. Try it while the patient is still in the lab if the echo is completely normal.

The murmur may be heard at the apex, but is typically *not loudest* at the apex.

The quality of the murmur has been also described as *groaning, squeaking, croaking,* and *buzzing*.

REFERENCES:

 Gardiner HM, Joffe HS. Genesis of Still's murmurs: a controlled Doppler echocardiographic study. *Br Heart J*. 1991;66:217–220.

Guntheroth WG. Innocent murmurs: a suspect diagnosis in non-pregnant adults. *Am J Cardiol*. 2009;104:735–737.

 Shub C. Echocardiography or auscultation? How to evaluate systolic murmurs. *Can Fam Physician*. 2003;49:163–167.

Advani N, Menahem S, Wilkinson JL. The diagnosis of innocent murmurs in childhood. *Cardiol Young*. 2000;10:340–342.

Darazs B, Hesdorffer CS, Butterworth AM, et al. The possible etiology of the vibratory systolic murmur. *Clin Cardiol*. 1987;10:341–346.

Wessel A, Beyer C, Pulss W, et al. False chordae tendineae in the left ventricle. Echo and phonocardiographic findings.[[Article in German] *Z Kardiol*. 1985;74:303–307.

Nothroff J, Suemenicht SG, Wessel A. Can fibrotic bands in the aortic arch cause innocent murmurs in childhood? *Cardiol Young*. 2001;11:643–646.

CARDIOPULMONARY MURMUR

“ *This is an innocent murmur that will not be solved by* ”
performing an echocardiogram.

QUESTION:

What is another name for the cardiopulmonary or cardiorespiratory murmur?

A. Cardiopneumatic.

B. Extracardial.

C. Systolic vesicular.

D. All of the above.

Description

This is a superficial sounding murmur (seemingly heard "halfway up" the stethoscope).

There are flowery descriptions of the nature of the murmur. It has been described as "bizarre," squealing, high pitched, blowing, and swishing, like the sound made by sipping hot soup, or like the puff of a steam locomotive. It is most commonly found in young patients and may disappear as they get older. As the multiple names imply, it may be heard at a border between the heart and the lungs. The murmur is short, and may start and stop abruptly. It may disappear during different phases of respiration.

It may not coincide with a particular phase of the cardiac cycle. It is usually localized, but the location where it is heard best varies from patient to patient. It is said to be most commonly heard at the apex, but can be localized to the left or right sternal borders, or to the left infrascapular area in the back. It will rarely transmit from where it is heard best—to the back or to the axilla.

• PRACTICAL TIP: A common circumstance where this murmur comes up for consideration is during daily routine cardiac auscultation. On first putting the stethoscope on the chest, it is not uncommon to form the auditory impression of a murmur. After a few respiratory cycles, it becomes clear that the examiner is hearing *breath* sounds, and the "murmur" is dismissed by the examiner.

ANSWER: D

SYSTOLIC EJECTION MURMURS

The flow pattern of continuous wave Doppler can help sort out a systolic ejection murmur by providing the following parameters with the EXCEPTION of:

A. Time of systolic peaking.

B. Onset in relation to the isovolumic period.

C. Ejection time.

D. Turbulent versus laminar nature.

The peak of a systolic Doppler flow signal through the aortic valve can be correlated with the auscultatory impression of whether an aortic murmur peaks early or late in systole. Systolic ejection murmurs *end before* the second heart sound. There is an auscultation "caveat" that may help the listener decide whether the murmur stops before the second heart sound (making it an ejection-type murmur).

This only works with loud murmurs where it is clear to the listener that the murmur is louder than the second heart sound. The caveat goes as follows: If the listener hears a second heart sound that is softer than the preceding systolic murmur, it means that the murmur STOPS before the second heart sound. This auscultatory impression can be confirmed by the Doppler flow pattern:

• Pulsed wave Doppler can show turbulence by exhibiting spectral broadening.
• Color flow Doppler can show turbulence with a variance map.

ANSWER: D

COLOR FLOW DOPPLER

A young dialysis patient with a systolic 2/6 murmur heard in the upper left sternal border in the recumbent position is referred for an echocardiogram. The murmur is inaudible in the seated position. An echocardiogram is performed. Which statement is FALSE?

A. Color flow Doppler will help in finding the cause of the murmur.

B. Color flow is comparable to an angiogram.

C. Color flow is a spatial display of real-time mean velocities.

D. A mosaic color pattern indicates turbulence.

Color flow Doppler is highly capable of detecting valvular regurgitation. It is an instantaneous spatial display of mean blood flow velocities—different from an angiogram. Regurgitant murmurs are commonly found by color flow Doppler without being heard on auscultation. Connecting color flow with a murmur is not always straightforward, but correlation of the color flow Doppler examination with auscultation is extremely valuable clinically.

Innocent flow murmurs may become audible in the recumbent position due to increased venous return. There is no color flow Doppler equivalent to a murmur caused by normal forward flow through the right cardiac chambers. Turbulent blood flow is displayed with a variance map on color flow, and by spectral broadening on pulsed wave Doppler.

PRACTICAL EXAMPLE: A sclerotic aortic valve may give rise to a prominent systolic ejection murmur, but there will be no significant gradient on pulsed and continuous wave Doppler.

Color flow Doppler is useful during the assessment of the severity of aortic stenosis. Multiple transducer positions are used to align the continuous wave Doppler beam with the stenotic jet. Color flow can help find the turbulent flow in the aorta in the right parasternal and suprasternal transducer positions during the "hunt" for the fastest aortic stenosis velocity.

BEDSIDE SCANNING TIP: Palpate for the thrill of the aortic stenosis murmur first, and place the transducer directly over that spot on the chest.

REFERENCE: Yoshida K, Yoshikawa J, Shakudo M, et al. Color Doppler evaluation of valvular regurgitation in normal subjects. *Circulation*. 1988;78:840–847.

ANSWER: B is wrong because C is correct.

NICOLADONI-BRANHAM SIGN

Renal patients with arteriovenous fistulas may have unusually prominent Doppler color flow patterns in the right atrium due to increased venous return. This can be altered by using a large blood pressure cuff to occlude the fistula during echocardiographic imaging.

During fistula occlusion, the color flow pattern will diminish. There should also be a reflex decrease in the heart rate (presumably due to decreased sympathetic tone).

REFERENCES: Velez-Roa S, Neubauer J, Wissing M, et al. Acute arteriovenous fistula occlusion decreases sympathetic activity and improves baroreflex control in kidney transplanted patients. *Nephrol Dial Transplant*. 2004;19:1606–1612.

Burchell HB. Observations on bradycardia produced by occlusion of an artery proximal to an arteriovenous fistula (Nicoladoni-Branham sign). *Med Clin North Am*. 1958; 42:1029–1035.

MURMUR IN THE BACK

QUESTION:

Which one of the following echocardiographic findings helps sort out the cause for a murmur heard in the back?

A. Mitral valve prolapse.

B. Hypertrophic cardiomyopathy.

C. Bicuspid aortic valve.

D. Pulmonic stenosis.

E. All of the above.

The mitral regurgitation jet of *anterior* mitral valve prolapse is directed opposite the culprit leaflet. It is therefore directed posteriorly and may be heard in the back in the interscapular region. Systolic anterior motion of the mitral valve in hypertrophic cardiomyopathy may direct the mitral regurgitation jet to the posterior left atrial wall.

Bicuspid aortic valve is associated with coarctation of the aorta. The murmur of coarctation is heard in the back. The jet of valvular pulmonic stenosis favors the left main branch of the pulmonary artery. The murmur is widely disseminated across chest and is also directed to the back.

QR 5.6: Posteriorly directed mitral regurgitation jet.

ANSWER: E

CHAPTER 6

ENDOCARDITIS

> *An echocardioGRAM is not a microSCOPE.*

QUESTION:

An echocardiogram is performed on a patient with suspected endocarditis. Which echocardiographic aspect of a suspected vegetation is LEAST useful?

A. Appearance.

B. Motion.

C. Location.

D. Temporal behavior.

E. Size.

Echocardiographic imaging of a vegetation does not equate to looking at the histology with a microscope. It is important to analyze all the echocardiographic features.

Echocardiographic *appearance* of a vegetation:

The word "shaggy" indicates an irregular shaped appearance. On M-mode, the lines made by reflections from a vegetation appear "stippled."

The gray scale density of vegetations is usually similar to the density of adjacent valve tissue. An unusually reflective calcific vegetation has probably been there for some time.

The *motion* of a vegetation is a high-frequency oscillation or "shimmering."

Location

Vegetations can attach to valves, supporting structures, endocardial surfaces, or to prosthetic material. They may be in the path of a regurgitant jet, with preference for the low-pressure atrial side in cases of mitral and tricuspid regurgitation.

Temporal echocardiographic equivalents of the clinical "call-to-action" of a *fever with a new murmur*:

1. New valvular regurgitation when there is no alternate explanation (such as progression of previous valvular disease, or another disorder, or cause such as traumatic injury).
2. Newly diagnosed dehiscence of a prosthetic ring may be the first manifestation of endocarditis. Rocking due to dehiscence is defined as >15 degree displacement of a prosthetic ring. This may *not* be present if <40% of the ring is dehisced. Evidence of abnormal regurgitation on color flow is more sensitive.

Vegetation *size* may not affect the decision to operate. There is a higher embolic risk with increasing size. A small vegetation may be the remnant of a larger one that has already "silently" embolized. Tricuspid vegetations tend to be large, and a size >2 cm *does* carry a worse prognosis.

Diagnosis of an abscess is difficult when the findings are subtle. Echocardiographic findings when abscess is present:

- Abnormally thickened or bright perivalvular reflections.
- Greater than 1 cm thickening of the aortic wall (in patients with no prior aortic surgery).
- Single or multiple intramyocardial echolucencies.
- Fistulas to other valves, or to the pericardial space.
- Color flow may show abnormal communications.

Definition

Pseudoaneurysm is an abscess that extends to the lumen of the aorta. Mitral valve aneurysm and eventual leaflet perforation may be due to "bacterial seeding" by a high-velocity regurgitation jet from an infected aortic valve.

Differential Diagnosis

Ruptured mitral and tricuspid valve chordae, and torn aortic leaflets may *look* like vegetations. Over time, thrombosis or pannus on a prosthesis can expand from the sewing ring to the lumen, but not to the rest of the annulus, giving the misleading appearance of a vegetation. Right atrial differential diagnostic dilemmas include pacemaker wires with fibrin strands and eustachian valves (that are often accompanied by a mobile Chiari network). Sterile Libman-Sacks vegetations are found in systemic lupus erythematosus. Antiphospholipid antibody syndrome is associated with sterile valvular vegetations.

FIGURE 6.1

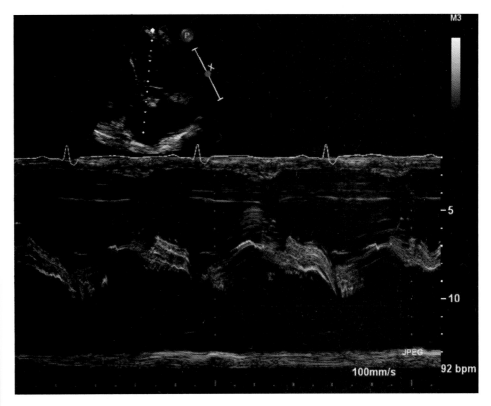

"Shaggy" tricuspid valve vegetation.

FIGURE 6.2

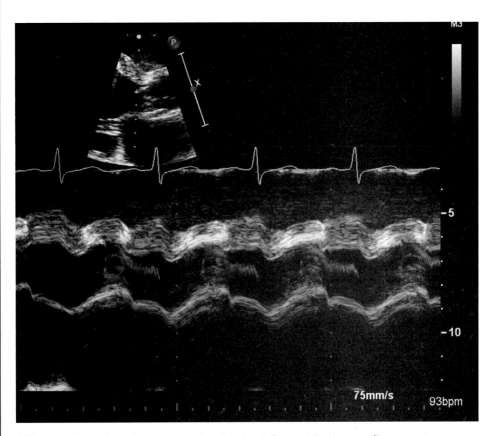

"Shaggy" aortic valve vegetation in the left ventricular outflow tract.

FIGURE 6.3

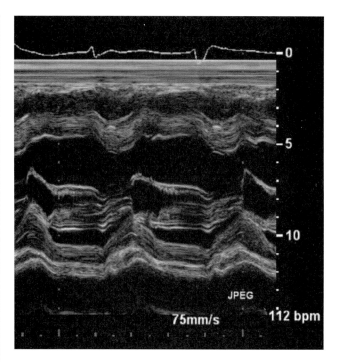

Mitral valve endocarditis—"shaggy" stippled appearance.

FIGURE 6.4

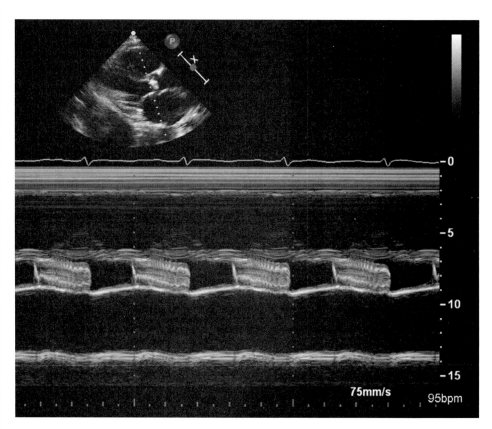

Aortic valve endocarditis—"shaggy" stippled appearance.

FIGURE 6.5

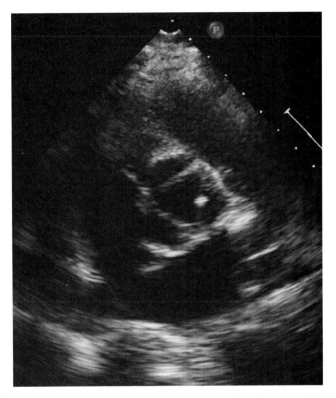

Normal nodules of Aranti on the aortic valve may become calcified and may be mistaken for a vegetation.

QR 6.1: Partial dehiscence of a prosthetic mitral ring.

QR 6.2: Endocarditis with perforation of the posterior mitral leaflet.

QR 6.3: Calcified vegetations on both the atrial and on the ventricular side of the mitral valve. The next time someone invokes the "real estate location rule" that vegetations favor the downstream, low-pressure side of a valve, show them these images.

QR 6.4a: Paravalvular mitral prosthesis regurgitation.

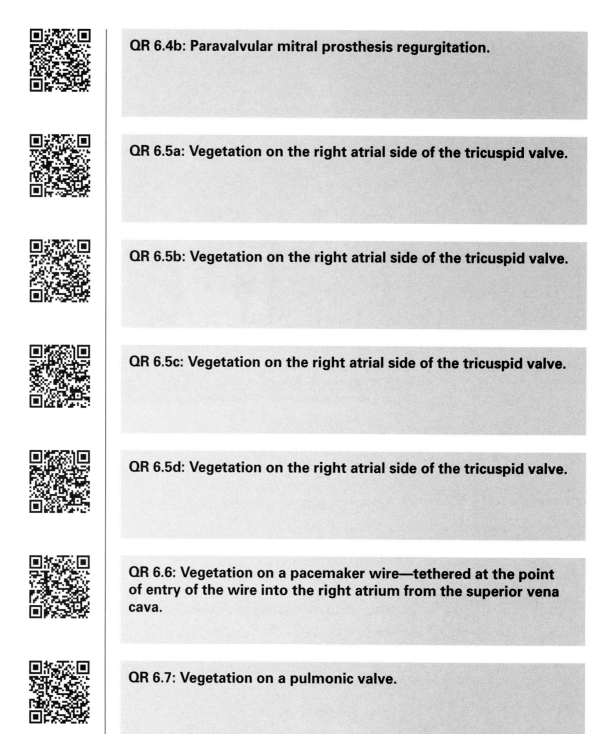

QR 6.4b: Paravalvular mitral prosthesis regurgitation.

QR 6.5a: Vegetation on the right atrial side of the tricuspid valve.

QR 6.5b: Vegetation on the right atrial side of the tricuspid valve.

QR 6.5c: Vegetation on the right atrial side of the tricuspid valve.

QR 6.5d: Vegetation on the right atrial side of the tricuspid valve.

QR 6.6: Vegetation on a pacemaker wire—tethered at the point of entry of the wire into the right atrium from the superior vena cava.

QR 6.7: Vegetation on a pulmonic valve.

QR 6.8: Aortic valve vegetation.

QR 6.9: Aortic root abscess.

QR 6.10: Abscess in the intervalvular fibrosa.

QR 6.11: Large Lambl's excrescence on the right coronary aortic cusp. Echocardiography cannot distinguish this from a papillary fibroelastoma, or from a small vegetation.

QR 6.12a: Pseudoaneurysm of the aorta in a patient with endocarditis.

QR 6.12b: Pseudoaneurysm of the aorta in a patient with endocarditis.

QR 6.13a: Pacemaker wire vegetations.

QR 6.13b: Pacemaker wire vegetations.

QR 6.14: Partial dehiscence of an aortic valve prosthesis may occur due to endocarditis.

QR 6.15: Normal eustachian valve.

QR 6.16a: Right atrial Chiari network should not be confused with vegetations.

QR 6.16b: Right atrial Chiari network should not be confused with vegetations.

QR 6.16c: Right atrial Chiari network should not be confused with vegetations.

QR 6.16d: Right atrial Chiari network should not be confused with vegetations.

QR 6.16e: Right atrial Chiari network should not be confused with vegetations.

QR 6.16f: Right atrial Chiari network should not be confused with vegetations.

QR 6.16g: Right atrial Chiari network should not be confused with vegetations.

QR 6.16h: Right atrial Chiari network should not be confused with vegetations.

QR 6.16i: Right atrial Chiari network should not be confused with vegetations.

QR 6.17: Systolic anterior motion of the mitral valve chordae should not be confused with vegetations.

REFERENCES:

 Li JS, Sexton DJ, Mick N, et al. Proposed modifications to the Duke criteria for the diagnosis of infective endocarditis. *Clin Infect Dis*. 2000;30:633–638.

Karalis DG, Bansal RC, Hauck AJ, et al. Transesophageal echocardiographic recognition of subaortic complications in aortic valve endocarditis. Clinical and surgical implications. *Circulation*. 1992;86:353–362. *Figure 1 illustrates the intervalvular fibrosa, and Figure 2 illustrates the complications.*

Rerkpattanapipat P, Wongpraparut N, Jacobs LE, et al. Cardiac manifestations of acquired immunodeficiency syndrome. *Arch Intern Med*. 2000;160:602–608.

Farrior JB, Silverman ME. A consideration of the differences between a Janeway's lesion and an Osler's node in infectious endocarditis. *Chest*. 1976;70:239–243. *The original comments by William Osler and Edward Janeway are presented, and the literature following their descriptions is reviewed. The diagnostic difference between the two is the tenderness that is associated with an Osler node but not with a Janeway lesion.*

Al-Refai MA, Oueida FM, Lui RC, et al. Impressive echocardiographic images of a rare pathology: Aneurysm of the mitral valve - Report of two cases and review of the literature. *J Saudi Heart Assoc*. 2013;25:47–51.

Zuily S, Regnault V, Selton-Suty C, et al. Increased risk for heart valve disease associated with antiphospholipid antibodies in patients with systemic lupus erythematosus: meta-analysis of echocardiographic studies. *Circulation*. 2011;124:215–224.

Alreja G, Lotfi A. Eustachian valve endocarditis: rare case reports and review of literature. *J Cardiovasc Dis Res*. 2011;2:181–185.

Fazlinezhad A, Fatehi H, Tabaee S, et al. Pseudoaneurysm of mitro-aortic intervalvular fibrosa during the course of mitral valve endocarditis with aorto-left ventricle outflow tract fistula. *J Saudi Heart Assoc*. 2012;24:201–204.

ANSWER: Probably E, technically D

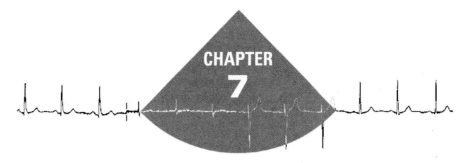

CHAPTER 7

HYPERTENSION AND PREOPERATIVE EVALUATION

RESISTANT HYPERTENSION

Which of the following resistant hypertensive patients will benefit most from an echocardiographic evaluation?

A. A hypertensive little old lady treated with multiple "industrial strength" antihypertensive agents.

B. A hypertensive with shirt size 18.

C. Snow White's friend Sneezy.

D. An elderly smoker with an incompressible radial pulse.

E. Papa John (likes to play dominoes with Little Caesar).

Patients with a *small* BMI being prescribed *large* doses of antihypertensive medications may be noncompliant. Patients with a large BMI may have sleep apnea and need a sleep study for confirmation. Overuse of pseudoephedrine is an example of drug-induced hypertension.

Pseudohypertension may require an arterial line to measure the true blood pressure. Patients with extensive arteriosclerosis may have easily imaged coronary arteries on echo. Volume overload hypertension due to excess dietary sodium and/or inadequate diuretic therapy results in volume expansion. There may be echocardiographic evidence of an increased stroke volume. Elevated right-side pressures may be found on the echocardiogram before the patient develops clinically detectable peripheral edema, or jugular venous distension.

Left atrial enlargement, diastolic dysfunction, and left ventricular hypertrophy are nonspecific echocardiographic findings that suggest cardiac end-organ damage from inadequately treated resistant hypertension.

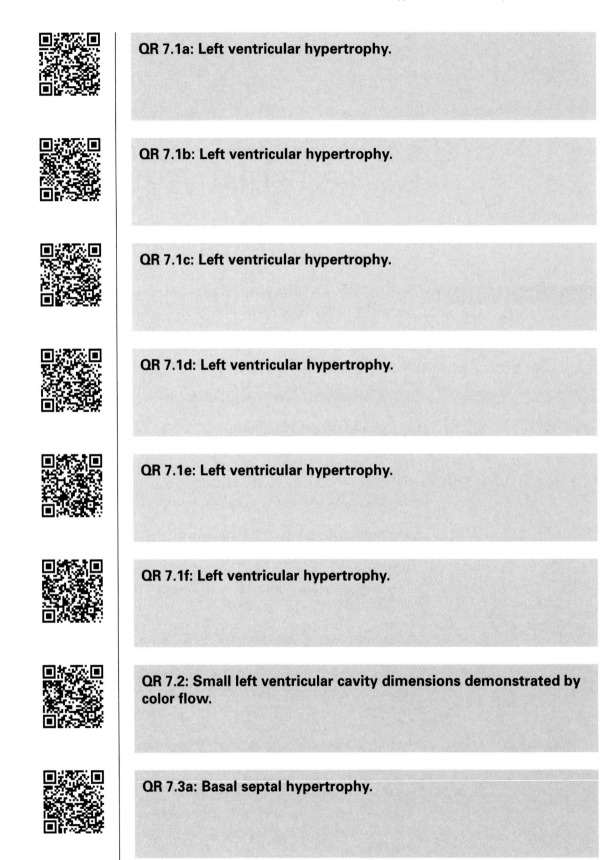

QR 7.1a: Left ventricular hypertrophy.

QR 7.1b: Left ventricular hypertrophy.

QR 7.1c: Left ventricular hypertrophy.

QR 7.1d: Left ventricular hypertrophy.

QR 7.1e: Left ventricular hypertrophy.

QR 7.1f: Left ventricular hypertrophy.

QR 7.2: Small left ventricular cavity dimensions demonstrated by color flow.

QR 7.3a: Basal septal hypertrophy.

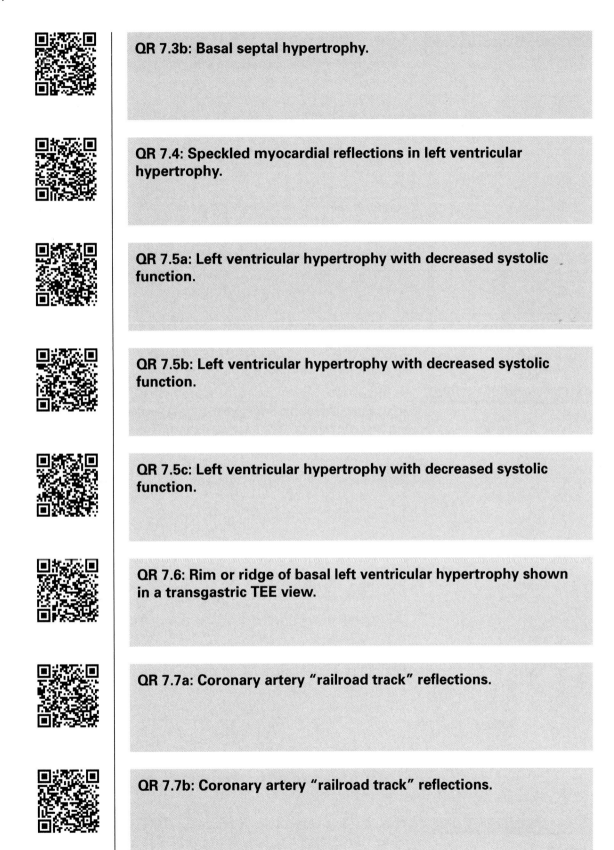

QR 7.3b: Basal septal hypertrophy.

QR 7.4: Speckled myocardial reflections in left ventricular hypertrophy.

QR 7.5a: Left ventricular hypertrophy with decreased systolic function.

QR 7.5b: Left ventricular hypertrophy with decreased systolic function.

QR 7.5c: Left ventricular hypertrophy with decreased systolic function.

QR 7.6: Rim or ridge of basal left ventricular hypertrophy shown in a transgastric TEE view.

QR 7.7a: Coronary artery "railroad track" reflections.

QR 7.7b: Coronary artery "railroad track" reflections.

REFERENCES:

Calhoun DA, Jones D, Textor S, et al. Resistant hypertension: diagnosis, evaluation, and treatment. A scientific statement from the American Heart Association Professional Education Committee of the Council for High Blood Pressure Research. *Hypertension*. 2008;51:1403–1419.

Faselis C, Doumas M, Papademetriou V. Common secondary causes of resistant hypertension and rationale for treatment. *Int J Hypertens*. 2011;2011, Article ID 236239. http://www.ncbi.nlm.nih.gov/pmc/articles/PMC3057025/pdf/IJHT2011-236239.pdf. Accessed October 15, 2013.

Beilin L, Mounsey P. The left ventricular impulse in hypertensive heart disease. *Br Heart J*. 1962;24:409–421. *The physical findings in this article correlate with pulsed wave Doppler findings in the left ventricular outflow.*

ANSWER: E (excess dietary sodium—pizza poisoning)

DOBUTAMINE STRESS ECHOCARDIOGRAPHY IN THE HYPERTENSIVE PATIENT

QUESTION:

A patient with end-stage renal disease undergoes dobutamine stress echo for preoperative clearance. Which of the following will affect interpretation of wall motion during dobutamine stress echo?

A. Severe systolic hypertension.

B. Left ventricular cavity obliteration.

C. Biphasic response.

D. All of the above.

Dobutamine stress echo is frequently performed for preoperative clearance in patients with end-stage renal disease. Uncontrolled hypertension may affect interpretation. Left ventricular cavity obliteration at peak stress may cause hypotension without underlying ischemia.

ANSWER: A and B

UTILITY OF THE ECHOCARDIOGRAM IN PREOPERATIVE CLEARANCE FOR VALVULAR REGURGITATION

QUESTION:

Which cardiac patient has the LOWEST risk of anesthetic complications during noncardiac surgery?

A. Severe aortic stenosis, or mitral stenosis, or pulmonic stenosis.

B. Pulmonary hypertension.

C. Unstable angina, or heart failure, or ventricular tachycardia.

D. Severe mitral regurgitation, or aortic regurgitation.

Severe valvular stenosis, pulmonary hypertension, unstable angina, heart failure, and malignant arrhythmias increase perioperative risk. Many anesthetic regimens reduce afterload, so both mitral and aortic regurgitation may hemodynamically improve during anesthesia.

When comparing aortic regurgitation and mitral regurgitation, there is a difference when it comes to afterload: The severity of both lesions is affected by changes in preload but aortic regurgitation is affected more significantly by changes in afterload. The best way to understand this is to first review what happens in diastole.

Diastolic filling is affected both in mitral regurgitation and in aortic regurgitation:

- In mitral regurgitation, diastolic filling is affected by the increased filling from the distended and overfilled left atrium.
- In aortic regurgitation, diastolic filling is affected by continuous filling from the aorta into the left ventricle.
- In aortic regurgitation, during diastole, the severity of the regurgitation will determine the degree of filling of the left ventricle.

In systole, the left ventricle in the patient with aortic regurgitation has to eject into an aorta that was not designed to accommodate the amount of stroke volume created by severe aortic regurgitation. In contrast, the left ventricle in the patient with mitral regurgitation "ejects" into the low impedance left atrium at the same time that it ejects into the aorta.

Echocardiographic Corollary

The presence of severe left ventricular dilatation is a useful marker of hemodynamically significant aortic regurgitation. As opposed to mitral regurgitation, progressive left ventricular dilatation does not beget more aortic regurgitation. If the left ventricle is getting progressively dilated, the existing aortic regurgitation is probably responsible.

Imaging Pitfall

The color flow display of mitral regurgitation in the left atrium *does* change dramatically with changes in afterload, because it reflects the left ventricular driving pressure. The color flow area also decreases dramatically after a stenotic aortic valve is replaced.

ANSWER: D

ABDOMINAL AORTIC ANEURYSM—PREOPERATIVE CLEARANCE

Dobutamine stress echo is frequently performed for preoperative clearance. Surgery for abdominal aortic aneurysm is risky, and preoperative clearance typically involves cardiac evaluation with dobutamine stress echo. A commonly asked question is whether it is safe to perform dobutamine stress echocardiography on a patient with marked aneurysmal distention of the abdominal aorta.

REFERENCES:

Pellikka PA, Roger VL, Oh JK, et al. Safety of performing dobutamine stress echocardiography in patients with abdominal aortic aneurysm > or = 4 cm in diameter. *Am J Cardiol*. 1996;77:413–416. *Ninety-eight patients with abdominal aortic aneurysms > or = 4 cm in diameter were identified. Records were reviewed to determine whether there was any evidence of aneurysm rupture or adverse vascular events as a result of the stress test. There was no case of aneurysm rupture or hemodynamic instability precipitated by dobutamine stress echocardiography. In addition, dobutamine stress echocardiography that was negative for ischemia identified patients at very low risk of perioperative cardiac events.*

Motreff P, Pierre-Justin E, Dauphin C, et al. Evaluation of cardiac risk before vascular surgery by dobutamine stress echocardiography. [Article in French] *Arch Mal Coeur Vaiss*. 1997;90:1209–1214. *Eighty-five patients with an aortic abdominal aneurysm or obstructive arterial disease underwent dobutamine stress echocardiography followed by coronary angiography. The only 2 non-fatal cardiac complications of peripheral surgery (3%) occurred after a positive dobutamine stress echo. This study confirms both the necessity of preoperative assessment of coronary risk and the efficacy of dobutamine stress echocardiography in this indication. Dobutamine stress echocardiography is a reliable alternative to isotopic methods. Its good predictive value justifies using coronary angiography only for patients with a positive result.*

Brooks MJ, Mayet J, Glenville B, et al. Cardiac investigation and intervention prior to thoraco-abdominal aneurysm repair: coronary angiography in 35 patients. *Eur J Vasc Endovasc Surg*. 2001;21:437–444. *There was a 40% prevalence of coronary artery disease, comparable to that of other patients undergoing arterial surgery. Non-invasive testing proved beneficial, both in screening low-risk patients and planning intervention in patients at higher risk.*

[pdf] Poldermans D, Arnese M, Fioretti PM, et al. Sustained prognostic value of dobutamine stress echocardiography for late cardiac events after major non-cardiac vascular surgery. *Circulation*. 1997;95:53–58.

CHAPTER 8

CARDIOMYOPATHIES

BROCKENBROUGH SIGN

A patient with *hypertrophic obstructive cardiomyopathy* shows the typical postextrasystolic pressure changes in the left ventricle and in the aorta. Which statements are true?

On the beat immediately following a premature ventricular contraction:

A. The left ventricular systolic pressure INcreases.

B. The systolic gradient between the left ventricle and the aorta INcreases.

C. The aortic systolic pressure DEcreases.

D. The aortic pulse pressure DEcreases.

E. All of the above are true.

Physical examination equivalent on palpation of the carotid pulse:

Palpating the carotid pulse may provide evidence of the systolic pressure drop. The amplitude of the very next beat following a premature ventricular contraction may be decreased. Normally, it would be increased.

Echocardiographic equivalent:

An echocardiographic technique to measure the left ventricular ejection time (LVET) in the postextrasystolic beat was shown to be more sensitive. LVET increased by >20 msec in 11 of 12 patients with IHSS.

FIGURE 8.1

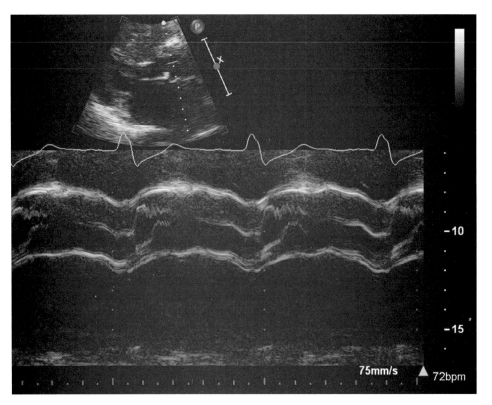

Mid-systolic closure of the aortic valve in hypertrophic cardiomyopathy.

FIGURE 8.2

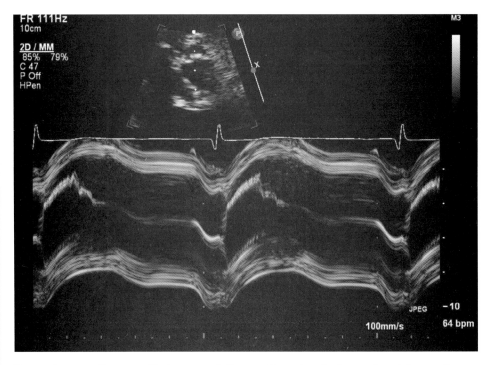

Premature or "tapered" closure of the aortic valve in hypertrophic cardio-myopathy may affect the second heart sound. The aortic component of the second heart sound may be misleadingly decreased or absent—potentially leading to confusion with valvular aortic stenosis during auscultation.

Brockenbrough EC, Braunwald E, Morrow AG. A hemodynamic technic for the detection of hypertrophic subaortic stenosis. *Circulation*. 1961;23:189–194.

 Kuijer PJ, van der Werf T, Meijler FL. Post-extrasystolic potentiation without a compensatory pause in normal and diseased hearts. *Br Heart J*. 1990;63: 284–286.

 White CW, Zimmerman TJ. Prolonged left ventricular ejection time in the post-premature beat. A sensitive sign of idiopathic hypertrophic subaortic stenosis. *Circulation*. 1975;52:306–312.

REFERENCES:

ANSWER: Although A, B, C, and D are all true; answer D is the only one necessary to understand and recognize.

CONTRADISTINCTION WITH VALVULAR AORTIC STENOSIS

In patients with valvular aortic stenosis, there is an INcrease in the pulse pressure following a premature beat. The post-extrasystolic murmur of valvular aortic stenosis gets audibly louder. The Doppler flow gets faster.

FIGURE 8.3

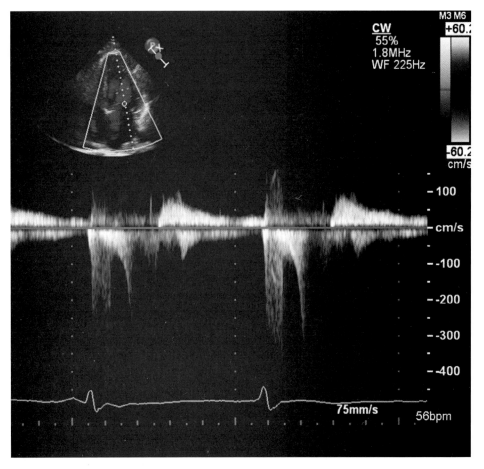

"Lobster claw" Doppler pattern in hypertrophic cardiomyopathy.

HYPERTROPHIC CARDIOMYOPATHY AND MITRAL REGURGITATION

  "   *Ejection....................Obstruction...............Regurgitation*   **"**

QUESTION: A college athlete with a family history of sudden death is referred for an echocardiogram because of a murmur. The echocardiogram shows a systolic jet with a peak velocity of 7 m per second. There is asymmetric septal hypertrophy. The septal myocardium has a speckled "ground glass" appearance. Systolic blood pressure is 126. Which interpretation of the findings is correct?

A. There is a $(7 \times 7 \times 4)$ 196 mmHg systolic gradient between the left ventricle and the aorta.

B. The left ventricular outflow gradient is 70 mmHg plus the estimated left atrial pressure.

C. The 7-m velocity is due to mitral regurgitation.

D. Answers B and C are correct.

Hypertrophic cardiomyopathy is well suited to echocardiographic evaluation. This case illustrates a potential source of error in interpretation of the Doppler flow. The problem arises during a typical sequence of left ventricular ejection followed by outflow obstruction. In hypertrophic cardiomyopathy, a left ventricular outflow gradient may be depressurized into the left atrium by mitral regurgitation.

Left ventricular ejection is hampered by left ventricular outflow obstruction with consequent systolic anterior motion of the mitral valve. Mitral leaflet coaptation may be affected by the systolic anterior displacement. This gives rise to mid-to-late systolic mitral regurgitation. The late systolic *regurgitant* Doppler signal appears *dagger shaped* and may get mistaken for the dagger-shaped *outflow* Doppler signal.

The left ventricular pressure (that determines the mitral regurgitation velocity) is the sum of the systolic pressure in the aorta plus the left ventricular outflow gradient. Left ventricular outflow gradients are dynamic, but they remain under 100 mmHg.

Consequently, Doppler velocities of left ventricular outflow gradients are <5 m per second. Normal mitral regurgitation velocities are 5 m per second, but can *increase* dramatically in hypertrophic cardiomyopathy. A 7 m per second blood flow velocity represents mitral regurgitation. It is too high to represent the gradient.

• TECHNICAL PITFALL: In order to measure a 7 m per second blood flow velocity, it is necessary to employ continuous wave Doppler.

Continuous wave Doppler creates range ambiguity errors. All blood velocities along the path of the continuous wave Doppler beam are recorded and superimposed. Both the mitral regurgitation and the left ventricular outflow velocity are recorded along the path of the same continuous wave Doppler beam. The fastest velocity is shown as the envelope of the Doppler signal. Slower velocities may, or may not, be displayed as a shadow within the fastest velocities.

It becomes technically difficult to directly measure the left ventricular outflow gradient, which would have a slower velocity than the mitral regurgitation.

The solution is an indirect determination of the gradient.

GRADIENT = LV systolic pressure minus the systemic blood pressure

Velocity is converted to pressure by the simplified Bernoulli equation: pressure $= 4V^2$.

The left ventricular systolic "driving" pressure is calculated as the mitral regurgitation velocity squared and multiplied by four. An estimated left atrial pressure is added to the "driving" pressure to give the left ventricular systolic pressure. The left ventricular outflow gradient can thus be "back calculated" by subtracting the systolic blood pressure from this calculated left ventricular systolic pressure.

FIGURE 8.4

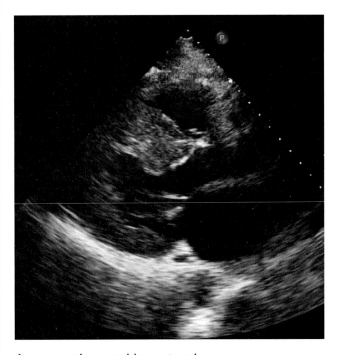

Asymmetric septal hypertrophy.

FIGURE 8.5

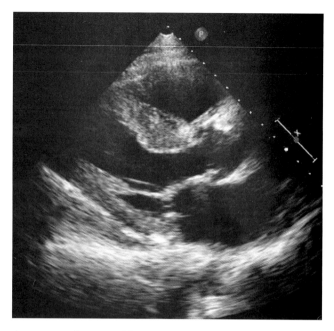

Asymmetric septal hypertrophy.

FIGURE 8.6

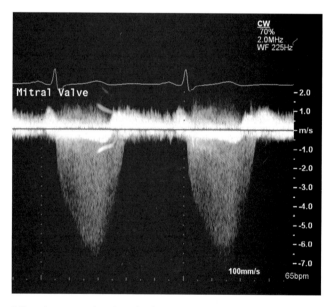

Mitral regurgitation in hypertrophic cardiomyopathy should not be mis-interpreted as an extreme intracavitary gradient. The stripes may be an indicator of a musical mitral regurgitation murmur on auscultation that increases with handgrip (rather than with Valsalva).

QR 8.1: High-velocity mitral regurgitation in hypertrophic obstructive cardiomyopathy.

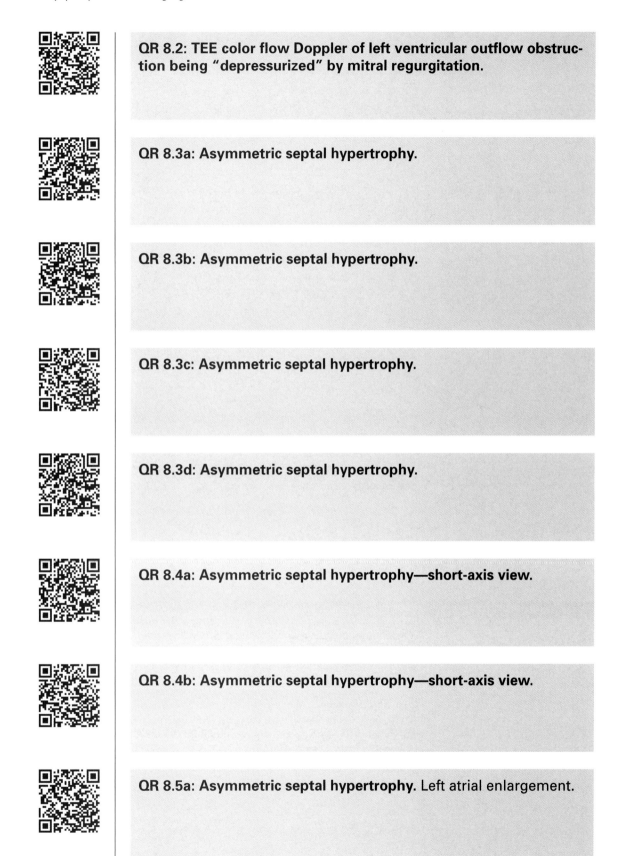

QR 8.2: TEE color flow Doppler of left ventricular outflow obstruction being "depressurized" by mitral regurgitation.

QR 8.3a: Asymmetric septal hypertrophy.

QR 8.3b: Asymmetric septal hypertrophy.

QR 8.3c: Asymmetric septal hypertrophy.

QR 8.3d: Asymmetric septal hypertrophy.

QR 8.4a: Asymmetric septal hypertrophy—short-axis view.

QR 8.4b: Asymmetric septal hypertrophy—short-axis view.

QR 8.5a: Asymmetric septal hypertrophy. Left atrial enlargement.

QR 8.5b: Asymmetric septal hypertrophy. Left atrial enlargement.

QR 8.5c: Asymmetric septal hypertrophy. Left atrial enlargement.

QR 8.6a: Severe asymmetric septal hypertrophy.

QR 8.6b: Severe asymmetric septal hypertrophy.

QR 8.7: Systolic anterior mitral leaflet motion with loss of leaflet coaptation.

REFERENCES:

Schwammenthal E, Nakatani S, He S, et al. Mechanism of mitral regurgitation in hypertrophic cardiomyopathy: mismatch of posterior to anterior leaflet length and mobility. *Circulation.* 1998;98:856–865. *Systolic anterior motion (SAM) produces greater mitral regurgitation if the posterior leaflet is limited in its ability to move anteriorly, participate in SAM, and coapt effectively.*

Yu EH, Omran AS, Wigle ED, Williams WG, Siu SC, Rakowski H. Mitral regurgitation in hypertrophic obstructive cardiomyopathy: relationship to obstruction and relief with myectomy. *J Am Coll Cardiol.* 2000;36:2219–2225. *Myectomy significantly reduces the degree of mitral regurgitation.*

ANSWER: D

BEDSIDE EXAMINATION IN HYPERTROPHIC CARDIOMYOPATHY WITH MITRAL REGURGITATION

QUESTION: **Which of the physical findings below is LEAST helpful (and most counter intuitive) for the above examination?**

A. The dynamic behavior of the murmur.

B. The pulse examination.

C. The neck vein examination.

D. The apical impulse.

E. The second heart sound.

There is a grade 3/6 systolic murmur, heard well at the upper left sternal border. The murmur begins after the first heart sound (ejection murmur comes first, followed by outflow obstruction and mitral regurgitation). It decreases with squatting and becomes louder on standing. It is also louder during the strain phase of a Valsalva maneuver. In contrast, the murmur of a ventricular septal defect (which can be heard in the same location) would get softer or disappear.

The murmur seems to last a little longer, and is a little louder in the mitral area at the apex (due to the associated mitral regurgitation). The radial pulse is brisk and brief (not the "parvus et tardus" pulse of aortic stenosis). The prominent, quick, tapping nature of the pulse actually suggests severe chronic aortic regurgitation, but there is no diastolic murmur on auscultation, and no aortic regurgitation on color flow Doppler.

As described by Bernheim over a hundred years ago, the jugular *venous* 'a' wave can be prominent and easy to identify in patients with *left* ventricular hypertrophy. The aortic component of the second heart sound is normal but the second heart sound is paradoxically split (indicating delayed aortic valve closure due to prolonged left ventricular ejection). There should be no left bundle branch block on the ECG to provide an alternate "electrical" explanation for this finding.

Palpation at the point of maximal impulse of the left ventricle reveals three distinct impulses. The first impulse is a palpable atrial gallop (S4). It is followed by a brisk early systolic impulse and another more subtle late systolic bump (this is affectionately known as the "triple ripple"). Amyl nitrite inhalation will increase the gradient.

FIGURE 8.7

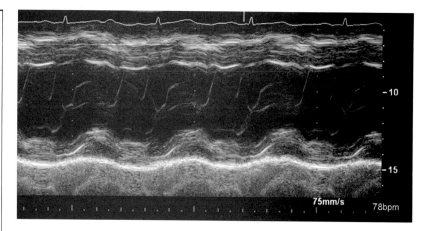

Systolic anterior motion of the mitral valve.

FIGURE 8.8

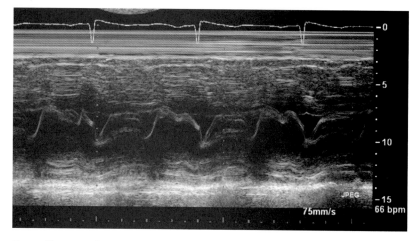

Systolic anterior motion of the mitral valve.

FIGURE 8.9

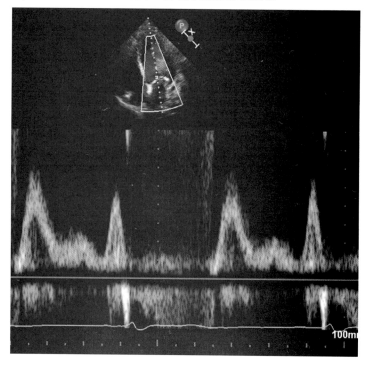

Mid diastolic forward transmitral flow into the left ventricle during diastasis is called an L wave.

REFERENCES:

 Keren G, Meisner JS, Sherez J, Yellin EL, Laniado S. Interrelationship of mid-diastolic mitral valve motion, pulmonary venous flow, and transmitral flow. *Circulation*. 1986;74:36–44.

 Henein MY, Xiao HB, Brecker SJ, Gibson DG. Bernheim "a" wave: obstructed right ventricular inflow or atrial cross talk? *Br Heart J*. 1993;69:409–413.

Huang MT, Goodman MA, Delaney TB. Pre-infarction angina secondary to calcific aortic stenosis with Bernheim's effect. *Clin Cardiol*. 1978;1:107–111.

Bernheim P.I.: De l'asystolie veineuse dans l'hypertrophie du coeur gauche par stenose concomitante du ventricule droit. *Rev Med*. 1910;30:785–801.

Lembo NJ, Dell'Italia LJ, Crawford MH, O'Rourke RA. Bedside diagnosis of systolic murmurs. *N Engl J Med*. 1988;318:1572–1578. *The murmur of hypertrophic cardiomyopathy was distinguished from other murmurs by*:

- *An increase in intensity with the Valsalva maneuver (65% and 96% specificity).*
- *During squatting-to-standing action (95% and 84% specificity).*
- *By a decrease in intensity during standing-to-squatting action (95% sensitivity and 85% specificity).*
- *Passive leg elevation (85% sensitivity and 91% specificity).*
- *Handgrip (85% sensitivity and 75% specificity).*

ANSWER: C

NONISCHEMIC CAUSES OF GIANT T-WAVE INVERSION ON THE ECG

Inverted T waves produced by myocardial ischemia are narrow and symmetric. The ST segment is described as coving, bowed, or concave, with a sharp symmetric downstroke.

Prominent, deeply inverted, *widely splayed* T waves can be found in:

- Apical hypertrophic cardiomyopathy. Takotsubo cardiomyopathy.
- Myocarditis. Pericarditis (later stages).
- Cerebrovascular disease. Subarachnoid bleeding. Elevated intracranial pressure.
- Pulmonary embolism. Severe right ventricular hypertrophy.
- Cocaine abuse.
- Pancreatitis. Acute abdomen.
- Early repolarization. Bundle branch block. Post pacemaker insertion. Complete heart block. Wolff–Parkinson–White syndrome.

QR 8.8: Apical left ventricular hypertrophy. This patient has giant T-wave inversions in the anterolateral precordial leads. There were no abnormalities on coronary angiography.

QR 8.9a: Apical left ventricular hypertrophy.

QR 8.9b: Apical left ventricular hypertrophy.

QR 8.10a: Spade-shaped contrast left ventriculogram in apical hypertrophy.

QR 8.10b: Spade-shaped contrast left ventriculogram in apical hypertrophy.

REFERENCES:

 Sakamoto T, Amano K, Hada Y, et al. Asymmetric apical hypertrophy: ten years experience. *Postgrad Med J*. 1986;62:567–570. *Echocardiography was essential for the diagnosis. Clinical complications have been infrequent and the prognosis seems good.*

Yamaguchi H, Ishimura T, Nishiyama S, et al. Hypertrophic nonobstructive cardiomyopathy with giant negative T waves (apical hypertrophy): ventriculographic and echocardiographic features in 30 patients. *Am J Cardiol*. 1979;44:401–412.

Drut R, Velasco Vela O, Maljar L. [Steinert's disease with cardiac arrhythmia. Morphological findings in the heart conduction system]. *Arch Inst Cardiol Mex*. 1975;45: 238–248. [Article in Spanish] *Myotonic dystrophy. ECG showed atrial flutter, complete A-V block, idioventricular rhythm, left bundle branch block; and giant, wide, negative T waves.*

Khairy P, Marsolais P. Pancreatitis with electrocardiographic changes mimicking acute myocardial infarction. *Can J Gastroenterol*. 2001;15:522–526.

Hayden GE, Brady WJ, Perron AD, Somers MP, Mattu A. Electrocardiographic T-wave inversion: differential diagnosis in the chest pain patient. *Am J Emerg Med*. 2002;20: 252–262.

LEFT VENTRICULAR HYPERTROPHY IN THE ATHLETE

QUESTION:

Which findings suggest that an elite male athlete has pathological left ventricular hypertrophy that should exclude him from further participation in intense competitive sports? More than one answer may be correct.

A. Dilated left ventricular cavity with an increased wall thickness.

B. Decrease in left ventricular cavity size and wall thickness after a 3-month period of deconditioning.

C. Small left ventricular cavity with 0.5 septum to end-diastolic cavity ratio.

D. Apical left ventricular hypertrophy with giant T-wave inversions in the anterolateral ECG leads.

The leading cause of sudden death during intense competitive sports in the young, asymptomatic athlete is hypertrophic cardiomyopathy. More than one-third of highly trained male athletes may increase their left ventricular cavity dimensions as part of the athletic conditioning process. There is a proportional but mild increase in left ventricular wall thickness. These adaptive changes tend to regress during athletic deconditioning.

In contrast, pathological hypertrophic cardiomyopathy is more likely to show disproportionate left ventricular wall thickening with a relatively small cavity. Pathological hypertrophy may affect variable regions of the left ventricle. Apical hypertrophy (with a markedly abnormal ECG) is one such example.

FIGURE 8.10

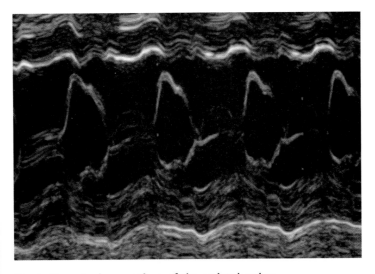

Systolic anterior motion of the mitral valve.

FIGURE 8.11

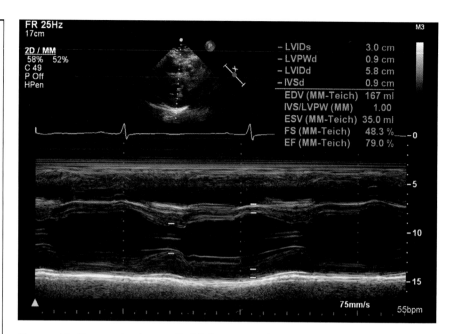

Normal left ventricular wall thickness and cavity dimensions.

QR 8.11: Concentric left ventricular hypertrophy.

QR 8.12: Left ventricular hypertrophy in a hypertensive patient. The left ventricular cavity dimensions are small. The cavity is likely to be more dilated in an elite athlete with the same degree of hypertrophy.

QR 8.13: Pathologic left ventricular hypertrophy with decreased mitral leaflet coaptation and consequent mitral regurgitation. This degree of mitral regurgitation is unlikely to be present in a normal athlete.

QR 8.14: Pathologic left ventricular hypertrophy with small left ventricular internal dimensions. The thickening of the interatrial septum in this case is due to unrelated lipomatous hypertrophy.

QR 8.15a: Severe left ventricular hypertrophy in a patient with amyloid heart disease.

QR 8.15b: Severe left ventricular hypertrophy in a patient with amyloid heart disease.

QR 8.15c: Severe left ventricular hypertrophy in a patient with amyloid heart disease.

QR 8.16a: Amyloid heart disease: Biventricular hypertrophy, systolic dysfunction, biatrial enlargement.

QR 8.16b: Amyloid heart disease: Biventricular hypertrophy, systolic dysfunction, biatrial enlargement.

QR 8.16c: Amyloid heart disease: Biventricular hypertrophy, systolic dysfunction, biatrial enlargement.

QR 8.16d: Amyloid heart disease: Biventricular hypertrophy, systolic dysfunction, biatrial enlargement.

QR 8.17: Amyloid heart disease: Preserved tricuspid annulus systolic excursion. Decreased lateral mitral annulus excursion.

QR 8.18: Nondiagnostic systolic anterior motion of the mitral chordae.

REFERENCES:

 Kholová I, Niessen HW. Amyloid in the cardiovascular system: a review. *J Clin Pathol*. 2005;58:125–133.

 Reinhold J, Rudhe U. Relation of the first and second heart sounds to events in the cardiac cycle. *Br Heart J*. 1957;19:473–485. *Auscultatory features of the first and second heart sounds in normal young people.*

Kaplan NM, Gidding SS, Pickering TG, et al. Task Force 5: systemic hypertension. *J Am Coll Cardiol*. 2005;45:1346–1348.

Recommendations from the above reference:

Before individuals commence training for competitive athletics, they should undergo careful assessment of BP and those with initially high levels (above 140/90 mm Hg) should have out-of-office measurements to exclude isolated office "white-coat" hypertension. Those with pre-hypertension (120/80 mm Hg up to 139/89 mm Hg) should be encouraged to modify lifestyle but should not be restricted from physical activity. Those with sustained hypertension should have echocardiography. Left ventricular hypertrophy (LVH) beyond that seen with "athletes' heart" should limit participation until BP is normalized by appropriate drug therapy.

The presence of stage 1 hypertension (140 to 159 mm Hg/90 to 99 mm Hg) in the absence of target organ damage (including LVH or concomitant heart disease) should not limit the eligibility for any competitive sport. Once having begun a training program, the hypertensive athlete should have BP remeasured every two to four months (or more frequently, if indicated) to monitor the impact of exercise.

Athletes with more severe hypertension (greater than or equal to 160/100 mm Hg), even without evidence of target organ damage such as LVH, should be restricted, particularly from high static sports, until their hypertension is controlled by either lifestyle modification or drug therapy.

All drugs being taken must be registered with appropriate governing bodies to obtain a therapeutic exemption.

When hypertension coexists with another cardiovascular disease, eligibility for participation in competitive athletics is usually based on the type and severity of the associated condition.

ANSWER: C and D

DILATED CARDIOMYOPATHY

    ❝   *The cardiomegaly may be striking and should be stricken*   ❞
(percussed).

QUESTION: **Which echocardiographic features are LEAST useful in the evaluation of dilated cardiomyopathy?**

A. Sphericity.

B. Wall thickness.

C. Lateral wall motion.

D. Speckled myocardial reflections.

E. Pericardial fluid.

Altered left ventricular geometry is manifested as increased short axis to long axis ratio. Increased wall thickness can be an adaptive process to keep myocardial stress from increasing. The lateral wall may be the "last man standing" in diffuse left ventricular wall hypokinesis. Myocardial infiltration may be manifested as a speckled or ground glass appearance. Small pericardial effusions with left ventricular *hypertrophy* are common in amyloid and in dialysis patients.

PHYSICAL EXAMINATION PEARLS

The first heart sound may be decreased on auscultation. Paradoxical splitting of S2 may be due to delayed left ventricular ejection. Several coughs may bring out a previously inaudible S3. *Percussion* may reveal the cardiomegaly by showing an increased area of cardiac dullness.

The art of percussion is as much tactile as it is auditory. A light tap is sufficient. It is not necessary to "percuss to the balcony." The total area of dullness to percussion in the normal heart is surprisingly small. Any dullness to percussion of the heart to the *right* of the sternum suggests cardiac enlargement.

Percussion of the heart should be performed from the right side of the patient. The left hand is placed on the chest when the examiner is right handed. The middle finger of the left hand is placed by separating it from the rest of the fingers and hand. It should be placed in the intercostal spaces rather than on top of the ribs. It should be bent in an arc so that only the distal two-thirds of the finger are in contact with the chest wall.

All soft tissue under the finger should be compressed firmly. The fingers of both hands should be as parallel to each other as possible.

One should strike at a 90-degree angle to prevent sideways displacement of the percussed finger (with resultant muffling of sounds). One should strike briskly with motion at the wrist only. The striking finger should be promptly removed to prevent muffling of the elicited percussion sound. The point of impact should be just proximal to the nail. Note: A true echocardiographer will never sneer at sending sound into the heart and analyzing the reflected vibrations.

FIGURE 8.12

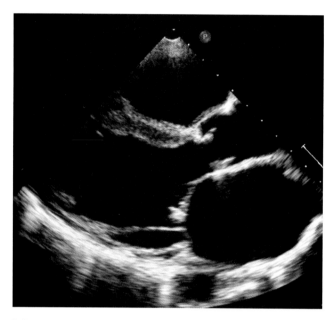

Dilated left atrium and left ventricle.

FIGURE 8.13

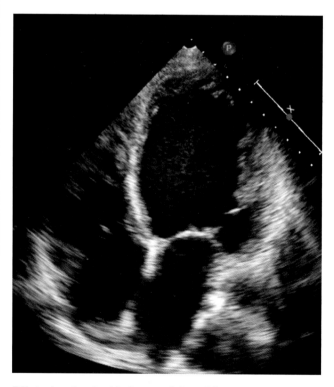

Dilated spherical left ventricle with spontaneous contrast in the left ventricular cavity.

FIGURE 8.14

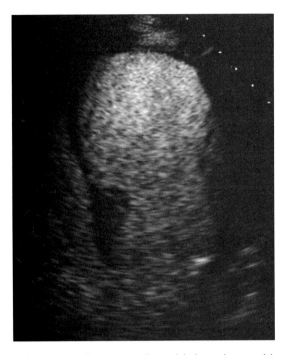

Dilated cardiomyopathy with basal septal hypertrophy.

QR 8.19: Biatrial enlargement with severe AV valve regurgitation.

FIGURE 8.15

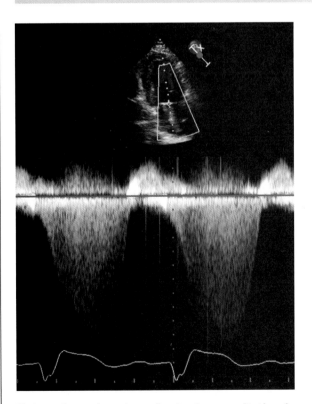

Delayed acceleration of mitral regurgitation in a patient with decreased systolic left ventricular function.

FIGURE 8.16

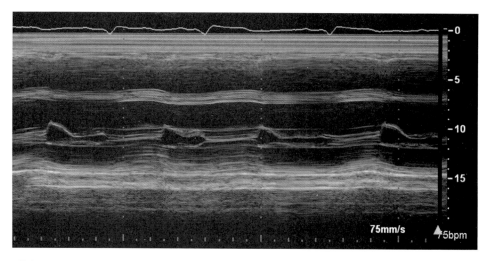

B bump—delayed mitral valve closure due to elevated end-diastolic pressures in severe systolic left ventricular dysfunction.

FIGURE 8.17

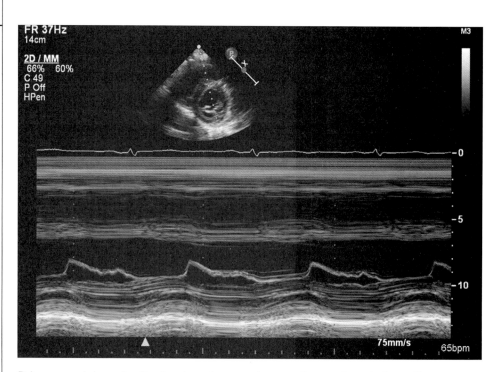

B bump—delayed mitral valve closure due to elevated end-diastolic pressures in severe systolic left ventricular dysfunction. The mitral component of first heart sound is typically *decreased* on auscultation in these patients.

FIGURE 8.18

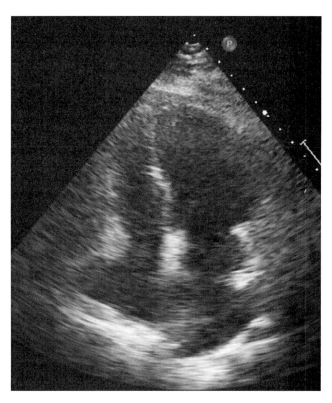

Three atrial suture line reflections in a heart transplant.

FIGURE 8.19

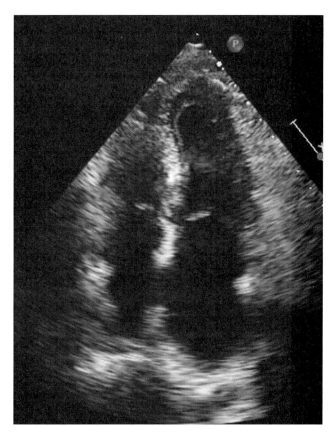

Three atrial suture line reflections in a heart transplant.

FIGURE 8.20

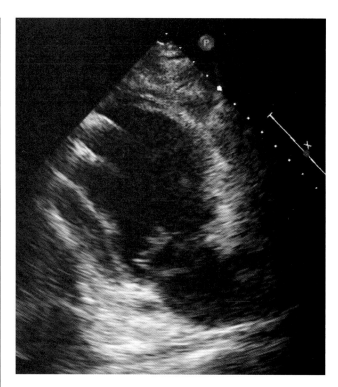

Apical left ventricular assist device.

FIGURE 8.21

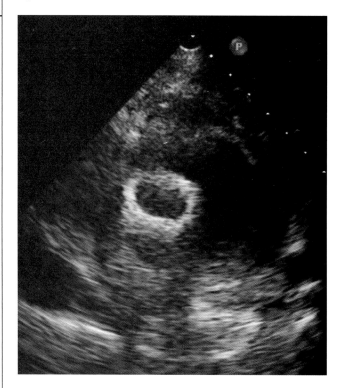

Apical left ventricular assist device.

QR 8.20: Early diastolic color flow propagation velocity.

QR 8.21: Ventricular assist device "pushing" blood into the ascending aorta. Continuous systolic and diastolic aortic regurgitation due to absence of forward stroke volume through the aortic valve.

FIGURE 8.22

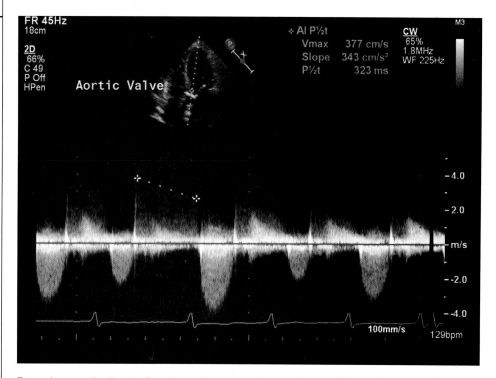

Doppler equivalent of pulsus alternans in a patient with aortic stenosis and dilated cardiomyopathy. Alternating strong and weak pulse amplitude during regular heart rhythm is called pulsus alternans. Very light palpation of the radial or femoral pulse should be used. The amount of pressure should be as light as the pressure created by blowing on the examiner's fingertips. The weak pulse may sometimes be too faint to feel. The tactile diagnosis can also be dramatically confirmed with a blood pressure cuff. On slowly deflating the cuff, the Korotkoff sounds are first heard at half the heart rate. With further lowering of the cuff pressure, the rate of Korotkoff sounds suddenly doubles.

FIGURE 8.23

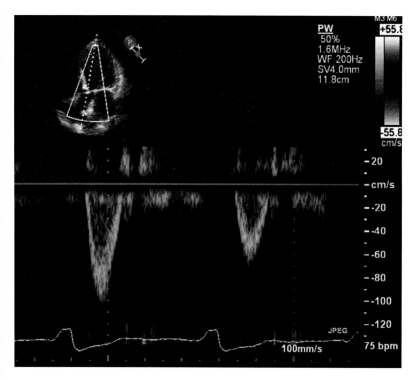

Abnormal Tei index and variable stroke volume in severe systolic left ventricular dysfunction.

QR 8.22a: Severely dilated, diffusely hypokinetic left ventricle.

QR 8.22b: Severely dilated, diffusely hypokinetic left ventricle.

QR 8.22c: Severely dilated, diffusely hypokinetic left ventricle.

QR 8.22d: Severely dilated, diffusely hypokinetic left ventricle.

QR 8.22e: Severely dilated, diffusely hypokinetic left ventricle.

QR 8.22f: Severely dilated, diffusely hypokinetic left ventricle.

QR 8.22g: Severely dilated, diffusely hypokinetic left ventricle.

QR 8.22h: Severely dilated, diffusely hypokinetic left ventricle.

QR 8.23: Dilated cardiomyopathy. Biatrial enlargement. Mitral prosthetic ring (not that obvious). Defibrillator wire in the right ventricle. Biatrial enlargement.

QR 8.24: Apical left ventricular wall akinesis on TEE giving the appearance of a "door knob turning."

QR 8.25: "Door knob turning" short axis view. Prominent false tendons.

QR 8.26: Severe dilatation, diffuse hypokinesis and akinesis, thin left ventricular walls. Small pericardial effusion.

QR 8.27a: Apical tethering of the mitral valve in dilated cardiomyopathy.

QR 8.27b: Apical tethering of the mitral valve in dilated cardiomyopathy.

QR 8.28: Decreased aortic leaflet opening due to the decreased stroke volume. Calcified papillary muscle tip due to apical tethering of the mitral valve.

QR 8.29: Decreased biventricular function. Biatrial enlargement.

QR 8.30: Thinning and increased reflectivity of the interventricular septum, indicating scarred, nonviable myocardium.

QR 8.31: Severely decreased biventricular systolic function.

QR 8.32: Mitral regurgitation in dilated cardiomyopathy.

QR 8.33: Left ventricular assist device "pushing" blood from the device to the ascending aorta.

QR 8.34: Right ventricular assist device "pushing" blood from the device to the pulmonary artery.

QR 8.35: Impella left ventricular assist device. Severe biventricular dysfunction. Biatrial enlargement. Loss of tricuspid leaflet opposition.

QR 8.36a: Impella left ventricular assist device.

QR 8.36b: Impella left ventricular assist device.

QR 8.37a: Apical left ventricular assist device. The aortic valve remains closed in systole.

QR 8.37b: Apical left ventricular assist device. The aortic valve remains closed in systole.

QR 8.38: Apical left ventricular assist device. Variable opening of the aortic valve from beat to beat. Sinus rhythm. No evident variability in mitral valve excursion from cycle to cycle.

REFERENCES:

 Yernault JC, Bohadana AB. Chest percussion. *Eur Respir J*. 1995;8:1756–1760.

Dressler W. Percussion of the sternum. I. Aid to differentiation of pericardial effusion and cardiac dilatation. *J Am Med Assoc*. 1960;173:761–764.

 Bedford DE. Auenbrugger's contribution to cardiology. History of percussion of the heart. *Br Heart J*. 1971;33:817–821.

 Yiu SF, Enriquez-Sarano M, Tribouilloy C, Seward JB, Tajik AJ. Determinants of the degree of functional mitral regurgitation in patients with systolic left ventricular dysfunction: a quantitative clinical study. *Circulation*. 2000;102:1400–1406.

Tei C, Ling LH, Hodge DO, et al. New index of combined systolic and diastolic myocardial performance: a simple and reproducible measure of cardiac function—a study in normals and dilated cardiomyopathy. *J Cardiol*. 1995;26:357–366. *Isovolumetric contraction time plus isovolumetric relaxation time divided by the ejection time provides a simple and reproducible Doppler index of combined systolic and diastolic myocardial performance in patients with primary myocardial systolic dysfunction.*

Weissler AM, Harris WS, Schoenfeld CD. Systolic time intervals in heart failure in man. *Circulation*. 1968;37:149–159.

ANSWER: E

RESTRICTIVE LEFT VENTRICULAR FILLING

QUESTION:

A patient with severe systolic left ventricular dysfunction presents with worsening dyspnea on exertion. There is a ventricular S3 gallop on auscultation. The ECG shows sinus tachycardia at a rate of 120. Blood pressure is 90/60. The echocardiogram shows a restrictive type 3 mitral inflow pattern. Which therapy is most appropriate at this time?

A. Diuretics.

B. Beta-blockers.

C. Vasodilators.

D. Digitalis.

E. Nesiritide.

A restrictive type 3 mitral inflow pattern indicates elevated left atrial pressures. Left ventricular filling takes place in early diastole. In this patient, it stops abruptly because of a rapid rise in left ventricular pressure, and as a result the ventricular S3 gallop is heard on auscultation.

Beta-blockers slow the heart rate and prolong diastole. They are indicated in the treatment of chronic compensated heart failure. They have been shown to prolong survival. In this case, prolonging diastole will not increase left ventricular stroke volume, since most of left ventricular filling takes place in early diastole with little contribution from the atrial contraction to left ventricular filling in late diastole. Decreasing the heart rate may actually decrease the cardiac output, which is calculated as stroke volume times the heart rate.

Loop diuretics do not prolong survival in heart failure, but they remain the treatment of choice for reducing left atrial and left ventricular filling pressures. The disappearance of a ventricular S3 gallop and a slowing of the heart rate indicate a return to a clinically stable form of compensated heart failure.

Nesiritide is an inotrope that has not been shown to provide long-term survival benefit. Digitalis has been relegated to a secondary role in the treatment heart failure. It may reduce the rate of readmission to hospitals for heart failure exacerbation, but digitalis therapy does not prolong long-term survival. Vasodilators such as ace inhibitors and angiotensin receptor blockers are valuable and will prolong survival in patients with heart failure. They may not be initially well tolerated in this case if the blood pressure is too low.

REFERENCE: Nihoyannopoulos P, Dawson D. Restrictive cardiomyopathies. *Eur J Echocardiogr.* 2009;10:iii23–iii33. *A restrictive left ventricular filling pattern does not mean that the patient has a restrictive cardiomyopathy.*

ANSWER: A

HYPEREOSINOPHILIA

" *Although the disorder is rare, the echocardiographic issues* **"**
illustrate a common dilemma during interpretation.

An echocardiogram of a young cancer patient shows a large thrombus in the left ventricle. The underlying left ventricular contractility is normal. Which test is most likely to confirm the diagnosis?

A. CBC with differential.

B. 24-hour urine 5-HIAA.

C. ANA.

D. Ferritin.

E. Serum protein electrophoresis.

F. Serum angiotensin converting enzyme.

If there is a thrombus in the left ventricle with no underlying wall motion abnormalities, check the CBC for hypereosinophilia.

Bonus Question

Match the echo and/or ECG description with the remaining choices:

Tricuspid and pulmonic leaflet thickening and retraction. (B. Carcinoid)

Mitral leaflet thickening. (C. Lupus-related Libman-Sacks endocarditis) (Alas, mitral leaflet thickening can also be seen in hypereosinophilic syndrome)

Heart "in molasses." (E. Myeloma-associated cardiac amyloidosis)

Echo-ECG discordance: Left ventricular hypertrophy on echo, but QRS voltage on the ECG is low. (also E. Amyloid infiltrative cardiomyopathy)

Heart block on ECG. (F. Cardiac sarcoidosis)

FIGURE 8.24

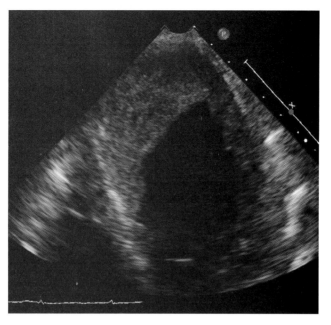

Large mural apical left ventricular thrombus.

QR 8.39a: Apical left ventricular thrombus with normal underlying left ventricular wall motion.

QR 8.39b: Apical left ventricular thrombus with normal underlying left ventricular wall motion.

QR 8.40: Apical left ventricular trabeculations may resemble a thrombus. The underlying left ventricular wall motion is normal.

REFERENCE:

Ommen SR, Seward JB, Tajik AJ. Clinical and echocardiographic features of hypereosinophilic syndromes. *Am J Cardiol*. 2000;86:110–113.

ANSWER TO THE FIRST QUESTION: A

VENTRICULAR NONCOMPACTION

QUESTION:

Prominent left ventricular trabeculations can be found on the echocardiogram of:

A. Noncompaction.

B. Hypertrophic cardiomyopathy.

C. Dilated cardiomyopathy.

D. All of the above.

Noncompaction has distinctive but not specific echocardiographic features. It is described as deep myocardial recesses with prominent trabecular outpouching. There is a bilayered appearance with non-compacted endocardial myocardium along with epicardial compacted myocardium.

MRI has a role following the echocardiographic examination. It provides the above morphological features, and may also demonstrate the presence of myocardial fibrosis. Alternate names for noncompaction: Spongy myocardium, persistent myocardial sinusoids, hyper-trabeculation.

Anatomic features of *normal* myocardial trabeculations that can be found during routine echocardiography:

1. Normal trabeculations protrude into the left ventricular cavity.
2. Their number is small (three or less).
3. Reflectivity is similar to the rest of the myocardium.
4. Normal trabeculations do not connect to adjacent myocardial segments.
5. They also do *not* favor the left ventricular apex.

FIGURE 8.25

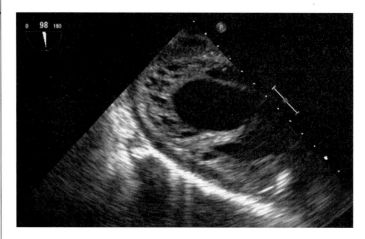

Noncompaction of the left ventricle.

QR 8.41: Noncompaction.

QR 8.42a: Noncompaction with severely decreased systolic left ventricular function.

QR 8.42b: Noncompaction with severely decreased systolic left ventricular function.

QR 8.42c: Noncompaction with severely decreased systolic left ventricular function.

QR 8.43: Apical left ventricular thrombus in noncompaction.

QR 8.44a: Cardiomyopathy with prominent trabeculations of the lateral left ventricular wall.

QR 8.44b: Cardiomyopathy with prominent trabeculations of the lateral left ventricular wall.

QR 8.45: Idiopathic cardiomyopathy with prominent biventricular trabeculations.

QR 8.46: Prominent left ventricular trabeculations with preserved systolic function.

REFERENCES:

  Jenni R, Oechslin E, Schneider J, Attenhofer Jost C, Kaufmann PA. Echocardiographic and pathoanatomical characteristics of isolated left ventricular non-compacton: a step towards classification as a distinct cardiomyopathy. *Heart.* 2001;86:666–671. *A two-layer structure is present with a compacted thin epicardial band and a much thicker noncompacted endocardial layer of trabecular meshwork with deep endomyocardial spaces. A maximal end-systolic ratio of noncompacted to compacted layers of >2 is diagnostic. Color Doppler shows deep perfused intertrabecular recesses.*

Jenni R, Oechslin EN, van der Loo B. Isolated ventricular non-compaction of the myocardium in adults. *Heart.* 2007;93:11–15. *Review article.*

Chin TK, Perloff JK, Williams RG, Jue K, Mohrmann R. Isolated noncompaction of left ventricular myocardium. A study of eight cases. *Circulation.* 1990; 82:507–513.

Shoji M, Yamashita T, Uejima T, et al. Electrocardiography characteristics of isolated non-compaction of ventricular myocardium in Japanese adult patients. *Circ J.* 2010;74:1431–1435.

ANSWER: D

EFFECT OF DRUGS AND PHYSICAL AGENTS ON THE HEART

“ *Amyloid, Carcinoid, Congestive Hepatopathy, End Stage Renal Disease, Radiation, Cocaine.* ”

QUESTION:

Which of the following echocardiographic findings should prompt a review of patient medications?

A. Dilated, diffusely hypokinetic left ventricle.

B. Dilated inferior vena cava.

C. Speckled myocardium AND a small pericardial effusion.

D. All of the above.

Congestive hepatopathy may affect hepatic drug metabolism. Answer C suggests cardiac amyloidosis, or end-stage renal disease. Both can affect drug metabolism. Normal doses of digitalis can be cardiotoxic. Valvular heart disease can be *caused* by drugs, by vasoactive substances, and by radiation.

QR 8.47a: Carcinoid tricuspid valve disease.

QR 8.47b: Carcinoid tricuspid valve disease.

QR 8.47c: Carcinoid pulmonic valve disease.

REFERENCES:

 Bhattacharyya S, Davar J, Dreyfus G, Caplin ME. Carcinoid heart disease. *Circulation*. 2007;116:2860–2865.

Pellikka PA, Tajik AJ, Khandheria BK, et al. Carcinoid heart disease. Clinical and echocardiographic spectrum in 74 patients. *Circulation*. 1993;87:1188–1196. *The broad spectrum of carcinoid heart disease is detailed in this large series. This includes not only right-sided valvular lesions but also left-sided involvement, pericardial effusion, and myocardial metastases.*

Pandya UH, Pellikka PA, Enriquez-Sarano M, et al. Metastatic carcinoid tumor to the heart: echocardiographic-pathologic study of 11 patients. *J Am Coll Cardiol.* 2002;40:1328–1332. *Metastatic carcinoid tumor involving the heart is uncommon but can be easily identified by echo if tumor size is ≥1.0 cm. In patients without valvular dysfunction, this may be may be the only manifestation of carcinoid heart disease.*

Jaworski C, Mariani JA, Wheeler G, Kaye DM. Cardiac complications of thoracic irradiation. *J Am Coll Cardiol.* 2013;61:2319–2328.

Crestanello JA, McGregor CG, Danielson GK, et al. Mitral and tricuspid valve repair in patients with previous mediastinal radiation therapy. *Ann Thorac Surg.* 2004;78:826–831. *Limited durability of repairs after mediastinal radiation suggests that valve replacement might be preferable.*

[pdf] Zanettini R, Antonini A, Gatto G, Gentile R, Tesei S, Pezzoli G. Valvular heart disease and the use of dopamine agonists for Parkinson's disease. *N Engl J Med.* 2007;356:39–46.

[pdf] Lange RA, Cigarroa JE, Hillis LD, Theodore E. Woodward award: cardiovascular complications of cocaine abuse. *Trans Am Clin Climatol Assoc.* 2004;115:99–111; discussion 112–114.

ANSWER: D

HEPATOJUGULAR REFLUX

This bedside physical examination sign remains valuable and is easy to do. It is also (more correctly) called the abdominojugular reflux. It is not a reflex. It correlates with left atrial pressure and can be performed during echocardiography. Transthoracic echocardiography does involve pressure on the abdomen with the transducer to obtain subcostal images. Doppler provides real-time changes in flow, and caval inflow can be demonstrated in many patients with Doppler.

Bedside Physical Examination Technique:

The examiner looks for neck vein distention (with or without pulsation) while firm pressure is exerted over the abdomen in the direction of the spinal column. Fifteen seconds of pressure on the abdomen are adequate for interpretation. The patient has to continue to breathe normally during the time that pressure is being exerted on the abdomen because an unintended Valsalva maneuver will create false-positive neck vein distention. An auscultatory equivalent of a positive hepatojugular reflux can also be sought: The first heart sound may get softer as pressure is being exerted on the abdomen of a patient with heart failure.

Hemodynamic Significance:

A positive test is thought to indicate an increased central blood volume. It should also correlate with echocardiographic findings of elevated left atrial pressure. Paraphrased from the original description in

1885: An impediment is created to the flow of blood, in either direction, through the inferior vena cava by this maneuver, especially when the liver is enlarged. With each systole an excessive reflux of blood takes place into the superior vena cava. Pulsation, as compared with distention or undulation, is merely one of degree of venous tension.

Hepatojugular reflux is not specific to any one disorder. It is a consequence of a right ventricle that cannot accommodate augmented venous return. Constrictive pericarditis, right ventricular infarction, and restrictive cardiomyopathy are common causes of a positive finding. Left ventricular failure may also induce the sign, but only when the pulmonary capillary wedge pressure is >15.

The one diagnosis NOT seen with hepatojugular reflux is cardiac tamponade. It was studied during right-sided cardiac catheterization by measuring changes in right atrial pressure. Bedside observation predicts the response during right-sided cardiac catheterization.

A positive sign has high sensitivity and specificity for predicting right atrial pressure >9 mmHg and right ventricular end-diastolic pressure >12 mmHg. In the absence of isolated right ventricular failure, seen in some patients with right ventricular infarction, a positive test suggests a pulmonary artery wedge pressure of 15 mmHg or greater.

QR 8.48: Saline contrast in the hepatic veins following injection into an arm vein in a patient with tricuspid regurgitation.

REFERENCES:

Wiese J. The abdominojugular reflux sign. *Am J Med*. 2000;109:59–61. *The sign is absent in patients with tamponade.*

Sochowski RA, Dubbin JD, Naqvi SZ. Clinical and hemodynamic assessment of the hepatojugular reflux. *Am J Cardiol*. 1990;66:1002. *Fifteen seconds of pressure are adequate for making the diagnosis.*

Ewy GA. The abdominojugular test: technique and hemodynamic correlates. *Ann Intern Med*. 1988;109:456. *A positive test correlates with a pulmonary artery wedge pressure of 15 mmHg or greater.*

Ducas J, Magder S, McGregor M. Validity of the hepatojugular reflux as a clinical test for congestive heart failure. *Am J Cardiol*. 1983;52:1299–1303. *An increase of 3 cm in the height of neck vein distention is a reasonable upper limit of normal.*

PERICARDIAL DISEASE

> **"** *Clinical and echocardiographic skills are equally important for* **"**
> *the diagnosis and management of pericardial disorders.*

The echocardiogram is a cornerstone in the clinical evaluation of pericardial diseases. The history, bedside examination, and electrocardiogram are equally important. The chest pain of pericarditis may be difficult to distinguish from ischemic pain. It may decrease on leaning forward; and worsen on lying back, on coughing, or on inspiration.

Radiation of pain to the *trapezius ridge* is a rare but useful distinguishing feature of pericardial pain. The neck vein examination may show jugular venous distention. More importantly, examination of neck vein pulsations by a skilled clinician provides findings that correlate with Doppler hemodynamics in constriction, or tamponade.

The pericardial rub is one of the instances in medicine where a physical finding makes the diagnosis. A pericardial knock is a triple rhythm of pericardial constriction. The electrocardiographic diagnosis of pericarditis is explicit, but subtle PR segment depression can be easily missed. PR segment elevation in aVR may be more obvious to the eye.

REFERENCES:

Spodick DH. Diagnostic electrocardiographic sequences in acute pericarditis. Significance of PR segment and PR vector changes. *Circulation*. 1973;48: 575–580.

Little WC, Freeman GL. Pericardial disease. *Circulation*. 2006;113:1622–1632.

Khandaker MH, Espinosa RE, Nishimura RA, et al. Pericardial disease: diagnosis and management. *Mayo Clin Proc*. 2010;85:572–593.

Peebles CR, Shambrook JS, Harden SP. Pericardial disease – anatomy and function. *Br J Radiol*. 2011;84(Spec No 3):S324–S337. *Overview of CT and MRI imaging of healthy and diseased pericardium.*

Maisch B, Seferovic PM, Ristic AD, et al. Guidelines on the diagnosis and management of pericardial diseases executive summary: the task force on the diagnosis and management of pericardial diseases of the European Society of Cardiology. *Eur Heart J*. 2004;25:587–610.

ECHOCARDIOGRAPHIC FINDINGS IN PERICARDIAL DISEASES ARE INFLUENCED BY ETIOLOGY

The etiology of most cases of acute pericarditis is idiopathic; and is usually assumed to be viral.

An effusion is not necessary for the clinical diagnosis of acute pericarditis. The history, physical examination, and ECG will usually suffice. Pericarditis can complicate myocardial infarction and can present as Dressler's syndrome. Renal failure patients have a spectrum of typical echocardiographic findings that may include pericardial abnormalities.

Rheumatological disorders have individual echocardiographic features that are also accompanied by pericardial involvement. Cancer patients may develop hemodynamically significant tamponade; even with long-standing effusions. Pericardial effusion in a young patient may be the initial manifestation of a malignant tumor. Trauma can cause tamponade. Aortic dissection can cause tamponade, but pericardiocentesis is potentially dangerous.

Unusual presentations of large pericardial effusions:

• Dysphagia due to esophageal compression.
• Hiccups due to diaphragmatic stimulation.
• Hoarseness due to recurrent laryngeal nerve compression.

Post open-heart effusions can be missed with echocardiography, and their hemodynamic importance may be misjudged because the pericardium is open.

REFERENCES:

Russo AM, O'Connor WH, Waxman HL. Atypical presentations and echocardiographic findings in patients with cardiac tamponade occurring early and late after cardiac surgery. *Chest*. 1993;104:71–78.

Ionescu A, Wilde P, Karsch KR. Localized pericardial tamponade: difficult echocardiographic diagnosis of a rare complication after cardiac surgery. *J Am Soc Echocardiogr*. 2001;14:1220–1223. *Two cases of localized pericardial tamponade after cardiac surgery. The diagnosis could not be made with transthoracic echocardiography. CT and transesophageal echocardiography were necessary. A high index of suspicion is crucial for reaching the correct diagnosis.*

Pepi M, Muratori M, Barbier P, et al. Pericardial effusion after cardiac surgery: incidence, site, size, and haemodynamic consequences. *Br Heart J*. 1994;72: 327–331.

COMMON CLINICAL QUESTIONS TO THE ECHOCARDIOGRAPHER

- Is there tamponade?
- Is there constriction?
- How thick is the pericardium?
- Is there tumor involvement of the heart?
- Is that a rub?

PERICARDIAL EFFUSION

QUESTION:

Echocardiography can determine the following aspects of a pericardial effusion EXCEPT:

A. Size.

B. Hemodynamic importance.

C. Content.

D. Presence or absence.

Although it is possible to detect fibrin in the pericardial space, echocardiography cannot reliably distinguish between a serous and a bloody effusion. Epicardial fat can usually be distinguished from fluid. Some "post open-heart" effusions may be difficult to identify. Large pericardial effusions may rarely be mistaken for pleural effusions. Pleural effusions adjacent to the right atrial free wall may be mistaken for loculated pericardial effusions.

REFERENCE:

Horowitz MS, Schultz CS, Stinson EB, et al. Sensitivity and specificity of echocardiographic diagnosis of pericardial effusion. *Circulation*. 1974;50:239. *More than 15 mL of fluid was always found when a posterior echo-free space persisted throughout the cardiac cycle between a flat pericardium relative to the epicardium. In the presence of such a posterior echo-free space, a large anterior echo-free space made a moderately large pericardial effusion likely. In the absence of this diagnostic posterior echo-free space, an anterior echo-free space had no diagnostic significance.*

ANSWER: C (some exceptions are noted above)

CARDIAC TAMPONADE

QUESTION:

Acute distention of the pericardium can cause hemodynamic compromise. Which abnormality does NOT cause pericardial pressure elevation?

A. Right ventricular infarction.

B. Acute pulmonary embolism.

C. Pulseless electrical activity.

D. Post open-heart effusion.

E. Low pressure tamponade.

Intrapericardial pressure rises when fluid accumulates faster than the pericardium can stretch. The intrapericardial pressure of low-pressure tamponade is, by definition, high enough to cause cardiac chamber compression. Pulseless electrical activity is found in myocardial rupture. The pericardium is generally left open after open-heart surgery.

FIGURE 9.1

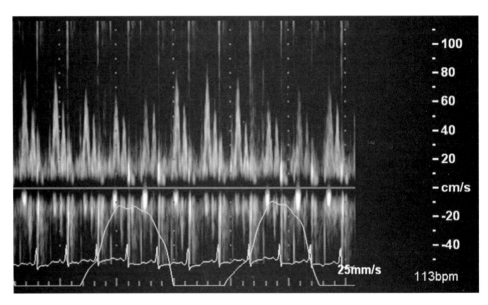

Inspiratory decrease in mitral inflow velocity in tamponade.

QR 9.1a: Large thrombus in the pericardial space following heart surgery.

QR 9.1b: Large thrombus in the pericardial space following heart surgery.

REFERENCES:

 Schiller NB, Botvinick EH. Right ventricular compression as a sign of cardiac tamponade: an analysis of echocardiographic ventricular dimensions and their clinical implications. *Circulation*. 1977;56:774.

Armstrong WF, Schilt BF, Helper DJ, et al. Diastolic collapse of the right ventricle with cardiac tamponade: an echocardiographic study. *Circulation*. 1982;65:1491. *Collapse of the right ventricular cavity in early diastole is abnormal. Conversely, normal motion of the right ventricular free wall is a reliable indicator that the effusion is exerting little effect on overall cardiac function.*

 Gillam LD, Guyer DE, Gibson TC, et al. Hydrodynamic compression of the right atrium: a new echocardiographic sign of cardiac tamponade. *Circulation*. 1983;68:294. *Right atrial inversion is initiated at end-diastole and continues through early systole.*

Himelman RB, Kircher B, Rockey DC, et al. Inferior vena cava plethora with blunted respiratory response: a sensitive echocardiographic sign of cardiac tamponade. *J Am Coll Cardiol*. 1988;12:1470.

Reddy PS, Curtiss EI, O'Toole JD, et al. Cardiac tamponade: hemodynamic observations in man. *Circulation*. 1978;58:265–272.

Sagristà-Sauleda J, Angel J, Sambola A, et al. Low-pressure cardiac tamponade: clinical and hemodynamic profile. *Circulation*. 2006;114:945–952.

Sagristà-Sauleda J, Angel J, Sambola A, et al. Hemodynamic effects of volume expansion in patients with cardiac tamponade. *Circulation*. 2008;117:1545–1549. *Volume expansion consistently causes a significant increase in intrapericardial pressure.*

ANSWER: D

PULSUS PARADOXUS

QUESTION:

What part of the cardiac cycle is hemodynamically best tolerated during cardiac tamponade?

A. Systole.

B. Diastole.

C. Late diastole and early systole.

D. Late systole and early diastole.

In the normal patient, examination of the jugular pulse will frequently show an inspiratory drop in the 'x' descent in systole. This is *preserved* in cardiac tamponade. Ventricular emptying into the great vessels (systole) remains unhampered. Tamponade is manifested with abnormal ventricular filling (diastole). There is inspiratory blunting of tricuspid inflow. An absent 'y' descent at the bedside confirms the hemodynamic compromise. Kussmaul sign is associated with pericardial constriction, but can be seen in cardiac tamponade. Increased inspiratory venous return cannot be completely accommodated by the right heart; and consequently, the jugular venous pressure increases.

• BAD NEWS The following abnormalities can create an absent 'y' descent (and mimic tamponade):

- Pulmonary embolism
- Right ventricular infarction
- Acute severe tricuspid regurgitation due to chest trauma.

Pulsus paradoxus may not be present (in spite of hemodynamic tamponade) in the following cases:

- Severe aortic regurgitation
- Atrial septal defect
- Mechanical ventilation with positive pressure breathing
- Left ventricular dysfunction

FIGURE 9.2

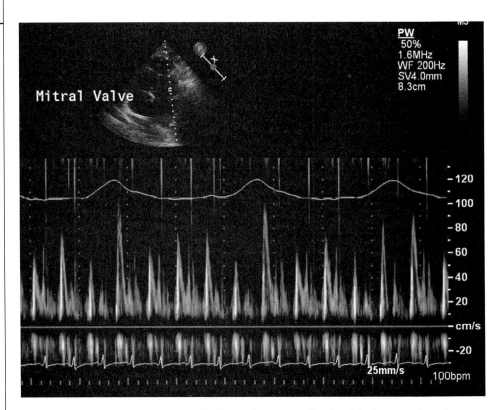

Respiratory variation in mitral inflow. Decreased mitral inflow on inspiration. The fastest early diastolic velocity is recorded in early expiration.

FIGURE 9.3

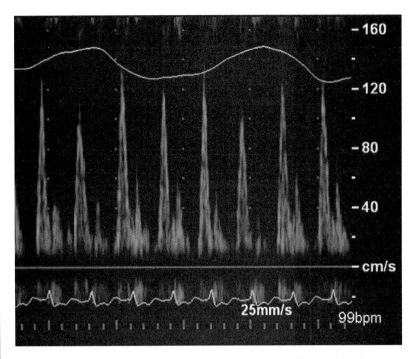

Inspiratory decrease in early diastolic mitral inflow velocity.

FIGURE 9.4

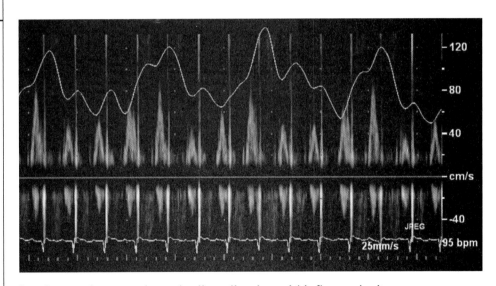

Inspiratory increase in early diastolic tricuspid inflow velocity.

FIGURE 9.5

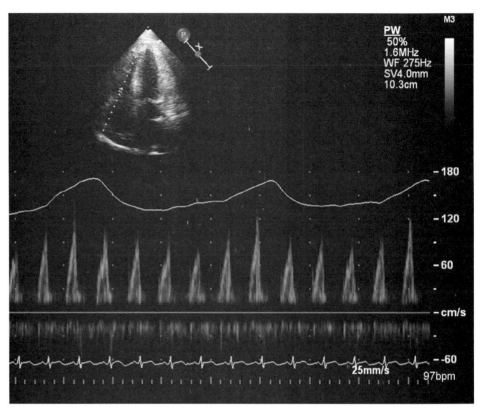

Inspiratory increase in diastolic tricuspid inflow velocity. There is fusion of the early and late diastolic waves (E-A fusion).

FIGURE 9.6

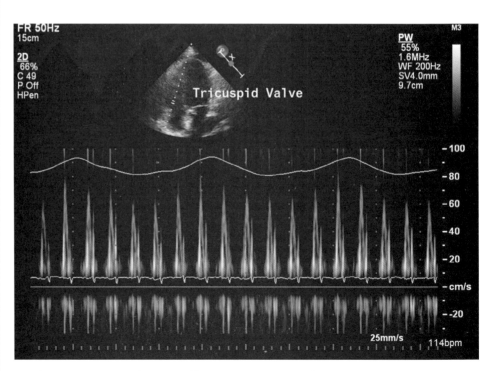

Inspiratory increase in early diastolic tricuspid inflow velocity.

FIGURE 9.7

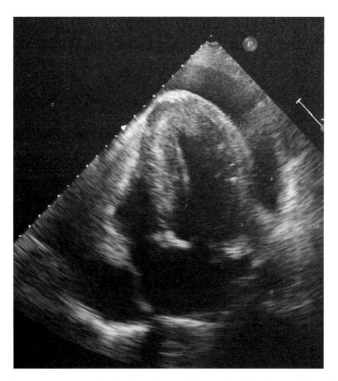

Large pericardial effusion with partial right atrial collapse.

QR 9.2: Large pericardial effusion with partial right atrial collapse.

QR 9.3: Pleural and pericardial effusion with partial right atrial collapse.

QR 9.4a: Partial right atrial collapse.

QR 9.4b: Partial right atrial collapse.

QR 9.5: Partial biatrial collapse.

QR 9.6: No right atrial collapse in this view. Fibrin in the pericardial space on the right ventricular epicardium.

QR 9.7a: Fibrin in the pericardial space.

QR 9.7b: Fibrin in the pericardial space.

QR 9.8: Fibrin in the pericardial space. Multiple views were needed to distinguish this from pleural fibrin.

QR 9.9: Saline contrast in the pericardial space during echo-guided pericardiocentesis.

QR 9.10a: Partial collapse of the right ventricular free wall.

QR 9.10b: Partial collapse of the right ventricular free wall.

QR 9.10c: Partial collapse of the right ventricular free wall.

QR 9.11: Exaggerated systolic right ventricular wall motion without diastolic inversion of the free wall. Aortic bioprosthesis.

QR 9.12: Pericardial effusion in a dialysis patient.

QR 9.13: Pericardial effusion in the transverse sinus between the left atrial appendage and the left upper pulmonary vein. This is not a persistent left superior vena cava.

QR 9.14a: Pericardial effusion in Dressler's syndrome following anterior myocardial infarction.

QR 9.14b: Pericardial effusion in Dressler's syndrome following anterior myocardial infarction.

QR 9.15a: Large pericardial effusion with swinging heart motion that can be responsible for an electrical alternans QRS pattern on the ECG.

QR 9.15b: Large pericardial effusion with swinging heart motion that can be responsible for an electrical alternans QRS pattern on the ECG.

QR 9.15c: Large pericardial effusion with swinging heart motion that can be responsible for an electrical alternans QRS pattern on the ECG.

QR 9.15d: Large pericardial effusion with swinging heart motion that can be responsible for an electrical alternans QRS pattern on the ECG.

QR 9.15e: Large pericardial effusion with swinging heart motion that can be responsible for an electrical alternans QRS pattern on the ECG.

QR 9.16: Pericardial effusion (not pleural) interposed between the descending aorta and the posterior left atrial wall.

QR 9.17: Large pleural effusion extending behind the descending aorta. Minimal pericardial effusion.

QR 9.18: Ascites on the abdominal side of the diaphragm.

QR 9.19: Large pericardial effusion that extends to the transverse sinus (behind the proximal ascending aorta).

QR 9.20: Pericardial fluid in the transverse sinus. Saline contrast in the superior vena cava and in the right branch of the pulmonary artery.

QR 9.21: Exaggerated excursion of the right ventricular free wall due to pericardial fluid. There is no diastolic inversion of the right ventricular wall.

QR 9.22: Questionable collapse of the basal right ventricular free wall. This should be confirmed in other views. Note: There is no right atrial inversion, and the pericardial effusion appears to be small.

QR 9.23a: Fibrin in the pleural space.

QR 9.23b: Fibrin in the pleural space.

QR 9.23c: Fibrin in the pleural space.

QR 9.23d: Fibrin in the pleural space.

QR 9.24: Pleural effusion extending behind the descending aorta. This helps distinguish it from the coexisting minimal pericardial effusion (only seen in systole in this case).

QR 9.25: Ascites can be mistaken for a pericardial cyst (diverticulum).

REFERENCES:

 Maier HC. Diverticulum of the pericardium with observations on mode of development. *Circulation.* 1957;16:1040–1045.

 Cosío FG, Martínez JP, Serrano CM, et al. Abnormal septal motion in cardiac tamponade with pulsus paradoxus. Echocardiographic and hemodynamic observations. *Chest.* 1977;71:787–788. *Pulsus paradoxus may be caused by competition of the ventricles for filling within a relatively rigid pericardial space.*

 Fowler NO. Cardiac tamponade. A clinical or an echocardiographic diagnosis? *Circulation.* 1993;87:1738–1741.

 D'Cruz IA, Cohen HC, Prabhu R, et al. Diagnosis of cardiac tamponade by echocardiography: changes in mitral valve motion and ventricular dimensions, with special reference to paradoxical pulse. *Circulation.* 1975;52:460–465.

 Settle HP Jr, Engel PJ, Fowler NO, et al. Echocardiographic study of the paradoxical arterial pulse in chronic obstructive lung disease. *Circulation.* 1980; 62:1297–1307.

 Shekerdemian L, Bohn D. Cardiovascular effects of mechanical ventilation. *Arch Dis Child.* 1999;80:475–480.

ANSWER: A

PERICARDIAL CONSTRICTION

" *A treatable cause of intractable right heart failure.* **"**

A patient with persistent symptoms and signs of heart failure is suspected of having undiagnosed pericardial constriction.

Which bedside examination finding is UNLIKELY to be present?

A. Elevated venous pressure.

B. Kussmaul sign.

C. Pericardial knock.

D. Blunted 'y' descent.

E. Systolic retraction of the apical impulse.

Prominent 'y' descent is a hallmark physical finding of constriction. When present, it is very striking to the trained eye. The neck veins collapse as if a trap door opened. You need to look and listen at the same time. The 'y' descent is seen in the neck just after the second heart sound is heard on auscultation. The 'y' descent is also out of phase with the palpated carotid impulse (an 'x' descent is simultaneous).

Pericardial constriction can be a difficult clinical and echocardiographic diagnosis. It may remain undiagnosed in patients with refractory right heart failure. There are characteristic clinical findings. Unfortunately, they may not be obvious because this is a rare disorder and clinicians rarely see patients with this conglomerate of bedside findings. Simply reading about them is not enough.

The echocardiographic diagnosis is also difficult and will be discussed below. In severe cases of pericardial constriction, the bedside findings may be very obvious. For example, elevated jugular venous pressure may be high enough to manifest itself as persistent jugular venous distention in the STANDING position.

The pericardial knock can manifest as an unusually loud early diastolic third heart sound. It gets louder on squatting. Even a relatively inexperienced clinician may recognize that there is a triple rhythm on auscultation. Brief but brisk early diastolic right ventricular filling (that halts with the knock) causes the prominent 'y' descent.

In constriction, the apical impulse may retract away from the palpating finger in systole. Kussmaul confused everybody. Kussmaul sign is characteristic, but not unique to constrictive pericarditis. The jugular veins paradoxically expand on inspiration in patients with constriction (normally, they collapse on inspiration).

An exaggerated (hence not paradoxical) drop in systolic blood pressure on inspiration (also described by the astute Kussmaul) is found in cardiac tamponade but further confuses, because it can also be present in constriction and is inappropriately called pulsus paradoxus. Kussmaul had his reasons for picking the name—the pulse went away, but he kept hearing the heart sounds.

REFERENCE: Fowler NO, Engel PJ, Settle HP, et al. The paradox of the paradoxical pulse. *Trans Am Clin Climatol Assoc.* 1979;90:27–37.

ECHOCARDIOGRAPHIC FINDINGS IN PERICARDIAL CONSTRICTION

The calcified pericardium "insulates" the heart from intrathoracic respiratory pressure changes and exaggerates respiratory interaction between the ventricles. A septal "bounce" is a respiratory phenomenon. It may be missed on a short digital loop and should be looked for in real time. A provocative maneuver such as a sniff may be necessary to demonstrate it.

Doppler examination of the hepatic veins provides the echocardiographic equivalent of the bedside jugular venous inspection. Reversal of hepatic blood flow in *expiration* is a useful sign that is best looked for in real time during the study. Biatrial enlargement may be striking (but non-specific). It is due to the chronic elevation in ventricular filling pressures. Transesophageal echocardiography, CT, or MRI may be better suited to evaluate pericardial thickness than transthoracic echocardiography. However, constriction may be also be caused by stiff pericardium that is not measurably thickened.

FIGURE 9.8

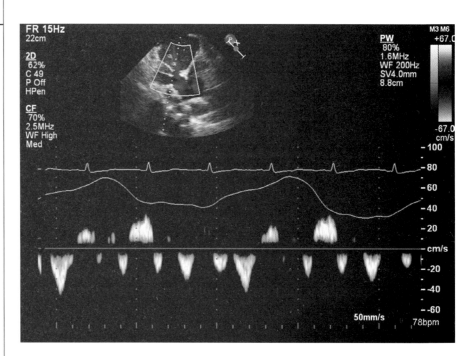

Expiratory reversal of hepatic vein flow in pericardial constriction.

FIGURE 9.9

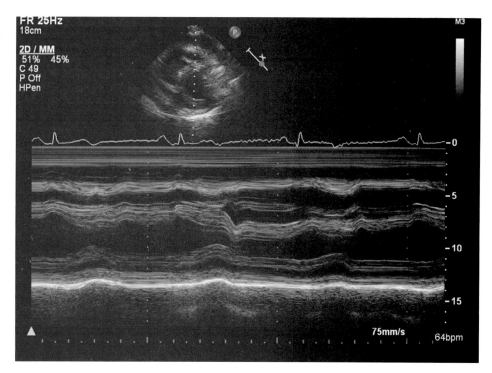

Respiratory "bounce" of the interventricular septum in pericardial constriction.

FIGURE 9.10

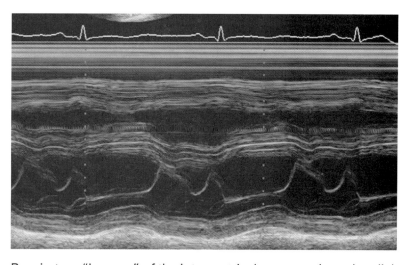

Respiratory "bounce" of the interventricular septum in pericardial constriction.

FIGURE 9.11

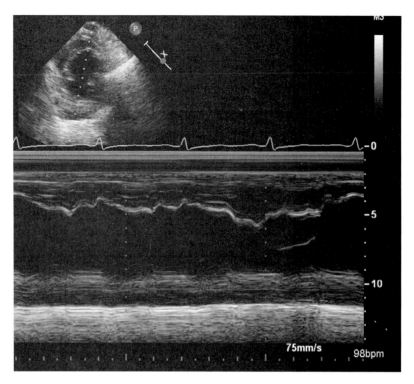

Respiratory "bounce" of the interventricular septum in pericardial constriction.

FIGURE 9.12

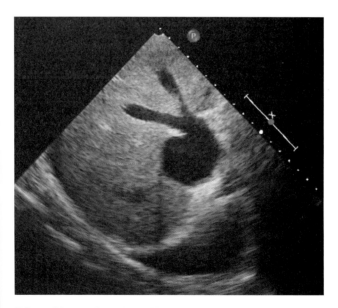

Dilated hepatic veins. "Bunny sign." In contrast, absence of hepatic venous congestion and IVC dilatation is strong evidence AGAINST the diagnosis of hemodynamically significant pericardial constriction.

QR 9.26a: Septal "bounce" in pericardial constriction.

QR 9.26b: Septal "bounce" in pericardial constriction.

QR 9.26c: Septal "bounce" in pericardial constriction.

QR 9.27: Normal motion of the interventricular septum (no "bounce") shown for comparison.

QR 9.28a: Pericardial thickness can be measured using echocardiography only when there is fluid on both sides of the pericardium.

QR 9.28b: Pericardial thickness can be measured using echocardiography only when there is fluid on both sides of the pericardium.

QR 9.28c: Pericardial thickness can be measured using echocardiography only when there is fluid on both sides of the pericardium.

QR 9.28d: Pericardial thickness can be measured using echocardiography only when there is fluid on both sides of the pericardium.

QR 9.28e: Pericardial thickness can be measured using echocardiography only when there is fluid on both sides of the pericardium.

QR 9.28f: Pericardial thickness can be measured using echocardiography only when there is fluid on both sides of the pericardium.

QR 9.29: Thick pericardium delineated by pleural and pericardial fluid.

QR 9.30: Left ventricular hypertrophy with biatrial enlargement.

QR 9.31a: Normal phasic decrease in the diameter of the inferior vena cava. This indicates that the right atrial pressures are normal and excludes significant pericardial constriction.

QR 9.31b: Normal phasic decrease in the diameter of the inferior vena cava. This indicates that the right atrial pressures are normal and excludes significant pericardial constriction.

QR 9.32: Dilated hepatic veins with prominent flow reversal (in blue). The reversal occurs on *expiration* in patients with pericardial constriction.

QR 9.33a: Fluoroscopic appearance of calcified pericardium.

QR 9.33b: Fluoroscopic appearance of calcified pericardium.

QR 9.33c: Fluoroscopic appearance of calcified pericardium.

REFERENCES:

 Boicourt OW, Nagle RE, Mounsey JP. The clinical significance of systolic retraction of the apical impulse. *Br Heart J*. 1965;27:379–391.

 el-Sherif A, el-Said G. Jugular, hepatic, and praecordial pulsations in constrictive pericarditis. *Br Heart J*. 1971;33:305–312.

Dal-Bianco JP, Sengupta PP, Mookadam F, et al. Role of echocardiography in the diagnosis of constrictive pericarditis. *J Am Soc Echocardiogr*. 2009;22:24–33. *The combination of exaggerated interventricular interdependence, relatively preserved left ventricular longitudinal deformation, and attenuated circumferential deformation is diagnostic.*

Ling LH, Oh JK, Tei C, et al. Pericardial thickness measured with transesophageal echocardiography: feasibility and potential clinical usefulness. *J Am Coll Cardiol*. 1997; 29:1317.

Oh JK, Tajik AJ, Appleton CP, et al. Preload reduction to unmask the characteristic Doppler features of constrictive pericarditis. A new observation. *Circulation*. 1997;95:796. *When the respiratory variation in Doppler mitral E velocity is blunted or absent during the evaluation of suspected constrictive pericarditis, repeat Doppler recording of mitral flow velocities after maneuvers to decrease preload is recommended to unmask the characteristic respiratory variation in mitral E velocity.*

Ha JW, Oh JK, Ling LH, et al. Annulus paradoxus: transmitral flow velocity to mitral annular velocity ratio is inversely proportional to pulmonary capillary wedge pressure in patients with constrictive pericarditis. *Circulation*. 2001;104:976. *The lateral expansion of the heart is limited by constricting pericardium, resulting in exaggerated longitudinal motion of the mitral annulus. The more severe the constriction, the more accentuated is the longitudinal motion.*

Sengupta PP, Mohan JC, Mehta V, et al. Accuracy and pitfalls of early diastolic motion of the mitral annulus for diagnosing constrictive pericarditis by tissue Doppler imaging. *Am J Cardiol*. 2004;93:886–890. *Mitral annular velocities help with diagnosis and differentiation of constrictive pericarditis in most cases, except in the presence of extensive annular calcification, left ventricular systolic dysfunction, or segmental nonuniformity in myocardial velocities.*

Rajagopalan N, Garcia MJ, Rodriguez L, et al. Comparison of new Doppler echocardiographic methods to differentiate constrictive pericardial heart disease and restrictive cardiomyopathy. *Am J Cardiol.* 2001;87:86. *Respiratory variation in the mitral inflow peak early velocity of ≥10% predicted constrictive pericarditis with 84% sensitivity and 91% specificity. Variation in the pulmonary venous peak diastolic flow velocity of ≥18% distinguished constriction with 79% sensitivity and 91% specificity. Using tissue Doppler echocardiography, a peak early velocity of longitudinal expansion of ≥8.0 cm/s differentiated patients with constriction from restriction with 89% sensitivity and 100% specificity. A slope of ≥100 cm/s for the first aliasing contour in color M-mode flow propagation predicted patients with constriction with 74% sensitivity and 91% specificity.*

Sengupta PP, Krishnamoorthy VK, Abhayaratna WP, et al. Disparate patterns of left ventricular mechanics differentiate constrictive pericarditis from restrictive cardiomyopathy. *JACC Cardiovasc Imaging.* 2008;1:29–38. *Deformation of the left ventricle is constrained in the circumferential direction in constriction, and in the longitudinal direction in restriction. Subsequent early diastolic recoil is also attenuated in each of the two directions, respectively, uniquely differentiating the abnormal diastolic restoration mechanics of these two entities.*

[pdf] Verhaert D, Gabriel RS, Johnston D, et al. The role of multimodality imaging in the management of pericardial disease. *Circ Cardiovasc Imaging.* 2010; 3:333–343.

ANSWER: D

PERICARDITIS

  "   *The term "friction rub" comes from the Department of*   **"**
Redundancy Department.

QUESTION: **Which statement about pericardial rubs is WRONG?**

A. The majority are "to and fro" biphasic.

B. The minority are monophasic—simulating a murmur.

C. They have variable auditory characteristics.

D. Rubs are evanescent—transient in nature.

On careful repeated auscultation, the majority of pericardial rubs are triphasic, and may get louder on inspiration. They are heard during atrial systole, ventricular systole, and in early diastole (coincident with early mitral inflow on echo). The best location for auscultation is adjacent to the left mid-sternal border (due to sound conduction via pericardiosternal ligaments, and due to direct contact of the pericardium with that part of the chest).

PRACTICAL TIPS: The three components are heard more easily at slower heart rates, but gentle exercise may make a rub *louder*. Held expiration may make a pericardial rub more audible, and exclude a pleural rub at the same time.

Leaning the patient forward, or completely face down, may make the rub more audible. Pericardial rubs can be very faint. A potentially useful technique consists of listening with the patient lying face down, chest propped up by leaning on their elbows. A less awkward approach is to have the patient stand, lean forward, and support the elbows on a table or a counter—the standing flexion position. This technique also makes it possible to increase the patient's heart rate by some form of upright exercise with immediate post-exercise stethoscope access while the rate is still fast.

Pericardial rubs have been described as:

Scratchy: Easily simulated by the sound you hear when you scratch your head three times.

Leathery: Like the sound made by sitting on a horse with new creaky saddle.

Crunchy: Similar to the sound of stepping on freshly fallen snow.

Superficial: Sounds like it is originating "half way up" the stethoscope.

Pleuropericardial rubs: The Means–Lerman scratch is a systolic sound heard in hyperthyroid patients presumably due to rubbing of hyperdynamic pericardium against the pleura. It mimics the systolic component of a pericardial rub.

QR 9.34: Pleuropericardial fibrin. Pleural effusion with fibrin in the pleural space adhering to the epicardial surface. This particular echocardiographic appearance can easily be mistaken for a large pericardial effusion.

REFERENCES:

 Weiss A, Luisada AA. The friction rubs of pericarditis. *Chest*. 1971;60:491–493.

 Tingle LE, Molina D, Calvert CW. Acute pericarditis. *Am Fam Physician*. 2007; 76:1509–1514.

 Sodeman WA. Acute pericarditis: its role in diagnostic interpretation. *Chest*. 1970;57:477–479.

TREATMENT OF PERICARDITIS

❝ *Short courses of treatment are more likely to result in relapse.* **❞**

● BAD NEWS: Steroid treatment of recurrent pericarditis may result in steroid dependence.

● GOOD NEWS: Colchicine is a better option compared to high dose steroids.

REFERENCES:

 Adler Y, Finkelstein Y, Guindo J, et al. Colchicine treatment for recurrent pericarditis. A decade of experience. *Circulation*. 1998;97:2183–2185.

Imazio M, Brucato A, Cumetti D, et al. Corticosteroids for recurrent pericarditis: high versus low doses: a nonrandomized observation. *Circulation*. 2008; 118:667–671.

Imazio M, Bobbio M, Cecchi E, et al. Colchicine as first-choice therapy for recurrent pericarditis: results of the CORE (COlchicine for REcurrent pericarditis) trial. *Arch Intern Med*. 2005;165:1987–1991.

Imazio M, Bobbio M, Cecchi E, et al. Colchicine in addition to conventional therapy for acute pericarditis: results of the COlchicine for acute PEricarditis (COPE) trial. *Circulation*. 2005;112:2012–2016.

Imazio M, Brucato A, Ferrazzi P, et al; COPPS Investigators. Colchicine reduces postoperative atrial fibrillation: results of the Colchicine for the Prevention of the Postpericardiotomy Syndrome (COPPS) atrial fibrillation substudy. *Circulation*. 2011,124.2290–2295.

ANSWER: A

SYSTEMIC LUPUS ERYTHEMATOSUS

QUESTION:

Which transthoracic echocardiographic findings are most likely to be abnormal in patients with systemic lupus erythematosus?

A. Tricuspid regurgitation velocity.

B. Left ventricular wall motion.

C. Lambl excrescences.

D. Libman–Sacks vegetations.

E. Pericardial fluid.

Libman–Sacks refers to sterile vegetations. They are more typical for SLE but less common than pericardial effusions. TEE is more sensitive in making this diagnosis. Pericardial effusions are very common in SLE. They are a consequence of a lupus flare with serositis. There may also be pleural effusions. Pulmonary hypertension is possible. Premature coronary artery disease can occur.

REFERENCES:

 Roman MJ, Salmon JE. Cardiovascular manifestations of rheumatologic diseases. *Circulation*. 2007;116:2346–2355.

 Knockaert DC. Cardiac involvement in systemic inflammatory diseases. *Eur Heart J*. 2007;28:1797–1804.

ANSWER: E

DIASTOLOGY

DIASTOLIC DYSFUNCTION FOR DUMMIES

QUESTION: **Which component of the sequence of progressive diastolic dysfunction is out of order?**

A. Active diastolic suction.

B. Impaired left ventricular relaxation.

C. Elevated left atrial pressure.

D. Pseudonormal mitral inflow pattern.

E. Impaired left ventricular filling.

F. I have no clue, but this sequence feels right.

ANOTHER QUESTION: **An elderly patient presents with heart failure but left ventricular systolic function is normal.**

Which statement is FALSE?

A. Diastole is an entire discipline with its own textbook and guidelines.

B. Diastole can be dramatic: flash pulmonary edema.

C. Diastole is difficult to understand.

D. Prognosis is good.

EASY QUESTION: **A middle-aged patient is referred for echocardiography to evaluate the recent onset of shortness of breath.**

Which echocardiographic finding is the most difficult to interpret in the context of the clinical presentation?

A. Severe aortic stenosis.

B. Mitral regurgitation with systolic flow reversal into the pulmonary veins.

C. Severely dilated, diffusely hypokinetic left ventricle.

D. Severe pulmonary hypertension.

E. Cardiac tamponade.

F. Increased atrial contribution to mitral inflow in *diastole*.

Assessment of diastolic left ventricular function is challenging because it is not simple.

The following (deliberately oversimplified) approach uses echocardiography to identify just two diastolic abnormalities: Impaired diastolic relaxation and elevated filling pressures.

ANSWER TO QUESTION ONE: F

ANSWER TO QUESTION TWO: D

ANSWER TO QUESTION THREE: Duh! (This is the diastole section)

REFERENCE:

 Mandinov L, Eberli FR, Seiler C, et al. Diastolic heart failure. *Cardiovasc Res.* 2000;45:813–825.

IMPAIRED DIASTOLIC RELAXATION

The process of aging (along with diseases such as hypertension, obstructive sleep apnea, and diabetes) causes the left ventricle to relax more slowly at the onset of diastole. Initially, this is simply a compensatory mechanism rather than an illness or disorder. Patients may remain asymptomatic, become progressively short of breath, or they may present with congestive heart failure.

Early diastolic left atrial pressure, and mean left atrial wedge pressure, are initially normal. Left atrial pressure begins to climb when this compensatory mechanism fails. For example, new onset atrial fibrillation with loss of atrial contraction and a rapid heart rate may manifest as palpitations followed by dyspnea, or in some cases, pulmonary edema.

FIGURE 10.1

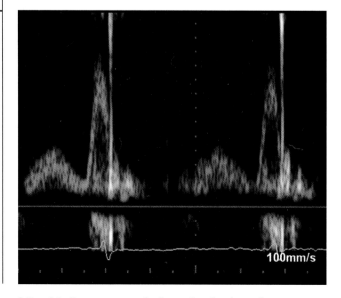

Mitral inflow pattern in impaired relaxation.

MITRAL INFLOW PATTERN

"   *A sucker is born every minute.*   **"**

The normal inflow pattern of a young healthy patient is brief because of brisk diastolic relaxation. The mechanism is dominated by the sucking action of the left ventricle. The left atrial pressure drops while the left ventricle fills.

As impaired diastolic relaxation results in increased atrial contribution to left ventricular filling, Doppler shows a slight delay in onset of mitral inflow (prolonged isovolumic relaxation time). The early diastolic inflow velocity is initially low—left ventricular filling gets delayed with proportionately more filling in late diastole.

The deceleration time of mitral inflow becomes prolonged. Flow continues *without a pause* in mid diastole (loss of diastasis).

FIGURE 10.2

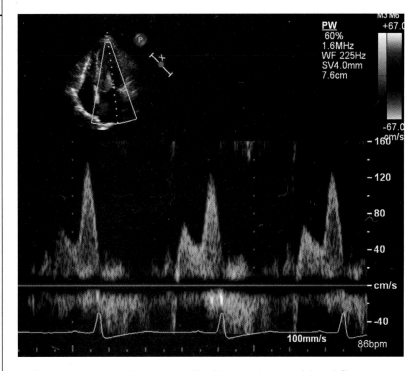

Left atrial contraction dramatically accelerates blood flow.

REFERENCE:

Ommen SR, Nishimura RA. A clinical approach to the assessment of left ventricular diastolic function by Doppler echocardiography: update 2003. *Heart.* 2003;89(Suppl 3):iii18–iii23.

FIGURE 10.3

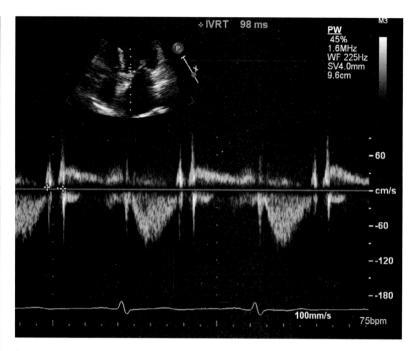

Isovolumic relaxation time is most useful at the bedside when it is extremely prolonged, or extremely short.

REFERENCES:

Scalia GM, Greenberg NL, McCarthy PM, et al. Noninvasive assessment of the ventricular relaxation time constant (tau) in humans by Doppler echocardiography. *Circulation.* 1997;95:151–155. *IVRT duration represents the physiological summation of diastolic myocardial function and the degree of preload compensation.*

Carroll JD, Hess OM, Hirzel HO, et al. Exercise-induced ischemia: the influence of altered relaxation on early diastolic pressures. *Circulation.* 1983;67:521–8. *During exercise there is a significant increase in cardiac output while maintaining normal diastolic pressures. During exercise-induced ischemia there is a dramatic rise in early diastolic pressures.*

Redfield MM, Jacobsen SJ, Burnett JC Jr, et al. Burden of systolic and diastolic ventricular dysfunction in the community: appreciating the scope of the heart failure epidemic. *JAMA.* 2003;289:194–202. *Figure 1 in this classic article presents the composite echocardiographic Doppler evaluation and classification of diastolic function.*

DYSPNEA

66 *The "sucker" becomes a "pusher."* **99**

Once relaxation becomes impaired, it does not return to normal. Left atrial blood gets pushed into the left ventricle by a progressively increasing left atrial pressure. The clinical price is DYSPNEA due to an adverse effect on pulmonary venous inflow. The echocardiographic price can be a misleading pseudonormal appearance.

RESTRICTIVE FILLING

Left ventricular ischemia, hypertrophy, or dilatation resists the increasing pressure. Severely decreased systolic left ventricular function results in elevated left atrial pressures. Diastolic filling is shifted back to early diastole with the price of elevated pressures. Early diastolic filling is cut off by rapidly rising left ventricular diastolic pressure. There is rapid inflow and a rapid halt. The late diastolic left ventricular pressure becomes high, minimizing left atrial contribution to filling.

FIGURE 10.4

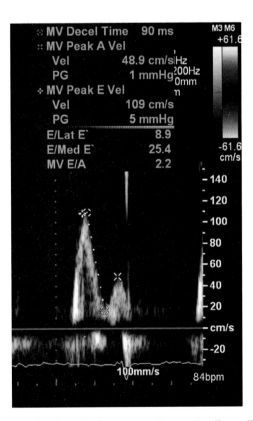

The E/E′ ratio between the early diastolic mitral filling velocity and the early diastolic mitral annulus tissue Doppler velocity is clinically very useful. It correlates with left ventricular filling pressures.

FIGURE 10.5

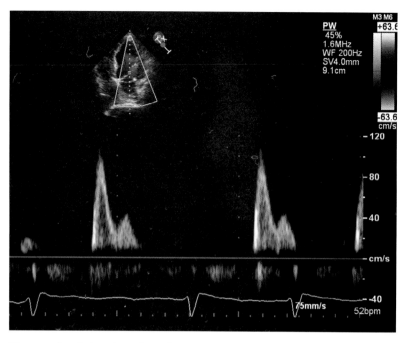

Short mitral deceleration time.

FIGURE 10.6

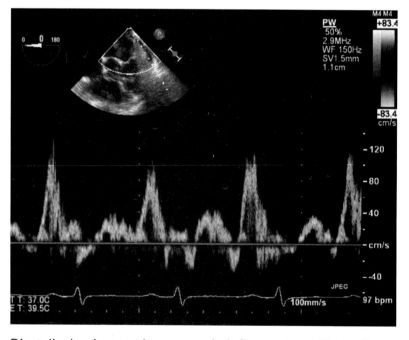

Diastolic dominant pulmonary vein inflow pattern. This pulmonary venous inflow pattern in a patient with a seemingly normal mitral inflow pattern indicates that left ventricular relaxation is actually abnormal.

REFERENCE: Keren G, Sherez J, Megidish R, et al. Pulmonary venous flow pattern—its relationship to cardiac dynamics. A pulsed Doppler echocardiographic study. *Circulation*. 1985;71:1105–1112.

FIGURE 10.7

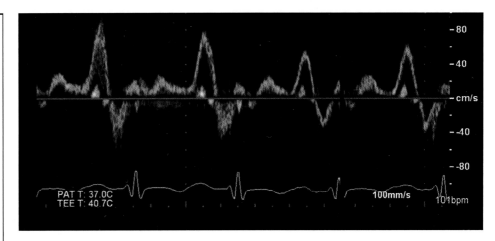

Diastolic dominant pulmonary venous inflow pattern. Elevated left atrial pressure.

QR 10.1a: Diastolic dominant right pulmonary vein inflow.

QR 10.1b: Diastolic dominant right pulmonary vein inflow.

REFERENCES:

Nagueh SF, Appleton CP, Gillebert TC, et al. Recommendations for the evaluation of left ventricular diastolic function by echocardiography. *Eur J Echocardiogr*. 2009;10:165–193.

Ommen SR, Nishimura RA, Appleton CP, et al. Clinical utility of Doppler echocardiography and tissue Doppler imaging in the estimation of left ventricular filling pressures: a comparative simultaneous Doppler-catheterization study. *Circulation*. 2000;102:1788–1794. *Mean left ventricular diastolic pressure was normal with E/E′ less than 8; and elevated with E/E′ greater than 15.*

Sohn DW, Kim YJ, Kim HC, et al. Evaluation of left ventricular diastolic function when mitral E and A waves are completely fused: role of assessing mitral annulus velocity. *J Am Soc Echocardiogr*. 1999;12:203–208. *A single diastolic mitral inflow wave (E-A fusion) is common in atrial fibrillation, which in turn, is common in diastolic dysfunction.*

Nagueh SF, Mikati I, Kopelen HA, et al. Doppler estimation of left ventricular filling pressure in sinus tachycardia. A new application of tissue Doppler imaging. *Circulation*. 1998;98:1644–1650. *The early diastolic mitral annulus velocity behaves as a relative load-independent index of left ventricular relaxation, which corrects the influence of relaxation on the transmitral E velocity; even in sinus tachycardia with complete merging of E and A velocities.*

THE SEEMING PARADOX OF THE S3 GALLOP

Young patients may have a normal S3 gallop on auscultation. Patients with decompensated heart failure have the same sounding S3 gallop, but the heart rate is increased. In both cases, Doppler shows abrupt halting of early mitral inflow. The difference is that the left ventricular end-diastolic pressure is *elevated* in the latter.

REFERENCE:

 Van de Werf F, Geboers J, Kesteloot H, et al. The mechanism of disappearance of the physiologic third heart sound with age. *Circulation*. 1986;73:877–84.

LEFT ATRIAL SIZE AND ELEVATED FILLING PRESSURES

Long-term diastolic dysfunction results in increased left atrial size. Left atrial enlargement indicates prior exposure to elevated filling pressures. A dilated left atrium does not help with the current state of events.

SERIOUS QUESTION:

What are two reasons to marry a man with an earring?

A. He has experienced pain.

B. He has bought jewelry.

Similarly, it can only be said that the *dilated* left atrium has "experienced the pain" of elevated pressure at some time in the past. Current pressure status is determined by Doppler.

Clinical pearl (speaking of jewelry): Normal left atrial size indicates no *prior* stretch.

Practical imaging caveats for the assessment of left atrial size: Left atrial enlargement may be dramatic. More subtle cases require more subtle measurement: Left atrial *volume* is a more accurate long-term "marker" than left atrial diameter or area. Age needs to be taken into account. Young people should have young (normal size) atria. Left atrial dilatation is quite common in the elderly. Body size must also be accounted for, by indexing left atrial size to body surface area.

REFERENCES:

 Abhayaratna WP, Seward JB, Appleton CP, et al. Left atrial size: physiologic determinants and clinical applications. *J Am Coll Cardiol*. 2006;47:2357–2363.

 Cameli M, Lisi M, Righini FM, et al. Novel echocardiographic techniques to assess left atrial size, anatomy and function. *Cardiovasc Ultrasound*. 2012;10:4.

SYSTOLIC–DIASTOLIC MISMATCH

Decreased systolic left ventricular function indicates some degree of *requisite* diastolic dysfunction.

• GOOD NEWS SCENARIO: Severe systolic dysfunction is associated with a restrictive filling pattern. A more favorable filling pattern in this case suggests better than expected functional capacity and better clinical prognosis.

• BAD NEWS SCENARIO: Mild-to-moderate systolic dysfunction is associated with a filling pattern of impaired relaxation. A restrictive filling pattern in this case is out of proportion to the degree of systolic dysfunction. It indicates volume overload, explains symptoms of dyspnea, and should be treated with diuretics and/or other antihypertensives if needed. Venodilation with "preemptive" nitroglycerin prior to exercise may reduce left atrial pressures and lessen or improve consequent exercise induced dyspnea.

FABRY DISEASE

This is a rare but treatable inherited deficiency of the enzyme alpha galactosidase A. Administration of the deficient enzyme may be curative. If it is misdiagnosed as hypertrophic cardiomyopathy causing symptomatic diastolic dysfunction; patients who could be treated effectively with medication – might instead be subjected to inappropriate invasive procedures such as alcohol septal ablation, or surgical septal myectomy.

REFERENCES:

 Sachdev B, Takenaka T, Teraguchi H, et al. Prevalence of Anderson-Fabry disease in male patients with late onset hypertrophic cardiomyopathy. *Circulation.* 2002;105:1407–11.

 Nakao S, Takenaka T, Maeda M, et al. An atypical variant of Fabry's disease in men with left ventricular hypertrophy. *N Engl J Med* 1995;333:288–93.

 Desnick RJ, Blieden LC, Sharp HL, et al. Cardiac valvular anomalies in Fabry disease: clinical, morphologic, and biochemical studies. *Circulation* 1976;54: 818–25.

 Pieroni M, Chimenti C, Ricci R, et al. Early detection of Fabry cardiomyopathy by tissue Doppler imaging. *Circulation* 2003:107:1978–84.

 Manson AL, Nudelman SP, Hagley MT, et al. Relationship of the third heart sound to transmitral flow velocity deceleration. *Circulation.* 1995;92:388–94.

PRECORDIAL EXAMINATION FOR THE DIASTOLOGIST

" *Reconciling physical and echo findings.* **"**

A loud atrial S4 gallop and/or a prominent mitral atrial filling wave on Doppler - may be palpable. Systolic retraction of the precordial impulse is found in pericardial constriction and in severe tricuspid regurgitation. The "triple ripple" of hypertrophic cardiomyopathy is distinctive when present; both on echo and on the physical examination.

REFERENCES:

Mounsey P. Precordial pulsations in relation to cardiac movement and sounds. *Br Heart J*. 1959;21:457–469. *See Figure 7. Severe left ventricular hypertrophy was associated with severe right atrial enlargement and a palpable right atrial beat. Echocardiography in the very elderly frequently shows severe left ventricular hypertrophy in association with severe tricuspid regurgitation.*

Mounsey P. Praecordial pulsations in health and disease. *Postgrad Med J*. 1968;44:134–139.

Mounsey P. The value of praecordial pulsations in the diagnosis of heart disease. *Postgrad Med J*. 1968;44:81-5. *By placing the whole palm of the hand on the chest - the examiner can imagine holding the surface of the heart in their hand.*

Shindler D. Post-it apexcardiography. *N Engl J Med*. 2004;351:1364. *A simple bedside examination technique can be used to reconcile tactile with visual diagnosis of a "triple ripple".*

THE VALSALVA MANEUVER

" *Decreased venous return can unmask diastolic dysfunction.* **"**

The purpose of this easily misunderstood, and sadly, too-rarely performed, maneuver is to alter venous return to the left atrium (decrease preload). It has to be performed properly. The patient closes the glottis (without a deep breath), contracts the diaphragm, and holds. Meanwhile, pulsed wave Doppler evaluation is performed at the mitral leaflet tips using the apical transducer position. During Valsalva *strain,* left atrial pressure *drops* and the mitral inflow pattern may change. Blood pressure response to the Valsalva maneuver can be used at the bedside in *systolic* heart failure.

REFERENCES:

 Robertson D, Stevens RM, Friesinger GC, et al. The effect of the Valsalva maneuver on echocardiographic dimensions in man. *Circulation*. 1977;55:596–602.

 Parisi AF, Harrington JJ, Askenazi J, et al. Echocardiographic evaluation of the Valsalva maneuver in healthy subjects and patients with and without heart failure. *Circulation*. 1976;54:921–927.

LEG RAISING

Raising the legs of a patient during the echocardiographic examination will have the opposite effect. Venous return (preload) will increase. Leg raising may also trigger a reflex bradycardia, which could affect the interpretation of the mitral inflow Doppler pattern.

REFERENCES:

Pozzoli M, Traversi E, Cioffi G, et al. Loading manipulations improve the prognostic value of Doppler evaluation of mitral flow in patients with chronic heart failure. *Circulation*. 1997;95:1222–1230.

Sato A, Koike A, Koyama Y, et al. Effects of posture on left ventricular diastolic filling during exercise. *Med Sci Sports Exerc*. 1999;3:1564–1569.

Percy RF, Conetta DA. Comparison of velocity and volumetric indexes of left ventricular filling during increased heart rate with exercise and amyl nitrite. *J Am Soc Echocardiogr*. 1994;7:388–393.

Lembo NJ, Dell'Italia LJ, Crawford MH, et al. Diagnosis of left-sided regurgitant murmurs by transient arterial occlusion: a new maneuver using blood pressure cuffs. *Ann Intern Med*. 1986;105:368–370. *Bedside maneuver: Transient arterial occlusion of both arms with blood pressure cuffs (inflated to 20 to 40 mm Hg above systolic pressure for 20 seconds) augments the intensity of the diastolic murmur of aortic regurgitation; as well as the intensity of systolic murmurs in mitral regurgitation and ventricular septal defect.*

TISSUE DOPPLER E′ VELOCITY

66   *E′ relaxes—E pushes.*   **99**

Once the early diastolic velocity decreases, it does not return to normal. Decreased E′ is permanent. Tissue Doppler does not pseudonormalize. The mitral E velocity can change with loading conditions but the E/E′ ratio will remain useful. Left atrial pressure can be estimated at the bedside by examining the patient for jugular venous distention, hepatojugular reflux, atrial S4 gallop, peripheral edema, pulmonary congestion (and by looking at the chest X-ray and at the BNP level).

REFERENCE:

Kasner M, Westermann D, Steendijk P, et al. Utility of Doppler echocardiography and tissue Doppler imaging in the estimation of diastolic function in heart failure with normal ejection fraction: a comparative Doppler-conductance catheterization study. *Circulation*. 2007;116:637–647.

PULMONARY VEIN FLOW PATTERNS

QUESTION:

Pulmonary vein inflow into the left atrium shows a flow pattern similar to the jugular veins. Which jugular venous wave does not have an equivalent in the pulmonary venous Doppler inflow pattern?

A. a wave.

B. x descent.

C. x′ descent.

D. v wave.

E. y descent.

QR 10.2a: Normal systolic dominant pulmonary vein inflow.

QR 10.2b: Normal systolic dominant pulmonary vein inflow.

QR 10.2c: Normal systolic dominant pulmonary vein inflow.

QR 10.3: Diastolic dominant pulmonary vein inflow pattern.

QR 10.4a: Diastolic dominant pulmonary vein inflow. Elevated left atrial pressure.

QR 10.4b: Diastolic dominant pulmonary vein inflow. Elevated left atrial pressure.

QR 10.4c: Diastolic dominant pulmonary vein inflow. Elevated left atrial pressure.

QR 10.4d: Diastolic dominant pulmonary vein inflow. Elevated left atrial pressure.

QR 10.5a: Right and left pulmonary veins in the apical four chamber view. The left pulmonary vein should not be confused with mitral regurgitation.

QR 10.5b: Right and left pulmonary veins in the apical four-chamber view. The left pulmonary vein should not be confused with mitral regurgitation.

QR 10.6: Unusually well-demonstrated pulmonary vein inflow into the left atrium.

REFERENCES:

 Braunwald E, Morrow AG. Origin of heart sounds as elucidated by analysis of the sequence of cardiodynamic events. *Circulation*. 1958;18:971–974. *See Figure 1 in the article.*

Pyhel HJ, Stewart J, Tavel ME. Clinical assessment of calibrated jugular pulse recording. *Br Heart J*. 1978;40:297–302. *Excellent discussion section.*

Constant J. Jugular wave recognition breakthrough: X' descent vs the X descent and trough. *Chest*. 2000;118:1788–1791. *The easiest way to recognize jugular waves at the bedside is by timing descents as being either systolic or diastolic according to their relation to either the patient's pulse or heart sounds.*

ANSWER: D (except when there is severe mitral regurgitation)

CLINICAL UTILITY OF THE TEI INDEX

The Tei index is also known as the MPI. The Doppler-derived myocardial performance index (MPI) is a measure of combined systolic and diastolic myocardial performance. It is clinically useful in heart failure and in coronary artery disease.

REFERENCES:

Parthenakis FI, Kanakaraki MK, Kanoupakis EM, et al. Value of Doppler index combining systolic and diastolic myocardial performance in predicting cardiopulmonary exercise capacity in patients with congestive heart failure: effects of dobutamine. *Chest*. 2002;121:1935–1941. *MPI correlates inversely with LV performance, reflects disease severity, and is a useful complimentary variable in the assessment of cardiopulmonary exercise performance in patients with heart failure.*

Bruch C, Schmermund A, Marin D, et al. Tei-index in patients with mild-to-moderate congestive heart failure. *Eur Heart J*. 2000;21:1888–1895. *This is a sensitive indicator of overall cardiac dysfunction in patients with mild-to-moderate congestive heart failure.*

Al-Mukhaini M, Argentin S, Morin JF, et al. Myocardial performance index as predictor of adverse outcomes following mitral valve surgery. *Eur J Echocardiogr*. 2003;4:128–134. *MPI is a useful predictor of increased risk of peri-operative death or congestive heart failure, in patients with moderate-severe mitral regurgitation undergoing corrective mitral valve surgery. In conjunction with left ventricular ejection fraction, it may be helpful in the pre-operative prognostication of these patients.*

Kato M, Dote K, Sasaki S, et al. Myocardial performance index for assessment of left ventricular outcome in successfully recanalised anterior myocardial infarction. *Heart*. 2005;91:583–588. *MPI can predict the left ventricular functional outcome after early successful recanalization of a patient's first anterior acute MI.*

INTRACARDIAC BLOOD VOLUME

" *Wet or dry?* **"**

QUESTION: **A trauma patient is undergoing a screening echo in the ER. Which statement below is FALSE?**

A. Apical images may be possible without need to turn the patient on their left side.

B. The normal-size right ventricle may be misrepresented as being dilated on an off-axis view.

C. Chamber size from two different imaging windows is more likely to represent the truth.

D. Short-axis images should be oval.

E. Transesophageal evaluation of wall motion provides better resolution.

Parasternal images often require that the patient be turned on the left side. TEE may *not* provide information about the true left ventricular apex in spite of the better resolution. Short-axis images should be round, not oval.

QR 10.7a: Left ventricular cavity obliteration.

QR 10.7b: Left ventricular cavity obliteration.

ANSWER: D (C needs to be done to avoid B)

VENTRICULAR TORSION

As echocardiographic tools such as tissue Doppler and strain become more familiar, our understanding of left ventricular function gets more sophisticated.

Left Ventricular Torsion:

There is systolic twisting like the wringing of a towel.

There is diastolic *untwisting* that creates diastolic suction.

Apical left ventricular aneurysm and apical right ventricular pacing will affect torsion.

REFERENCES:

 Esch BT, Warburton DE. Left ventricular torsion and recoil: implications for exercise performance and cardiovascular disease. *J Appl Physiol*. 2009;106: 362–369.

 Bethell HJ, Nixon PG. Examination of the heart in supine and left lateral positions. *Br Heart J*. 1973;35:902–907. *Technical validation of physical findings obtained in the left lateral decubitus position. The atrial gallop of diastolic dysfunction can be heard and palpated in this position.*

 Greenbaum RA, Ho SY, Gibson DG, et al. Left ventricular fibre architecture in man. *Br Heart J*. 1981;45:248–263.

Nakatani S. Left ventricular rotation and twist: why should we learn? *J Cardiovasc Ultrasound*. 2011;19:1–6.

Zaglavara T, Pillay T, Karvounis H, et al. Detection of myocardial viability by dobutamine stress echocardiography: incremental value of diastolic wall thickness measurement. *Heart*. 2005;91:613–617. *Measurement of diastolic left ventricular wall thickness helps predict myocardial viability.*

Derumeaux G, Ovize M, Loufoua J, et al. Assessment of nonuniformity of transmural myocardial velocities by color-coded tissue Doppler imaging: characterization of normal, ischemic, and stunned myocardium. *Circulation*. 2000;101:1390–1395.

Steeds RP. Echocardiography: frontier imaging in cardiology. *Br J Radiol*. 2011;84:S237–S245.

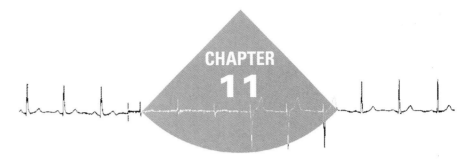

ARRHYTHMIAS AND NEUROLOGICAL DISORDERS

LEFT ATRIAL APPENDAGE

There is bidirectional blood flow in and out of the normal left atrial appendage (LAA). In normal sinus rhythm, there is rapid emptying of the appendage following the atrial contraction. There is subsequent reversal of the direction of flow with filling of the LAA. Normal LAA *emptying* velocities have been reported as 46 +/– 18 cm/s. Normal LAA *filling* velocities have been reported as a close 46 +/– 17 cm/s. In an individual patient, the velocities may be different because the duration of filling and emptying may be different.

LAA velocities may progressively decrease in atrial fibrillation to the point of becoming unmeasurable. Left atrial size, left ventricular systolic and diastolic function, and presence and severity of valvular regurgitation help in the interpretation. The most dramatic oscillation in LAA velocities is found in atrial flutter (as long as mechanical LAA function remains preserved).

FIGURE 11.1

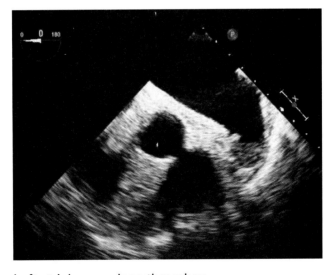

Left atrial appendage thrombus.

FIGURE 11.2

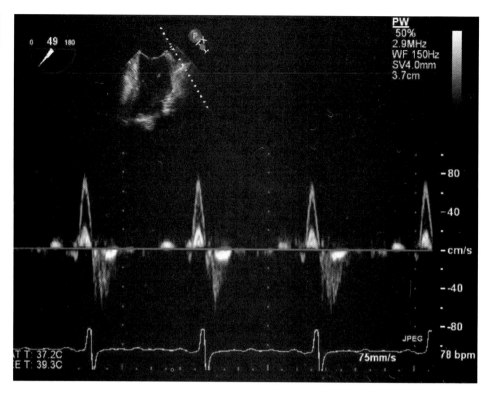

Normal left atrial appendage—emptying with the atrial contraction and filling with left ventricular contraction.

FIGURE 11.3

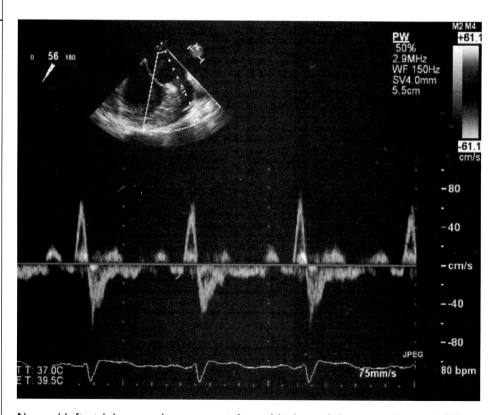

Normal left atrial appendage—emptying with the atrial contraction and filling with left ventricular contraction.

FIGURE 11.4

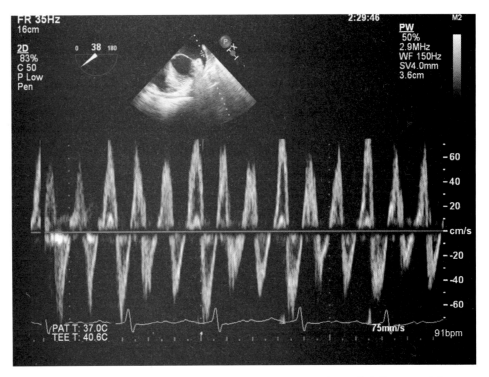

Doppler flow patterns in the left atrial appendage in atrial flutter with preserved velocities.

FIGURE 11.5

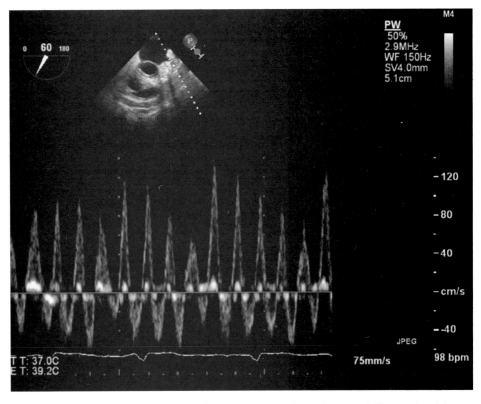

Doppler flow patterns in the left atrial appendage in atrial flutter in this patient have remained fast throughout the cardiac cycle.

FIGURE 11.6

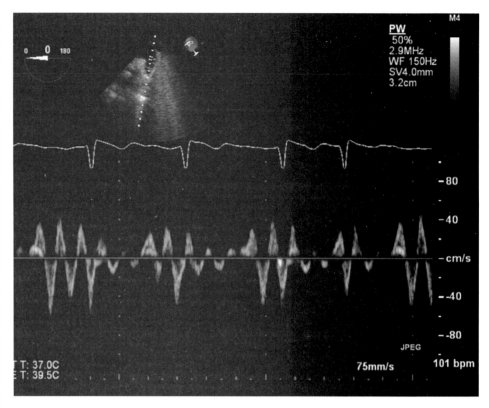

Doppler flow patterns in the left atrial appendage in atrial flutter and fibrillation.

FIGURE 11.7

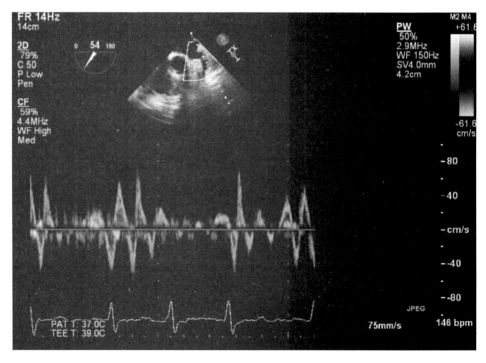

Doppler flow patterns in the left atrial appendage in atrial flutter and fibrillation.

FIGURE 11.8

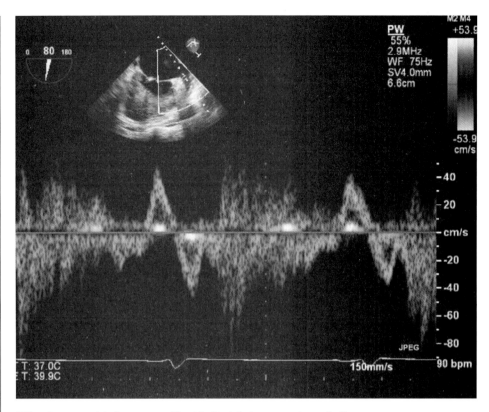

Mitral regurgitation can affect left atrial appendage inflow.

FIGURE 11.9

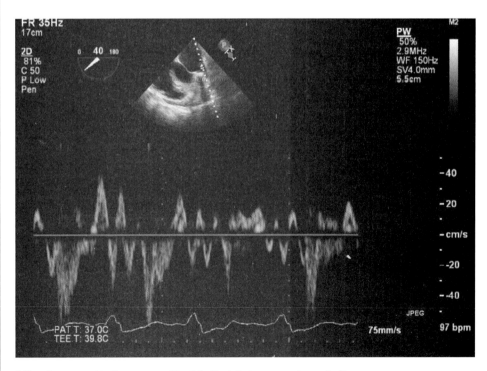

Mitral regurgitation can affect left atrial appendage inflow.

FIGURE 11.10

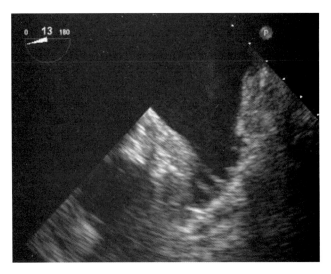

Normal trabeculations in the left atrial appendage.

FIGURE 11.11

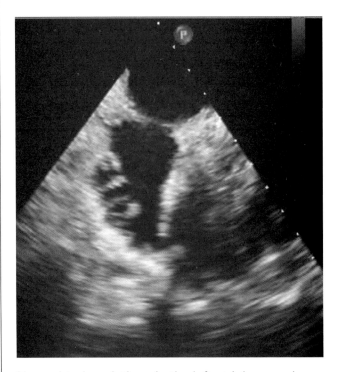

Normal trabeculations in the left atrial appendage.

REFERENCES:

 Chue CD, de Giovanni J, Steeds RP. The role of echocardiography in percutaneous left atrial appendage occlusion. *Eur J Echocardiogr.* 2011;12:i3–i10.

Nucifora G, Faletra FF, Regoli F, et al. Evaluation of the left atrial appendage with real-time 3-dimensional transesophageal echocardiography: implications for catheter-based left atrial appendage closure. *Circ Cardiovasc Imaging.* 2011;4:514–523.

FIGURE 11.12

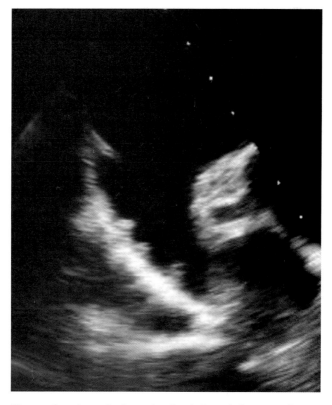

Normal trabeculations in the left atrial appendage.

FIGURE 11.13

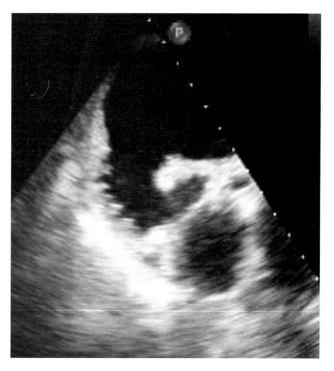

Normal trabeculations in the left atrial appendage.

FIGURE 11.14

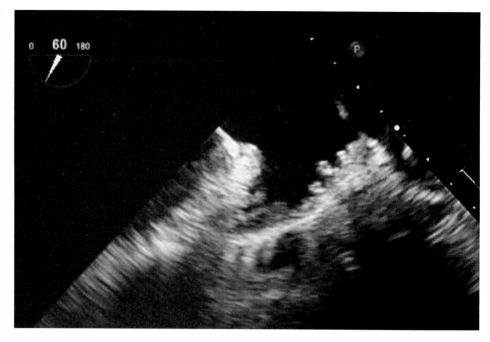

Normal trabeculations in the left atrial appendage.

FIGURE 11.15

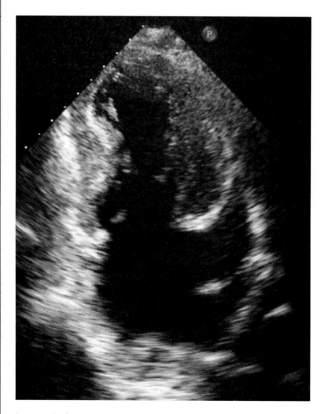

Large left atrial appendage.

FIGURE 11.16

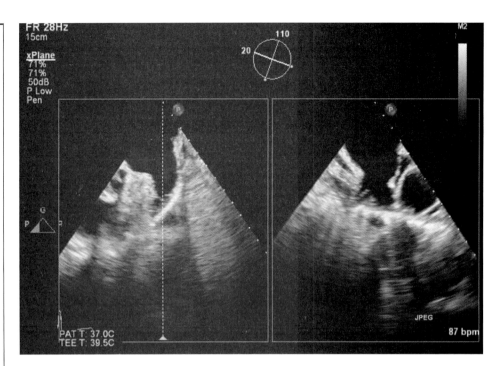

Bilobed left atrial appendage.

FIGURE 11.17

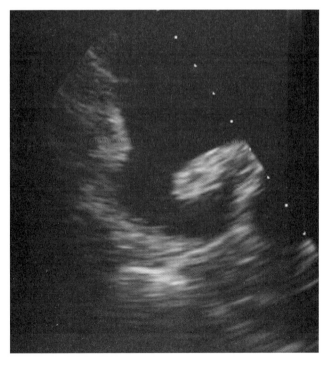

Sharply angled left atrial appendage.

REFERENCE: Freixa X, Tzikas A, Basmadjian A, et al. The chicken-wing morphology: an anatomical challenge for left atrial appendage occlusion. *J Interv Cardiol.* 2013;26:509–514.

FIGURE 11.18

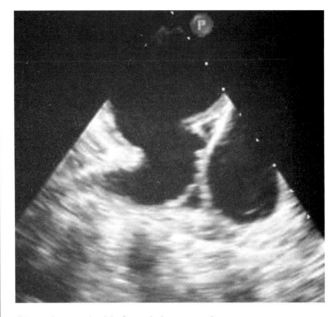

Sharply angled left atrial appendage.

FIGURE 11.19

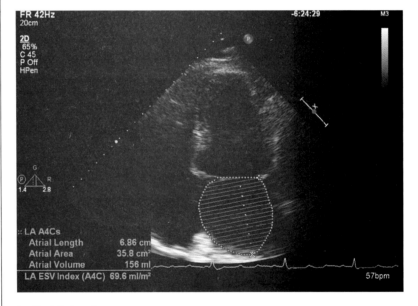

Left atrial volume.

QR 11.1: Left atrial appendage thrombus.

QR 11.2: Left atrial appendage thrombus located at the far part of the appendage with "shimmering" oscillations and discrete borders. A separate ultrasound artifact located closer to the opening appears more hazy, and less mobile.

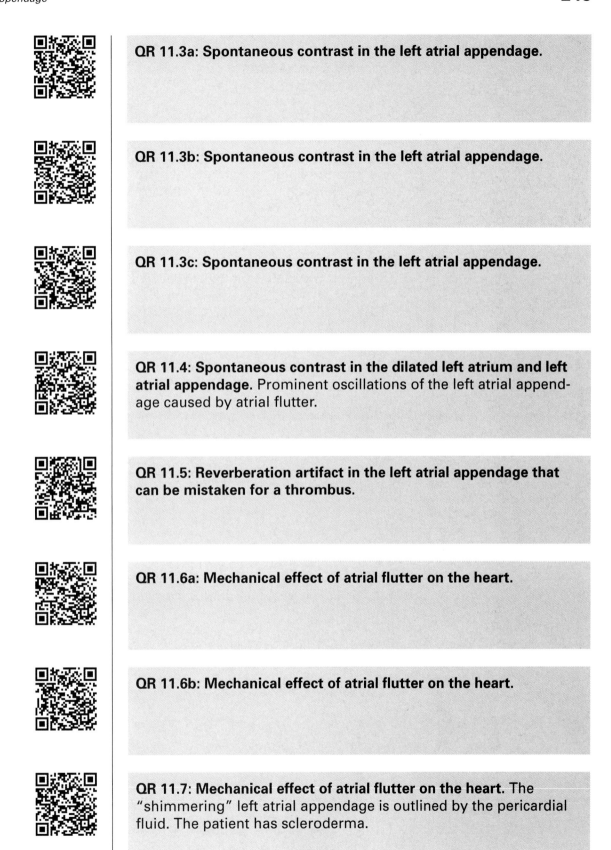

QR 11.3a: Spontaneous contrast in the left atrial appendage.

QR 11.3b: Spontaneous contrast in the left atrial appendage.

QR 11.3c: Spontaneous contrast in the left atrial appendage.

QR 11.4: Spontaneous contrast in the dilated left atrium and left atrial appendage. Prominent oscillations of the left atrial appendage caused by atrial flutter.

QR 11.5: Reverberation artifact in the left atrial appendage that can be mistaken for a thrombus.

QR 11.6a: Mechanical effect of atrial flutter on the heart.

QR 11.6b: Mechanical effect of atrial flutter on the heart.

QR 11.7: Mechanical effect of atrial flutter on the heart. The "shimmering" left atrial appendage is outlined by the pericardial fluid. The patient has scleroderma.

QR 11.8: Variable aortic leaflet opening (and variable stroke volume) in atrial flutter.

QR 11.9: Triangular-shaped left atrial appendage. A ridge created by folded atrial tissue separates it from the left pulmonary vein (located below the ridge on this image).

QR 11.10: Normal left atrial appendage contractility with prominent trabeculations and a reverberation artifact.

QR 11.11a: Left atrial appendage that was sewn closed during heart surgery.

QR 11.11b: Left atrial appendage that was sewn closed during heart surgery.

QR 11.12: Left atrial appendage that was only partly closed during heart surgery. Atrial flutter. Paravalvular mitral prosthesis regurgitation.

QR 11.13: Biatrial enlargement in atrial flutter.

REFERENCES:

Antonielli E, Pizzuti A, Palinkas A, et al. Clinical value of left atrial appendage flow for prediction of long-term sinus rhythm maintenance in patients with nonvalvular atrial fibrillation. *J Am Coll Cardiol*. 2002;39:1443–1449. *High LAA flow velocity identifies patients with greater likelihood to remain in sinus rhythm for 1 year after successful cardioversion. Low LAA velocity is of limited value in identifying patients who will relapse into atrial fibrillation.*

The Stroke Prevention in Atrial Fibrillation Investigators Committee on Echocardiography. Transesophageal echocardiographic correlates of thromboembolism in high-risk patients with nonvalvular atrial fibrillation. *Ann Intern Med.* 1998;128:639–647. *In high-risk patients with atrial fibrillation, subsequent rates of thromboembolism are correlated with dense spontaneous echocardiographic contrast, thrombus of the atrial appendage, and aortic plaque.*

Sanders P, Morton JB, Morgan JG, et al. Reversal of atrial mechanical stunning after cardioversion of atrial arrhythmias: implications for the mechanisms of tachycardia-mediated atrial cardiomyopathy. *Circulation.* 2002;106:1806–1813.

Manning WJ, Silverman DI, Katz SE, et al. Impaired left atrial mechanical function after cardioversion: relation to the duration of atrial fibrillation. *J Am Coll Cardiol.* 1994;23:1535–1540. *Recovery of left atrial mechanical function is related to the duration of atrial fibrillation before cardioversion. Atrial mechanical function is greater immediately and at 24 h and 1 week after cardioversion in patients with "brief" compared with "prolonged" atrial fibrillation. In all groups, atrial mechanical function increases over time, ultimately achieving similar levels. Full recovery of atrial mechanical function, however, is achieved within 24 h in patients with brief atrial fibrillation, within 1 week in patients with moderate-duration atrial fibrillation, and within 1 month in patients with prolonged atrial fibrillation.*

Klein AL, Grimm RA, Murray RD, et al. Use of transesophageal echocardiography to guide cardioversion in patients with atrial fibrillation. *N Engl J Med.* 2001;344:1411–1420.

Weigner MJ, Caulfield TA, Danias PG, et al. Risk for clinical thromboembolism associated with conversion to sinus rhythm in patients with atrial fibrillation lasting less than 48 hours. *Ann Intern Med.* 1997;126:615–620.

Wong CK, White HD, Wilcox RG, et al. New atrial fibrillation after acute myocardial infarction independently predicts death: the GUSTO-III experience. *Am Heart J.* 2000;140:878–885.

Packer DL, Keelan P, Munger TM, et al. Clinical presentation, investigation, and management of pulmonary vein stenosis complicating ablation for atrial fibrillation. *Circulation.* 2005;111:546–554. *This post-procedural complication is diagnosable with TEE. Patients are very symptomatic, but the symptoms may be misdiagnosed as bronchitis. Most present with dyspnea on exertion as the initial manifestation over the course of 1–3 months. Pleuritic chest pain is a late manifestation. Hemoptysis is uncommon.*

Subramaniam B, Riley MF, Panzica PJ, et al. Transesophageal echocardiographic assessment of right atrial appendage anatomy and function: comparison with the left atrial appendage and implications for local thrombus formation. *J Am Soc Echocardiogr.* 2006;19:429–433.

Bălăceanu A. Right atrium thrombosis in nonvalvular permanent atrial fibrillation. *J Med Life.* 2011;4:352–355.

Manning WJ, Weintraub RM, Waksmonski CA, et al. Accuracy of transesophageal echocardiography for identifying left atrial thrombi. A prospective, intraoperative study. *Ann Intern Med.* 1995;123:817–822.

Fatkin D, Loupas T, Low J, et al. Inhibition of red cell aggregation prevents spontaneous echocardiographic contrast formation in human blood. *Circulation.* 1997;96:889–896. *Protein-mediated red cell aggregation is the mechanism of spontaneous echo contrast in human blood. Both red cells and plasma proteins are required to produce low flow–related echogenicity. Individual red cells are normally prevented from aggregating by the repulsive electrostatic effects of their negative surface charge. Plasma proteins, particularly fibrinogen, are able to overcome these electrostatic forces and facilitate aggregation of cells at low shear rates by the formation of cross-bridges between the cells. Variegated echodensity with circular flow patterns is produced by the relatively higher velocity pulmonary venous inflow mixing with static, echogenic blood in the left atrium.*

LONG QT SYNDROMES

The electrocardiographic patterns of long QT syndromes include:

1. Wide T waves.
2. Notched T waves.

The clinical presentation of syncope with long QT syndrome:

1. Syncope with exertion.
2. Syncope with loud sounds.
3. Syncope at rest.

Role of echocardiography in syncope with suspected long QT syndrome:

Echocardiography establishes the "structural integrity" of the left ventricle by ruling out a cardiomyopathy as a potential (possibly alternative) cause of arrhythmia.

REFERENCES:

Wexler RK, Pleister A, Raman S. Outpatient approach to palpitations. *Am Fam Physician.* 2011;84:63–69.

Brenyo AJ, Huang DT, Aktas MK. Congenital long and short QT syndromes. *Cardiology.* 2012;122:237–247.

LEFT BUNDLE BRANCH BLOCK

" *Chicken vs. Egg.* **"**

A patient with left bundle branch block may have a pacemaker/defibrillator. It is sometimes difficult to sort out what came first. It may not be possible to determine whether the wall motion abnormality represents abnormal electrical activity of the myocardium, or whether the abnormal electrical activity of the myocardium is due to underlying cardiomyopathy. Many patients with cardiomyopathy meet criteria for biventricular pacing when the QRS complex is wide.

QR 11.14: Dilated cardiomyopathy with a wide QRS. Abnormal septal motion due to the bundle branch block. Lateral wall contractility is preserved.

QR 11.15a: Dilated cardiomyopathy with paradoxical motion of the interventricular septum due to bundle branch block.

QR 11.15b: Dilated cardiomyopathy with paradoxical motion of the interventricular septum due to bundle branch block.

REFERENCE: Xiao HB, Lee CH, Gibson DG. Effect of left bundle branch block on diastolic function in dilated cardiomyopathy. *Br Heart J*. 1991;66:443–447. *Left bundle branch block prolongs mitral regurgitation by increasing pre-ejection and relaxation times. This directly impairs diastolic function by shortening the time available for the left ventricle to fill.*

DEFIBRILLATORS

QUESTION: **A patient undergoes echocardiography following implantation of a defibrillator. Which of the following echocardiographic findings will indicate that not only will prognosis be improved, but also that the patient's quality of life will improve?**

A. Asymmetric septal hypertrophy.

B. Left ventricular aneurysm.

C. Dilated diffusely hypokinetic left ventricle.

D. Wire in the coronary sinus.

The SCD-HeFT trial showed that quality of life does not necessarily improve following implantation of an ICD. Echocardiography is a tomographic technique. It does not demonstrate the complete path of a pacemaker or defibrillator wire even with three-dimensional imaging. A wire in the coronary sinus on an echocardiogram indicates the presence of a biventricular pacemaker. Biventricular pacemakers are advanced by way of the coronary sinus to the lateral left ventricular wall. When the QRS complex on the electrocardiogram is wide, there may be an indication for inserting a biventricular pacemaker. Biventricular pacing can improve symptoms of heart failure.

FIGURE 11.20

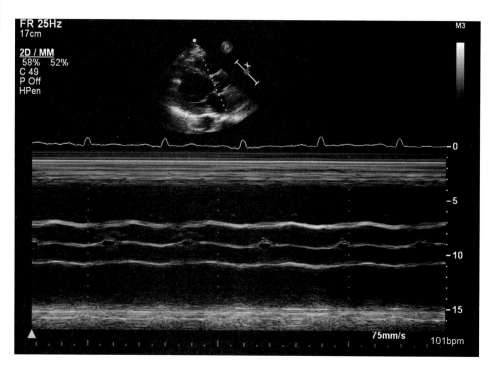

Minimal forward stroke volume in a patient with an apical left ventricular assist device, which is doing most of the ejecting from the left ventricular cavity in systole. This is an indication of minimal residual systolic left ventricular function.

QR 11.16: Pacemaker wire.

QR 11.17: Pacemaker wire in the coronary sinus manifested as a reverberation artifact in the pleural effusion.

QR 11.18: Chiari network in the right atrium.

QR 11.19: Chiari network and a pacemaker wire in the right atrium.

REFERENCES:

Chapa DW, Lee HJ, Kao CW, et al. Reducing mortality with device therapy in heart failure patients without ventricular arrhythmias. *Am J Crit Care.* 2008; 17:443–452.

Cleland JG, Daubert JC, Erdmann E, et al.Cardiac Resynchronization-Heart Failure (CARE-HF) Study Investigators. The effect of cardiac resynchronization on morbidity and mortality in heart failure. *N Engl J Med.* 2005;352:1539–1549. *In patients with heart failure and cardiac dyssynchrony, cardiac resynchronization improves symptoms and the quality of life; and reduces complications and the risk of death. These benefits are in addition to those afforded by standard pharmacologic therapy. The implantation of a cardiac-resynchronization device should routinely be considered in such patients.*

Bristow MR, Saxon LA, Boehmer J, et al. Comparison of Medical Therapy, Pacing, and Defibrillation in Heart Failure (COMPANION) Investigators. Cardiac-resynchronization therapy with or without an implantable defibrillator in advanced chronic heart failure. *N Engl J Med.* 2004;350:2140–2150. *In patients with advanced heart failure and a prolonged QRS interval, cardiac-resynchronization therapy decreases the combined risk of death from any cause or first hospitalization and, when combined with an implantable defibrillator, significantly reduces mortality.*

Young JB, Abraham WT, Smith AL, et al. Multicenter InSync ICD Randomized Clinical Evaluation (MIRACLE ICD) Trial Investigators. Combined cardiac resynchronization and implantable cardioversion defibrillation in advanced chronic heart failure: the MIRACLE ICD Trial. *JAMA.* 2003;289:2685–2694. *Cardiac resynchronization improved quality of life, functional status, and exercise capacity in patients with moderate to severe HF, a wide QRS interval, and life-threatening arrhythmias. These improvements occurred in the context of underlying appropriate medical management without proarrhythmia or compromised ICD function.*

Zhang Q, Yu CM. Clinical implication of mechanical dyssynchrony in heart failure. *J Cardiovasc Ultrasound.* 2012;20:117–123.

Suffoletto MS, Dohi K, Cannesson M, et al. Novel speckle-tracking radial strain from routine black-and-white echocardiographic images to quantify dyssynchrony and predict response to cardiac resynchronization therapy. *Circulation.* 2006;113:960–968.

Penicka M, Bartunek J, De Bruyne B, et al. Improvement of left ventricular function after cardiac resynchronization therapy is predicted by tissue Doppler imaging echocardiography. *Circulation.* 2004;109:978–983.

ANSWER: D

SYNCOPE

"   *Autonomic Dysfunction vs. Sympathetic Activation.*   **"**

Favorite CCU rounds question:

QUESTION ONE:

Which is a more important prognostic marker during acute myocardial infarction?

A. Ventricular tachycardia.

B. Sinus tachycardia.

"   *Echo Can Show that the "Tank is Empty".*   **"**

QUESTION TWO:

Which clinical syndrome can cause hypotension and possibly syncope with echocardiographic evidence of small left ventricular internal dimensions?

A. Hypertrophic cardiomyopathy.

B. Dialysis related hypotension.

C. Chronic fatigue syndrome.

D. Postural tachycardia syndrome.

Clinical use of echocardiography in syncope:

Left ventricular cavity obliteration needs to be demonstrated with multiple two-dimensional views.

Left atrial pressure estimation helps with diuretic management.

Doppler can estimate left ventricular stroke volume.

Aortic stenosis can be identified and quantitated.

QR 11.20: Small left ventricular internal dimensions with systolic cavity obliteration.

REFERENCES:

Nerheim P, Birger-Botkin S, Piracha L, et al. Heart failure and sudden death in patients with tachycardia-induced cardiomyopathy and recurrent tachycardia. *Circulation.* 2004;110:247–252. *Tachycardia-induced cardiomyopathy develops slowly and appears reversible by left ventricular ejection fraction improvement, but recurrent tachycardia causes rapid decline in left ventricular function and development of heart failure. Sudden death is possible.*

Morillo CA, Klein GJ, Thakur RK, et al. Mechanism of 'inappropriate' sinus tachycardia. Role of sympathovagal balance. *Circulation*. 1994;90:873–877.

ANSWER TO QUESTION ONE: B

ANSWER TO QUESTION TWO: All are correct

ARRHYTHMOGENIC RIGHT VENTRICULAR CARDIOMYOPATHY

QUESTION:

What echocardiographic findings have been reported in arrhythmogenic right ventricular cardiomyopathy?

A. Sacculations of the right ventricular free wall.

B. Dilatation of the right ventricle and right ventricular outflow.

C. Myocardial thinning and dyskinesis.

D. Thickening and hyperreflectivity of the moderator band.

E. All of the above.

Arrhythmogenic right ventricular cardiomyopathy (dysplasia) is a predominantly right ventricular disorder. Pathology shows replacement of myocardial fibers with fatty, fibrous, or fibrofatty tissue.

FIGURE 11.21

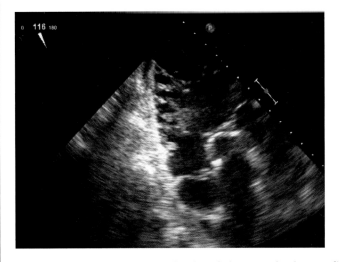

Prominent trabeculations in the right ventricular outflow.

FIGURE 11.22

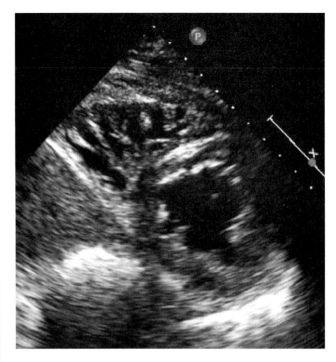

Prominent trabeculations in the right ventricular cavity.

REFERENCES:

[pdf] Hulot JS, Jouven X, Empana JP, et al. Natural history and risk stratification of arrhythmogenic right ventricular dysplasia/cardiomyopathy. *Circulation.* 2004;110:1879–1884.

[pdf] Lakdawala NK, Givertz MM. Dilated cardiomyopathy with conduction disease and arrhythmia. *Circulation.* 2010;122:527–534. *Diagnostic considerations in various inflammatory, infectious, genetic, and infiltrative cardiomyopathies.*

ANSWER: E

ECHOCARDIOGRAPHIC FINDINGS IN THE STROKE PATIENT

QUESTION ONE: **Which of the following statements is FALSE?**

A. Systolic left ventricular dysfunction can occur in patients with subarachnoid hemorrhage.

B. The left ventricular wall motion abnormality found during a stroke corresponds to a particular coronary artery distribution.

C. Stress-induced (Takotsubo) cardiomyopathy can occur in association with a stroke.

Left ventricular wall motion abnormalities in stroke patients (with no coronary artery disease) may be due to catecholamine surges. They may be patchy and typically do NOT follow a single coronary artery distribution.

QUESTION TWO:

Transesophageal echocardiography (TEE) is generally more sensitive than transthoracic echo in finding the cause of a stroke. Which one of the causes listed below may be found on transthoracic and NOT on TEE?

A. Aortic atheromas.

B. Papillary fibroelastoma.

C. Patent foramen ovale (PFO).

D. Left atrial appendage thrombus.

A foramen ovale may be intermittently patent. Transthoracic echo with cough and Valsalva may demonstrate a right to left saline shunt. These maneuvers are less effective with the sedated TEE patient. See the next section.

FIGURE 11.23

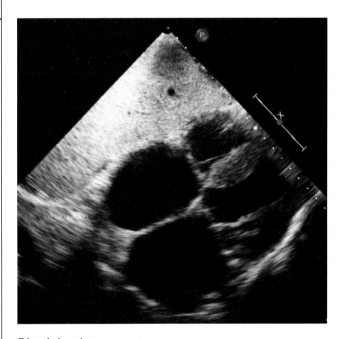

Biatrial enlargement.

QR 11.21: Patent foramen ovale shown by color flow.

QR 11.22a: Sometimes an unconventional view can demonstrate a patent foramen ovale with color flow.

QR 11.22b: Sometimes an unconventional view can demonstrate a patent foramen ovale with color flow.

QR 11.23a: Patent foramen ovale shown by saline contrast.

QR 11.23b: Patent foramen ovale shown by saline contrast.

QR 11.23c: Patent foramen ovale shown by saline contrast.

QR 11.23d: Patent foramen ovale shown by saline contrast.

QR 11.24: Atrial septal aneurysm.

QR 11.25a: Residual interatrial communication in a patient with a stroke following attempted device closure of a patent foramen ovale.

QR 11.25b: Residual interatrial communication in a patient with a stroke following attempted device closure of a patent foramen ovale.

QR 11.26: Lambl's excrescence on the ventricular side of the aortic valve in a patient with dilated cardiomyopathy.

QR 11.27a: Lambl's excrescences on the aortic valve.

QR 11.27b: Lambl's excrescences on the aortic valve.

QR 11.27c: Lambl's excrescences on the aortic valve.

QR 11.28: Papillary fibroelastoma on the aortic valve. The motion has been described as "shimmering."

QR 11.29: Papillary fibroelastoma in the left ventricular outflow below the aortic valve.

QR 11.30a: Large serpiginous thrombus in the right atrium.

QR 11.30b: Large serpiginous thrombus in the right atrium.

QR 11.31a: Large thrombus in the left pulmonary vein of a lung cancer patient.

QR 11.31b: Large thrombus in the left pulmonary vein of a lung cancer patient.

QR 11.32a: Apical ballooning—stress induced—Takotsubo cardiomyopathy.

QR 11.32b: Apical ballooning—stress induced—Takotsubo cardiomyopathy.

QR 11.32c: Apical ballooning—stress induced—Takotsubo cardiomyopathy.

REFERENCES:

 Wittstein IS, Thiemann DR, Lima JA, et al. Neurohumoral features of myocardial stunning due to sudden emotional stress. *N Engl J Med*. 2005;352:539–548.

 Richard C. Stress-related cardiomyopathies. *Ann Intensive Care*. 2011;1:39.

 Samuels MA. The brain-heart connection. *Circulation*. 2007;116:77–84.

ANSWER TO QUESTION ONE: B

ANSWER TO QUESTION TWO: C

INTERMITTENTLY PATENT FORAMEN OVALE

QUESTION: Which of the following can be a useful adjunct in establishing the presence of a PFO during agitated saline injection?

A. Cough.

B. Valsalva maneuver.

C. Pulsed wave Doppler.

D. Color flow Doppler

E. All of the above.

A foramen ovale can be intermittently patent. Intravenous saline contrast injection may *not* demonstrate a right to left shunt in some PFO cases without the help of a provocative maneuver. A transient flurry of saline contrast bubbles may be elicited with a cough or a Valsalva maneuver.

It is uncomfortable for the patient to intentionally cough or bear down during TEE. It may not even be possible in the heavily sedated patient. Color flow Doppler is easily done during TEE. It may demonstrate left to right flow across a foramen ovale.

TECHNICAL HINT: You can use your *hearing* to detect a saline contrast shunt. Pulsed wave Doppler may be used to provide auditory (rather than visual) evidence of a PFO. Pulsed wave Doppler at the mitral leaflet tips (with the transducer positioned at the apex) may detect audible "plinks" of saline contrast (use low gain settings, and turn up the speaker volume).

 QR 11.33a: Patent foramen ovale demonstrated by intravenous agitated saline.

 QR 11.33b: Patent foramen ovale demonstrated by intravenous agitated saline.

 QR 11.33c: Patent foramen ovale demonstrated by intravenous agitated saline.

QR 11.33d: Patent foramen ovale demonstrated by intravenous agitated saline.

QR 11.33e: Patent foramen ovale demonstrated by intravenous agitated saline.

QR 11.33f: Patent foramen ovale demonstrated by intravenous agitated saline.

QR 11.34: Patent foramen ovale demonstrated by color flow Doppler.

QR 11.35: Right atrial thrombus in a patient with patent foramen ovale and paradoxical embolism.

QR 11.36a: Atrial septal aneurysm.

QR 11.36b: Atrial septal aneurysm.

QR 11.36c: Atrial septal aneurysm.

QR 11.36d: Atrial septal aneurysm.

QR 11.36e: Atrial septal aneurysm.

QR 11.36f: Atrial septal aneurysm.

QR 11.36g: Atrial septal aneurysm.

QR 11.36h: Atrial septal aneurysm.

QR 11.36i: Atrial septal aneurysm.

QR 11.37a: Atrial septal aneurysm seen intermittently, simulating a left atrial mass.

QR 11.37b: Atrial septal aneurysm seen intermittently, simulating a left atrial mass.

QR 11.37c: Atrial septal aneurysm seen intermittently, simulating a left atrial mass.

REFERENCES:

Mas JL, Arquizan C, Lamy C, et al. Patent Foramen Ovale and Atrial Septal Aneurysm Study Group. Recurrent cerebrovascular events associated with patent foramen ovale, atrial septal aneurysm, or both. *N Engl J Med*. 2001;345:1740–1746.

Mügge A, Daniel WG, Angermann C, et al. Atrial septal aneurysm in adult patients. A multicenter study using transthoracic and transesophageal echocardiography. *Circulation*. 1995;91:2785–2792.

Messé SR, Silverman IE, Kizer JR, et al. Quality Standards Subcommittee of the American Academy of Neurology. Practice parameter: recurrent stroke with patent foramen ovale and atrial septal aneurysm: report of the Quality Standards Subcommittee of the American Academy of Neurology. *Neurology*. 2004;62:1042–1050.

Ghosh S, Ghosh AK, Ghosh SK. Patent foramen ovale and atrial septal aneurysm in cryptogenic stroke. *Postgrad Med J*. 2007;83:173–177.

Furie KL, Kasner SE, Adams RJ, et al. American Heart Association Stroke Council, Council on Cardiovascular Nursing, Council on Clinical Cardiology, and Interdisciplinary Council on Quality of Care and Outcomes Research. Guidelines for the prevention of stroke in patients with stroke or transient ischemic attack: a guideline for healthcare professionals from the American Heart Association/American Stroke Association. *Stroke*. 2011;42:227–276.

Kerr AJ, Buck T, Chia K, et al. Transmitral Doppler: a new transthoracic contrast method for patent foramen ovale detection and quantification. *J Am Coll Cardiol*. 2000; 36:1959–1966.

ANSWER: E

TRANSPULMONARY SALINE CONTRAST SHUNT

" *Better late than Botalli.* **"**

TEE in a patient with hepatic cirrhosis shows transpulmonary passage of agitated saline. The contrast enters the left atrium after five cardiac cycles. Which of the following is true?

A. There is an unroofed coronary sinus.

B. Repeated agitated saline injections may result in less transpulmonary passage of the bubbles.

C. There are no neurological implications.

D. PFO has been ruled out.

Pulmonary arteriovenous malformations can be found in patients with cirrhosis. They are also found in patients with congenital heart diseases palliated with the Glenn shunt. The neurological implication is that cerebral arteriovenous malformations may coexist with pulmonary arteriovenous malformations. PFO (described by Botalli) can coexist.

The appearance of contrast on the left side of the heart within two to three cardiac cycles indicates a transatrial shunt. Conversely, late contrast appearance after say, five cardiac cycles, has two possible explanations. First, it may be an intermittently PFO. Second, it may represent transpulmonary passage.

When this happens during a TEE, it is important to image the pulmonary veins. The mechanism of a small transpulmonary shunt is presumed to be a small arteriovenous connection. Repeated agitated saline injections may indeed result in less transpulmonary passage of the bubbles as these pulmonary arteriovenous connections become saturated and obstructed by the contrast bubbles.

A prominent transpulmonary saline contrast shunt may be found in the following conditions, EXCEPT:

A. Hepatic cirrhosis.

B. Glenn shunt.

C. Cerebral arteriovenous malformations.

D. Unroofed coronary sinus.

QR 11.38: Transpulmonary saline contrast shunt entering the left atrium from the left upper pulmonary vein.

REFERENCES:

Xie MX, Yang YL, Cheng TO, et al. Coronary sinus septal defect (unroofed coronary sinus): echocardiographic diagnosis and surgical treatment. *Int J Cardiol.* 2013;168:1258–1263.

 Sperling DC, Cheitlin M, Sullivan RW, et al. Pulmonary arteriovenous fistulas with pulmonary hypertension. *Chest.* 1977;71:753–757. *X-rays and pulmonary angiograms in two cases.*

Hagen PT, Scholz DG, Edwards WD. Incidence and size of patent foramen ovale during the first 10 decades of life: an autopsy study of 965 normal hearts. *Mayo Clin Proc.* 1984 Jan;59:17–20. *The incidence and size of the patent foramen ovale were studied in 965 autopsy specimens of human hearts, which were from subjects who were evenly distributed by sex and age. Neither incidence nor size of the defect was significantly different between male and female subjects. The overall incidence was 27.3%, but it progressively declined with increasing age from 34.3% during the first three decades of life to 25.4% during the 4th through 8th decades and to 20.2% during the 9th and 10th decades. Among the 263 specimens that exhibited patency in the study, the foramen ovale ranged from 1 to 19 mm in maximal potential diameter (mean, 4.9 mm). In 98% of these cases, the foramen ovale was 1 to 10 mm in diameter. The size tended to increase with increasing age, from a mean of 3.4 mm in the first decade to 5.8 mm in the 10th decade of life.*

Guchlerner M, Kardos P, Liss-Koch E, et al. PFO and right-to-left shunting in patients with obstructive sleep apnea. *J Clin Sleep Med.* 2012;8:375–380.

McCarthy K, Ho S, Anderson R. Defining the morphologic phenotypes of atrial septal defects and interatrial communications. *Images Paediatr Cardiol.* 2003;5:1–24.

ANSWER TO QUESTION ONE: B

ANSWER TO QUESTION TWO: D

CONGENITAL HEART DISEASE

VENTRICULAR SEPTAL DEFECT

Echocardiographic diagnosis of a small restrictive perimembranous ventricular septal defect requires the following, EXCEPT?

A. Continuous wave Doppler.

B. Color flow Doppler.

C. Demonstration of the actual defect on two-dimensional (2D) echo.

D. Stethoscope.

Doppler is required to confirm the presence of a perimembranous ventricular septal defect. The parasternal view yields distinctive Doppler findings. There is a turbulent high-velocity *systolic* Doppler flow pattern directed *toward* the parasternal transducer. The origin is close to the tricuspid valve chordae. Demonstration of a small defect with 2D may not be possible in some cases (even with the use of nonstandard views). Auscultation remains a valuable resource. Small color flow jets may be missed in some cases where the murmur is well heard. In these cases, a ventricular septal defect may be easier to hear on auscultation than to find with echo. Mechanism of closure: The tricuspid septal leaflet chordae may seal the defect by becoming thicker. In some cases, an aneurysm is created in the process and can be demonstrated with 2D echo.

QR 12.1: Color flow Doppler pattern typically found with a restrictive perimembranous ventricular septal defect. The flow convergence is frequently misleading. It appears to originate in the aorta, even though it is originating in the left ventricle.

QR 12.2: A high-velocity (4 m/s or greater) systolic flow *toward* the parasternal transducer (shown here in red) is due to a ventricular septal defect. Tricuspid regurgitation (shown here in blue) and pulmonic stenosis (not present) would be directed *away* from the parasternal transducer.

QR 12.3: Continuous wave Doppler demonstrates that the jet is systolic, high velocity, and directed toward the transducer.

QR 12.4: Normal patient. Common question in the echo lab: "Is this color flow evidence of a ventricular septal defect?" Aliasing of color flow in the left ventricular outflow may wrongly suggest flow convergence of a ventricular septal defect to an inexperienced observer. The direction of flow in a small ventricular septal defect with normal pulmonary pressures is from left to right. Lesson: if you see something for the first time on an echo, keep looking for it in subsequent studies. If it is normal, you will find it again in another normal patient.

FIGURE 12.1

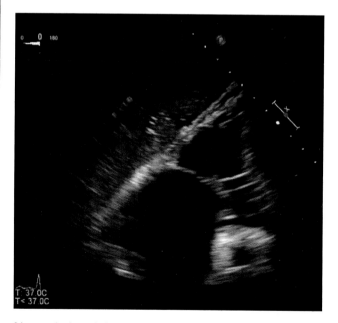

Normal chordal attachments of the tricuspid valve to the interventricular septum.

QR 12.5a: Muscular ventricular septal defect.

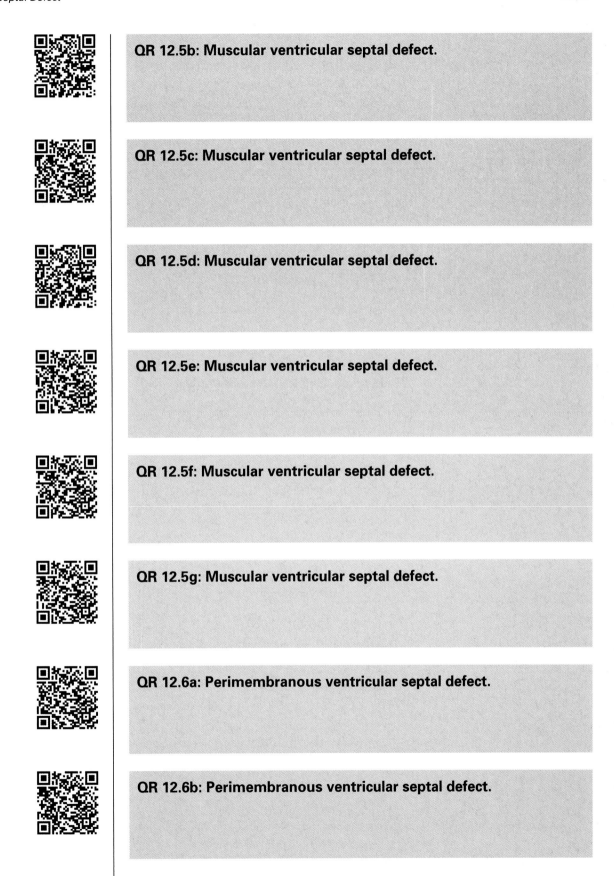

QR 12.5b: Muscular ventricular septal defect.

QR 12.5c: Muscular ventricular septal defect.

QR 12.5d: Muscular ventricular septal defect.

QR 12.5e: Muscular ventricular septal defect.

QR 12.5f: Muscular ventricular septal defect.

QR 12.5g: Muscular ventricular septal defect.

QR 12.6a: Perimembranous ventricular septal defect.

QR 12.6b: Perimembranous ventricular septal defect.

QR 12.6c: Perimembranous ventricular septal defect. The defect is obvious on color flow and audible on auscultation. Two-dimensional echo does *not* show small defects. The most common perimembranous type is adjacent to the tricuspid valve, but may also be adjacent to the aortic valve. Caution: High-velocity flow from the left ventricle may cross the tricuspid valve into the right atrium, and get *misdiagnosed* by the echocardiographer as severe pulmonary hypertension! A rare and distinct shunt from the left ventricle directly to the right atrium is called a Gerbode defect. It has the same diagnostic pitfall, a high (4–5 m) systolic Doppler velocity.

QR 12.7: Aneurysm created by tricuspid valve tissue in a healed ventricular septal defect.

QR 12.8: Overriding aorta. Healed subaortic ventricular septal defect with tricuspid tissue aneurysm.

REFERENCES:

 Farru O, Duffau G, Rodriguez R. Auscultatory and phonocardiographic characteristics of supracristal ventricular septal defect. *Br Heart J.* 1971;33: 238–245. *Extensive description of the bedside findings in this rare form of ventricular septal defect.*

Gościniak P, Larysz B, Baraniak J, et al. The Gerbode defect—a frequent echocardiographic pitfall. *Kardiol Pol.* 2012;70:1191–1193.

Tehrani F, Movahed MR. How to prevent echocardiographic misinterpretation of Gerbode type defect as pulmonary arterial hypertension. *Eur J Echocardiogr.* 2007;8:494–497. *The absence of other signs or symptoms of right ventricular overload; careful review of the jet direction; and estimation of the pulmonary arterial diastolic pressure using the pulmonary regurgitation jet can avoid this echocardiographic mistake.*

Xhabija N, Prifti E, Allajbeu I, et al. Gerbode defect following endocarditis and misinterpreted as severe pulmonary arterial hypertension. *Cardiovasc Ultrasound.* 2010;8:44.

Can I, Krueger K, Chandrashekar Y, et al. Gerbode-type defect induced by catheter ablation of the atrioventricular node. *Circulation.* 2009;119:e553–e556. *The diagnosis should be considered in cases of a new murmur, or worsening heart failure, after an AV node ablation procedure.*

ANSWER: C

ECHO DURING HEART CATHETERIZATION

Which diagnosis can be facilitated by using echocardiography DURING cardiac catheterization?

A. Sinus of Valsalva aneurysm.

B. Ventricular septal defect.

C. Atrial septal defect (ASD).

D. Mitral regurgitation.

The package inserts of echocardiographic contrast agents warn not to administer it to patients with known or suspected right-to-left, bidirectional, or transient right to left shunts, and not to give it by intra-arterial injection. However, imaging with ultrasound during a standard radiologic contrast left ventriculogram performed in the catheterization laboratory may help in the localization of the left-to-right shunt of a ventricular septal defect.

ANSWER: B

SECUNDUM ATRIAL SEPTAL DEFECT

Which statement is true?

A. Echocardiography is frequently the only abnormal diagnostic modality in adults with secundum ASD.

B. Patent foramen ovale and ASD are frequently confused on echocardiography.

C. Associated valvular pulmonic stenosis does not affect the echocardiographic findings of secundum ASD.

D. Undiagnosed ASD may be found during an echocardiogram for new onset atrial fibrillation.

Patients with secundum ASD have an abnormally split second heart sound and a pulmonic flow murmur. Fixed splitting of the second heart sound can be easily identified (after some practice). The electrocardiogram (ECG) shows variable stages of right bundle branch block, from incomplete to complete. Chest X-ray will show right heart enlargement, dilated pulmonary artery, and pulmonary vascular plethora. Some ASD patients suffer from recurrent pulmonary infections, which may have prompted the X-ray. A previously undiagnosed ASD may also present for the first time as atrial fibrillation. Patent foramen ovale does not dilate the right heart chambers. In the adult with secundum ASD, there is echocardiographic dilatation of the right atrium and the right ventricle.

Valvular pulmonic stenosis alters the echocardiographic findings. It is associated with ASD. In cases of combined severe pulmonic stenosis and ASD, the right ventricle becomes hypertrophic rather than dilated.

Note about the fixed splitting of the second heart sound: Once pulmonary hypertension develops in patients with ASD, there are changes in the auscultatory findings. The pulmonic component of the second heart sound becomes louder. The split second heart sound simulates going *up* the musical scale. The more faint aortic closure sound is followed by a louder pulmonic closure sound. An early systolic pulmonary ejection click (that gets louder on inspiration) may become audible in the upper left sternal border.

QR 12.9a: Secundum atrial septal defect.

QR 12.9b: Secundum atrial septal defect.

QR 12.10: Large secundum atrial septal defect. The color flow outlines the rim.

QR 12.11: Primum atrial septal defect.

QR 12.12: Negative contrast effect in the contrast-filled right atrium. This is due to left to right blood flow across a secundum ASD. The shunt is primarily from left to right, but some contrast bubbles are crossing from the right atrium to the left atrium.

QR 12.13: Intact atrial septum: Flow from the inferior vena cava into the right atrium creates a negative contrast effect.

QR 12.14: Secundum atrial septal defect in a neonate.

QR 12.15a: Secundum atrial septal defect.

QR 12.15b: Secundum atrial septal defect.

QR 12.15c: Secundum atrial septal defect.

QR 12.15d: Secundum atrial septal defect.

QR 12.16: Iatrogenic fenestration in the membrane of the fossa ovalis created by a previous electrophysiology procedure. The right cardiac chamber dimensions have remained normal because the shunt is hemodynamically insignificant.

QR 12.17: Increased pulmonary artery flow in a patient with a secundum atrial septal defect. There was no pulmonic valve stenosis.

QR 12.18: Intact atrial septum with negative contrast in the right atrium from inferior cava inflow. The Eustachian valve should not be mistaken for the atrial septum in this case.

QR 12.19: Normal caval inflow may be mistaken to be an atrial septal defect.

QR 12.20a: Atrial septal defect closure device.

QR 12.20b: Atrial septal defect closure device.

REFERENCES:

O'Toole JD, Reddy PS, Curtiss EI, et al. The mechanism of splitting of the second heart sound in atrial septal defect. *Circulation.* 1977;56:1047–1053. *The study includes patients with pulmonary hypertension and atrial fibrillation.*

Gilliam PM, Deliyannis AA, Mounsey JP. The left parasternal impulse. *Br Heart J.* 1964;26:726–736. *The abnormal left parasternal impulse as a clinical sign of right heart disease: A steady heave is found in pulmonary hypertension and pulmonary stenosis, as opposed to the more tumultuous hyperdynamic lift of atrial septal defect.*

ANSWER: D

ATRIOVENTRICULAR (AV) SEPTAL DEFECTS

66 *Abnormalities of the atrioventricular valves associated with* **99**
variable deficiencies of adjacent septal tissue.

QUESTION:

Which anatomical abnormality is LEAST likely to be present in the various forms of AV septal defect?

A. Cleft.

B. Gooseneck.

C. Straddling.

D. Overriding.

Patients with Down syndrome may have an AV septal defect.

The AV valves may each have lateral, superior, and inferior components. Mitral valve regurgitation due to a *cleft* is easily found with color flow Doppler. The cleft itself may be more difficult to demonstrate with 2D echo. A useful 2D and M-mode clue is the presence of chordal attachments from the abnormal mitral valve to the interventricular septum. The left ventricular outflow may be narrowed giving rise to a radiological appearance termed *gooseneck* deformity. Chordal attachments may *straddle* the interventricular septum.

They may attach to the interventricular crest, straddle the crest, and attach to the right ventricle, or appear to float over the interventricular crest. This is the anatomic basis of the Rastelli classification. Overriding is found in (unrelated) tetralogy of Fallot where the aorta appears to hover over the interventricular septum.

QR 12.21: AV canal defect.

QR 12.22: AV canal defect with a dilated hypertrophic right ventricle due to severe pulmonary hypertension.

QR 12.23: AV canal defect manifested as an intermittent connection of the mitral valve chordae to the interventricular septum at the left ventricular outflow.

REFERENCES:

 Tandon R, Moller JH, Edwards JE. Unusual longevity in persistent common atrioventricular canal. *Circulation*. 1974;50:619–626. *Excellent diagrams with photographs of pathological findings*.

Fraisse A, Massih TA, Kreitmann B, et al. Characteristics and management of cleft mitral valve. *J Am Coll Cardiol*. 2003;42:1988–1993.

Becker AE, Ho SY, Caruso G, et al. Straddling right atrioventricular valves in atrioventricular discordance. *Circulation*. 1980;61:1133–1141.

ANSWER: D

SINUS VENOSUS ATRIAL SEPTAL DEFECT

This is a defect of the infolding of the atrial roof where it normally separates the superior vena cava from the right upper pulmonary vein. It can only be diagnosed when the rim of the fossa ovalis is present. The defect overrides the rim. The superior vena cava overrides the defect and has a biatrial connection. It is interatrial but is considered extracardiac from an embryologic perspective. It is frequently missed on transthoracic echo in the adult. The right atrium and right ventricle are dilated. Transesophageal echo is usually necessary in the adult to identify the abnormal right pulmonary venous drainage, and to demonstrate the defect.

REFERENCES:

Van Praagh S, Carrera ME, Sanders SP, et al. Sinus venosus defects: unroofing of the right pulmonary veins – anatomic and echocardiographic findings and surgical treatment. *Am Heart J*. 1994;128:365–379.

 al Zaghal AM, Li J, Anderson RH, et al. Anatomical criteria for the diagnosis of sinus venosus defects. *Heart*. 1997;78:298–304.

 Anderson RH, Brown NA, Webb S. Development and structure of the atrial septum. *Heart*. 2002;88:104–110.

Schleich JM, Dillenseger JL, Houyel L, et al. A new dynamic 3D virtual methodology for teaching the mechanics of atrial septation as seen in the human heart. *Anat Sci Educ*. 2009;2:69–77.

Sharma VK, Radhakrishnan S, Shrivastava S. Three-dimensional transesophageal echocardiographic evaluation of atrial septal defects: a pictorial essay. *Images Paediatr Cardiol*. 2011;13:1–18.

D-TRANSPOSITION OF THE GREAT VESSELS

"   *With unoperated D-TGA you D-ie.*   **"**

With L-TGA you L-ive.

QUESTION: **How will the echocardiographic images in a newborn baby with uncorrected D-TGA compare to the standard images in the adult?**

A. The anatomic left ventricle will be in its usual position on the echo.

B. A great vessel that bifurcates will take off from this ventricle.

C. The atria will still receive blood normally and connect to their respective ventricles normally.

D. In the parasternal view, the aortic valve will be way on top of the screen (coronary ostia may help identify it).

E. The great vessels may look parallel rather than intertwining.

F. All of the above.

This disorder is easier to understand anatomically than L-TGA, but the adult echocardiographer does not get to scan an uncorrected D-TGA adult patient. The anatomic description of the disorder is as follows: ventriculoarterial discordance with atrioventricular concordance. The surgical repairs help to understand the anatomy. At birth, blood flows in two parallel circuits and needs to be redirected. Switch procedures redirected blood at the *atrial* level from 1959 until 1975. Since 1976, the *arterial* switch has become the preferred surgical mode of redirection. Associated defects serve to keep the baby alive, but some will make surgical repair more difficult (ventricular septal defects, outflow obstruction). Bedside examination will reveal a loud second heart sound. It may be loud enough to be palpable.

QR 12.24a: Mustard repair of D-TGA.

QR 12.24b: Mustard repair of D-TGA.

QR 12.25: Mustard procedure—severely dilated systemic ventricle.

QR 12.26: Mustard procedure—Doppler inflow.

QR 12.27a: Fontan operation. Single ventricle. Three-chamber heart.

QR 12.27b: Fontan operation. Single ventricle. Three-chamber heart.

REFERENCES:

 Liebman J, Cullum L, Belloc NB. Natural history of transposition of the great arteries. Anatomy and birth and death characteristics. *Circulation.* 1969;40:237–262.

 Trusler GA, Mustard WT, Fowler RS. The role of surgery in the treatment of transposition of the great vessels. *Can Med Assoc J.* 1964;91:1096–1100.

Senning A. Surgical correction of transposition of the great vessels. *Surgery.* 1959;45:966–980.

Jatene AD, Fontes VF, Paulista PP, et al. Anatomic correction of transposition of the great vessels. *J Thorac Cardiovasc Surg.* 1976 Sep;72:364–370.

Rashkind WJ, Miller WW. Creation of an atrial septal defect without thoracotomy. A palliative approach to complete transposition of the great arteries. *JAMA.* 1966;196:991–992.

Rastelli GC, McGoon DC, Wallace RB. Anatomic correction of transposition of the great arteries with ventricular septal defect and subpulmonary stenosis. *J Thorac Cardiovasc Surg.* 1969;58:545–552.

 Wilkinson JL, Acerete F. Terminological pitfalls in congenital heart disease. Reappraisal of some confusing terms, with an account of a simplified system of basic nomenclature. *Br Heart J.* 1973;35:1166–1177.

 Kilner PJ. Imaging congenital heart disease in adults. *Br J Radiol.* 2011;84 (Spec No 3):S258–S268.

Carey LS, Elliott LP. Complete transposition of the great vessels. Roentgenographic findings. *Am J Roentgenol Radium Ther Nucl Med.* 1964;91:529–543. *Egg on a string sign: in the PA view—the configuration of the heart has the shape of an egg tilted so the long axis lays in a oblique position. The pole with the least convexity is upwards and to the right. The pole with the greatest convexity is downwards and to the left the cardiac apex. The aortic knob and the pulmonary "mogul" are lined up one behind the other in this PA view, resulting in a narrow great vessel pedicle—hence, the egg is on a string.*

ANSWER: F

L-TRANSPOSITION OF THE GREAT VESSELS

"   *Atrio-ventricular and ventriculo-arterial discordance.*   **"**

An echocardiogram is performed on an adult with progressive shortness of breath. Color flow Doppler shows severe "mitral" regurgitation. Which of the findings below indicates congenitally corrected L-TGA?

A. Loss of fibrous continuity between the "mitral" valve and the aortic valve in the parasternal long axis view.

B. The "mitral" valve in the apical four-chamber view is more apically displaced than the "tricuspid" valve.

C. In the parasternal view: the aortic valve will be way on top of the screen (coronary ostia may help identify it).

ANATOMICAL RULES IN TRANSPOSITION

There are several useful rules to sort out echocardiographic findings.

Rule: The AV valve goes with the ventricle. It is possible to identify the right ventricle on most echocardiographic examinations. The right ventricle has an infundibulum. This is manifested on echo as lack of fibrous continuity between the AV valve and the semilunar valve.

Corollary: If the ventricle has an infundibulum, the AV valve of that ventricle is tricuspid. The left ventricle has no infundibulum, so the AV valve and the semilunar valve are in fibrous continuity.

Corollary Two: If the ventricle has no infundibulum, the AV valve of that ventricle is anatomically mitral.

Rule: The branching pattern of the great vessels helps in their identification.

Corollary: The pulmonary artery bifurcates. The aorta gives rise to the coronary ostia and shows the branching pattern at the arch.

Rule: The semilunar artery goes with the great vessel.

Corollary: If the great vessel bifurcates, it is a pulmonic valve. If the great vessel gives rise to coronary ostia, it is an aortic valve.

Rule: The suprahepatic segment of the inferior vena cava empties into the right atrium.

Corollary: The right atrium is identified as the chamber that receives this vein in the subcostal view. A saline contrast injection into a lower extremity vein can help.

QR 12.28: Congenitally corrected transposition (L-TGA) in an adult. The left atrium (identified by the narrow based appendage) connects to a dilated (anatomic right) ventricle (identified by the apically displaced tricuspid valve).

QR 12.29: Congenitally corrected transposition (L-TGA) in an adult. There is fibrous continuity between the venous AV valve (anatomic mitral) and the pulmonic valve.

QR 12.30: Lack of fibrous continuity between the systemic AV valve on the bottom of the screen (anatomic tricuspid) and the aortic valve (with coronary ostia) on the top of the screen. The aortic closure sound is loud and palpable because of the proximity to the chest wall.

QR 12.31: Systemic ventricle with an infundibulum (hence the lack of fibrous continuity between the AV valve and the aortic valve). Pacemaker wire in the venous ventricle (anatomic left ventricle, where there is fibrous continuity between the venous anatomic mitral and the pulmonic valve).

REFERENCES:

Presbitero P, Somerville J, Rabajoli F, et al. Corrected transposition of the great arteries without associated defects in adult patients: clinical profile and follow up. *Br Heart J*. 1995;74:57–59.

Prieto LR, Hordof AJ, Secic M, et al. Progressive tricuspid valve disease in patients with congenitally corrected transposition of the great arteries. *Circulation*. 1998;98:997–1005.

de la Cruz MV, Berrazueta JR, Arteaga M, et al. Rules for diagnosis of arterio-ventricular discordances and spatial identification of ventricles. Crossed great arteries and transposition of the great arteries. *Br Heart J*. 1976;38:341–354.

Shinebourne EA, Macartney FJ, Anderson RH. Sequential chamber localization – logical approach to diagnosis in congenital heart disease. *Br Heart J*. 1976;38: 327–340.

Warnes CA. Transposition of the great arteries. *Circulation*. 2006;114:2699–2709.

ANSWER: A and B (C is present in both L-TGA and in unoperated D-TGA)

PULMONIC VALVE STENOSIS

QUESTION: **Which of the following statements about patients with pulmonic valve stenosis is WRONG?**

A. Like all other right-side auscultatory findings, a pulmonic stenosis ejection click gets louder on inspiration.

B. High Doppler flow velocity of an associated ventricular septal defect indicates mild pulmonic stenosis.

C. Tricuspid regurgitation velocity increases with pulmonic stenosis severity.

D. In pulmonic stenosis, the pulmonic valve opens prematurely in late diastole.

E. A dilated right ventricle suggests an alternate diagnosis.

F. The loudness of the systolic pulmonic stenosis murmur correlates with severity.

Valve opening: In pulmonic valve stenosis, the atrial contraction will open the stenotic valve *a crack* in late diastole and it will then remain open until the end of systole, closing at the beginning of next diastole. The reason is that in isolated valvular pulmonic stenosis the right ventricle becomes muscular and stiff, but does not dilate. Atrial contraction elevates the pressure in this noncompliant right ventricle above the relatively low pulmonary artery diastolic pressure and the valve opens and stays ajar. The appearance of partly open stenotic pulmonic leaflets is fused leaflets that dome with a circular orifice like a short windsock or a volcano.

Auscultation: The ejection click of valvular pulmonic stenosis is an *exception* to the useful clinical rule that right-side murmurs increase on inspiration. The loudness of an ejection click is determined by the distance the pulmonic valve travels before stopping short with a resulting click. On inspiration, the right heart fills more because of the negative intrathoracic pressure. A doming stenotic pulmonic valve travels less during inspiration than it does when the heart is smaller in expiration. Examining the patient during held expiration will also make the ejection click more audible.

The loudness of the systolic pulmonic stenosis murmur does correlate with severity. It may be harsh and sound like someone is clearing their throat. It may radiate to the back.

Pitfalls: The right heart chambers become dilated in patients with ASDs, not in patients with isolated valvular pulmonic stenosis. It is a common echocardiographic misinterpretation that patients with dilated right heart chambers have pulmonic stenosis because of the increased blood flow in the pulmonary artery from the shunt.

Tricuspid regurgitation velocity indicates right ventricular "driving" pressure, or in other words, the pressure gradient between the right ventricle and the right atrium in systole. The right ventricular systolic pressure is equal to the pulmonary artery systolic pressure *plus* the pulmonary stenosis gradient.

In patients with an associated restrictive ventricular septal defect, the Doppler velocity indicates the interventricular gradient. As the right ventricular pressure rises in worsening pulmonic stenosis, the velocity of the ventricular septal defect *decreases*.

FIGURE 12.2

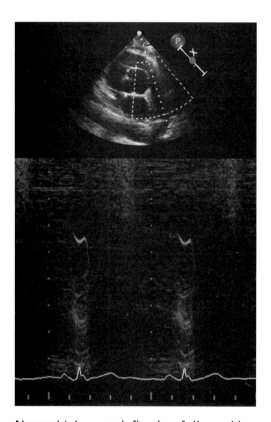

Normal 'a' wave deflection followed by pulmonic leaflet opening in systole.

REFERENCES:

 Craige E, Schmidt RE. Precordial movements over the right ventricle in normal children. *Circulation*. 1965;32:232–240.

 Schmidt RE, Craige E. Precordial movements over the right ventricle in children with pulmonary stenosis. *Circulation*. 1965;32:241–250.

Koretzky ED, Moller JH, Korns ME, et al. Congenital pulmonary stenosis resulting from dysplasia of valve. *Circulation*. 1969;40:43–53. *Pulmonic stenosis can be due to three distinct, markedly thickened, immobile cusps. In such cases, there is no commissural fusion and no dome-shaped deformity of the valve.*

ANSWER: A

PERSISTENT LEFT SUPERIOR VENA CAVA

❝ *An impressive "blink of an eye" echocardiographic diagnosis.* **❞**

A 24-year-old baseball player has a syncopal episode. Routine echocardiogram is performed. The reading echocardiographer makes an instant (albeit irrelevant to the syncope) diagnosis from the first parasternal long-axis image (see Figure 12.3).

Which statement is true?

A. Physical examination will be completely normal.

B. ECG will be abnormal.

C. Chest X-ray will provide the diagnosis.

D. Intravenous contrast study should be done.

You will amaze all your friends and colleagues. Just remember to scrutinize the size of the coronary sinus in the first few seconds of looking at the parasternal long-axis echocardiographic image. There IS a subtle physical exam abnormality. On physical examination, the internal jugular venous *pulsations* are easier to examine on the left side of the neck.

Lack of other clinical clues: There are no symptoms associated with persistent left superior vena cava (PLSVC). There are no ECG abnormalities. There are no chest X-ray abnormalities. However, an impressive "blink of an eye" echocardiographic diagnosis can be expected. An experienced echocardiographer (and the reader of this book):

FIRST: makes the diagnosis of a congenital "abnormality" in the first few seconds of looking at the study!

SECOND: confirms the diagnosis by starting an intravenous line in the LEFT arm and injecting agitated saline that arrives first in the dilated coronary sinus and then empties into the right atrium.

Additional echocardiographic views are helpful: Coronary sinus dilatation can be confirmed in the apical images but nonstandard views may be needed.

Confirmation is by injection of agitated saline contrast into the left arm, which then travels down a PLSVC.

Don't take the wrong turn at Albuquerque.

Importance of making the diagnosis: Problems are caused by physicians (unaware of the anatomy) advancing a catheter, or a wire, where it does not belong. Pacemakers are routinely implanted on the LEFT side of the chest. The prospect of taking a wrong turn with a pacemaker wire looms with every procedure. There may be patients with *known* PLSVC who may not want the right side of their chest occupied by a pacemaker box. For example, someone who pitches a baseball, swings a tennis racquet, or braces a shotgun on the right shoulder may insist that a pacemaker be placed on the left side of the chest.

Technical aspects of purposely advancing a pacemaker wire through a PLSVC: After the left subclavian vein is punctured for permanent pacemaker insertion, the guide wire would take a left-sided downward course to the coronary sinus and from there it would enter the right atrium. The right ventricular pacemaker lead tip deflects away from the tricuspid annulus, making advancement difficult. It is necessary to manually reshape the stylet into a U. With considerable manipulation, one can form a loop in the right atrium using the right atrial free wall for support, and cross the tricuspid valve to advance the pacemaker wire into the right ventricle.

Implications for cardioplegia: In patients undergoing cardioplegia for open-heart surgery, it is important to diagnose PLSVC because the cardioplegia will become ineffective and therefore potentially dangerous for the patient.

• BAD NEWS: Retrograde cardioplegia is hampered by the presence of a PLSVC that results in excessive runoff of solution into the PLSVC and the right atrium.

• GOOD NEWS: It is possible to technically modify the procedure, and it has been possible to perform cardioplegia in patients with PLSVC (using only retrograde cardioplegia).

Common misconceptions: There are misconceptions when it comes to a second superior vena cava on the left side of the chest. This is simply an extra-systemic vein (it is NOT a pulmonary vein). There is NO arteriovenous shunt. It does not require intervention. A dilated coronary sinus may be mistaken for: The descending thoracic aortic aorta, a localized pericardial effusion, or a pericardial cyst.

FIGURE 12.3

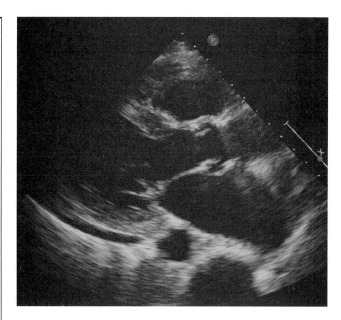

Dilated coronary sinus. Small pericardial effusion. Descending aorta behind the left atrium.

FIGURE 12.4

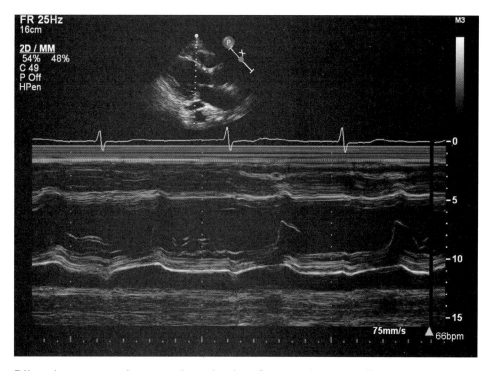

Dilated coronary sinus can be mistaken for a pericardial effusion on M-mode.

FIGURE 12.5

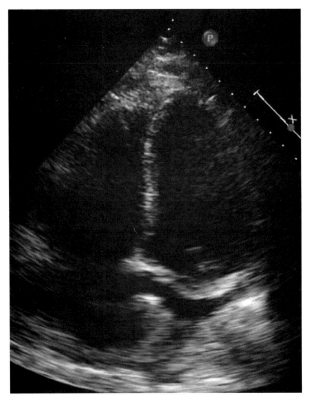

Normal size coronary sinus draining into the right atrium.

QR 12.32: Parasternal long-axis view showing a dilated coronary sinus.

QR 12.33: TEE sweep from the right atrial cavity to the dilated coronary sinus.

QR 12.34a: Saline contrast in the left SVC between the left pulmonary vein and the left atrial appendage.

QR 12.34b: Saline contrast in the left SVC between the left pulmonary vein and the left atrial appendage.

QR 12.34c: Saline contrast in the left SVC between the left pulmonary vein and the left atrial appendage.

QR 12.35a: Dilated coronary sinus under the mitral annulus.

QR 12.35b: Dilated coronary sinus under the mitral annulus.

QR 12.35c: Dilated coronary sinus under the mitral annulus.

QR 12.35d: Dilated coronary sinus under the mitral annulus.

QR 12.36: Dilated coronary sinus shown on a modified apical four-chamber view that scans for the coronary sinus below the posterior mitral annulus. There is a pacemaker wire in the right ventricle. This patient also has an apical left ventricular aneurysm.

QR 12.37: A dilated coronary sinus can easily be mistaken for a loculated pericardial effusion, or a pericardial cyst.

QR 12.38: Normal coronary sinus appearance in a patient with left ventricular hypertrophy. The descending aorta is also shown.

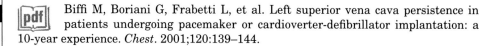

QR 12.39: Venous flow *towards* the heart on the *left* side of the chest.

REFERENCES:

 Biffi M, Boriani G, Frabetti L, et al. Left superior vena cava persistence in patients undergoing pacemaker or cardioverter-defibrillator implantation: a 10-year experience. *Chest*. 2001;120:139–144.

 Ramos N, Fernández-Pineda L, Tamariz-Martel A, et al. Absent right superior vena cava with left superior vena cava draining to an unroofed coronary sinus. *Rev Esp Cardiol*. 2005;58:984–987. *Once in a lifetime echo: A patient with a dilated coronary sinus undergoes saline contrast injection into the left arm vein. The saline contrast goes from the left arm vein to the LEFT atrium.*

Kong PK, Ahmad F. Unroofed coronary sinus and persistent left superior vena cava. *Eur J Echocardiogr*. 2007;8:398–401.

Rose AG, Beckman CB, Edwards JE. Communication between coronary sinus and left atrium. *Br Heart J*. 1974;36:182–185.

ANSWER: D

SCIMITAR CHEST X-RAY

QUESTION:

A chest X-ray performed to evaluate recurrent pulmonary infections shows a "scimitar sign." Which statement is true?

A. Desaturated venous blood is draining into the systemic circulation.

B. There is no shunt.

C. Saturated blood drains into the venous system.

Pulmonary veins may drain abnormally into locations other than the left atrium. The scimitar X-ray sign indicates partial anomalous *infracardiac* pulmonary venous return.

REFERENCES:

Espinola-Zavaleta N, Játiva-Chávez S, Muñoz-Castellanos L, et al. Clinical and echocardiographic characteristics of scimitar syndrome. *Rev Esp Cardiol*. 2006;59:284–288. *Scimitar X-ray sign in infracardiac anomalous pulmonary venous drainage.*

Snellen HA, Albers FH. The clinical diagnosis of anomalous pulmonary venous drainage. *Circulation*. 1952;6:801–816. *Snowman (Figure 8) X-ray sign in supracardiac anomalous pulmonary venous drainage.*

ANSWER: C

EBSTEIN'S ANOMALY OF THE TRICUSPID VALVE

An asymptomatic 50-year-old patient is found to have a Wolf–Parkinson–White pattern on a routine ECG. Which statement is FALSE?

A. An intermittent pattern is prognostically more favorable.

B. Initial diagnosis over age 40 is prognostically more favorable.

C. No prior syncope is prognostically more favorable.

D. Ebstein's anomaly should be routinely sought with echocardiography.

Ebstein's anomaly should *probably* not be routinely sought with echocardiography in every patient with newly diagnosed Wolf–Parkinson–White pattern on ECG (unless the P waves are dramatically large). Although this is a rare abnormality, the possibility that it is present may also come up when there is massive cardiomegaly on the chest X-ray in an asymptomatic adult. The lungs are clear and the pulmonary artery shadow is small. Auscultation may reveal four distinct heart sounds that "mimic a slow-moving train."

QR 12.40a: Ebstein's abnormality of the tricuspid valve.

QR 12.40b: Ebstein's abnormality of the tricuspid valve.

Attenhofer Jost CH, Connolly HM, Dearani JA, et al. Ebstein's anomaly. *Circulation*. 2007;115:277–285. *Excellent overview*.

Shiina A, Seward JB, Tajik AJ, et al. Two-dimensional echocardiographic-surgical correlation in Ebstein's anomaly: preoperative determination of patients requiring tricuspid valve plication vs. replacement. *Circulation*. 1983;68:534–544.

ANSWER: D

DISEASES OF THE AORTA

PALPABLE CAROTID THRILLS

QUESTION: **An echocardiogram was performed for suspected aortic valve disease after the referring physician noted a palpable carotid thrill. The aortic valve appeared normal on the echocardiogram. What is another cause for a carotid thrill?**

A. Trauma.

B. Congenital arteriovenous malformation.

C. Prior catheterization.

D. All of the above.

There are rare causes of palpable carotid artery thrills. A 22-year-old man developed shortness of breath after lifting weights and then developed acute heart failure due to rupture of an aneurysm of the right sinus of Valsalva into the right ventricle. The patient developed dyspnea, tachycardia, wide pulse pressure, bounding carotid and peripheral pulses, pulmonary crackles, and prominent continuous precordial murmur with thrill. Transesophageal echocardiogram with Doppler examination confirmed the diagnosis (*Am J Med Sci*. 2006 Feb; 331(2):100–102).

A 42-year-old man presented with a palpable thrill in the cervical region and headache. He had a shotgun injury 10 years before presentation. Diagnosis of a high output traumatic arteriovenous fistula between the right common carotid artery and the internal jugular vein was made arteriographically. A neighboring traumatic aneurysm on the common carotid artery and a 9 mm diameter fistula tract required surgery. At the operation, ligation of the tract and aneurysmorrhaphy were performed and the patient was discharged on the third postoperative day (*Vasa*. 2004;33(1):46–48).

A congenital carotid–jugular aneurysm was responsible for severe heart failure in a 2-day old baby. The child recovered after surgery. The signs suggesting an arteriovenous fistula (a continuous murmur and thrill, hyperdynamic circulation) may be absent, as in this case, when the child is in severe cardiac failure. The signs should be sought when the circulation improves (*Arch Fr Pediatr*. 1979;36(5):502–507). Amusement park injuries include carotid artery dissections, which can present as a palpable carotid thrill (*Ann Emerg Med*. 2002;39(1):65–72).

Iatrogenic vertebral arteriovenous fistulas have been reported following angiographic procedures and percutaneous internal jugular and subclavian venous catheterizations performed for routine hemodynamic monitoring. It may be possible to obliterate the thrill by pressure on the common carotid artery in some patients (*Surgery* 1980;87:343–346).

Thrills that are palpated at various locations on the chest wall have other, more commonly recognized causes. Aortic stenosis, pulmonic stenosis, and ventricular septal defect may give rise to a palpable thrill at the upper sternal area. The thrill of aortic stenosis may be more readily palpable over the carotid arteries. The thrill of a patent ductus arteriosus may be palpable in systole and in diastole. Increased blood flow in the pulmonary artery due to an atrial septal defect (even without associated pulmonic stenosis) may also give rise to a faint thrill at the upper left sternal border.

Mitral regurgitation may give rise to a palpable apical *systolic* thrill. Mitral stenosis may give rise to a palpable apical *diastolic* thrill.

REFERENCE: Evans W, Lewes D. The carotid shudder. *Br Heart J*. 1945;7:171–172. *Palpable vibration at the peak of the carotid pulse in combined aortic stenosis and aortic regurgitation.*

ANSWER: D

SINUS OF VALSALVA ANEURYSM

QUESTION: **A 60-year-old patient with history of a loud SYSTOLIC childhood murmur (that spontaneously disappeared), has been followed for several years for a soft, blowing, high pitched, 2/6 DIASTOLIC decrescendo murmur. He is now in the emergency room being intubated for sudden onset of pulmonary edema.**

An astute cardiologist (who just finished reading this book) puts a stethoscope on the patient's chest, listens briefly, and announces the urgent diagnosis of ruptured sinus of Valsalva aneurysm. What was the new auscultatory finding that provided this diagnosis?

A. Austin Flint murmur.

B. Graham Steell murmur.

C. The old systolic murmur came back.

D. Continuous murmur.

The clinical hallmark of a ruptured sinus of Valsalva aneurysm is the new finding of a continuous murmur. Sinus of Valsalva aneurysm refers to aneurysmal dilatation of the proximal portion of the ascending aorta. Sinus of Valsalva aneurysms can rupture. The rupture usually connects to the right ventricular outflow tract. It may alternatively connect to the right atrium.

In contradistinction to aortic dissection, a ruptured of Valsalva aneurysm does not typically empty into the pericardium. If there is no pericardial effusion, there is no tamponade. Patients can survive the acute rupture of a sinus of Valsalva, but they develop fulminant congestive heart failure and present with flash pulmonary edema.

REFERENCES:

 Feigl D, Feigl A, Edwards JE. Mycotic aneurysms of the aortic root. A pathologic study of 20 cases. *Chest*. 1986;90:553–557.

 Lavall D, Schäfers HJ, Böhm M, et al. Aneurysms of the ascending aorta. *Dtsch Arztebl Int*. 2012;109:227–233.

ANSWER: D

MARFAN SYNDROME

QUESTION:

Which of the following echocardiographic findings does NOT help in the diagnosis of Marfan syndrome?

A. Annuloaortic ectasia.

B. Mitral valve prolapse.

C. Dilated pulmonary artery.

D. Mitral annular calcium.

E. Pericardial effusion.

Cardiovascular evidence of Marfan syndrome:

• Dilatation of the aorta involving at least the sinus of Valsalva.
• Mitral valve prolapse.
• Mitral annular calcification below age 40.
• Pulmonary artery dilatation below age 40 (in the absence of pulmonic stenosis).

Annuloaortic ectasia refers to the pear-shaped appearance of the dilated sinus of Valsalva and the proximal aorta.

FIGURE 13.1

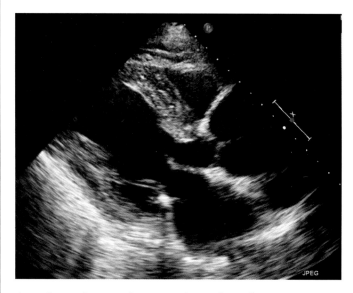

Annuloaortic ectasia: pear-shaped aortic root.

FIGURE 13.2

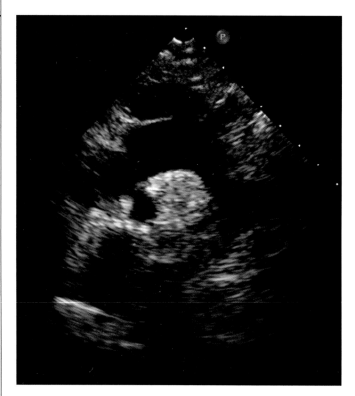

Normal aortic arch.

QR 13.1: Mildly dilated sinus of Valsalva with stretching of the aortic leaflets.

QR 13.2a: Aneurysm of the proximal ascending aorta.

QR 13.2b: Aneurysm of the proximal ascending aorta.

QR 13.2c: Aneurysm of the proximal ascending aorta.

QR 13.2d: Aneurysm of the proximal ascending aorta.

QR 13.3: Aneurysm of the descending aorta.

REFERENCE:

 Dean JC. Marfan syndrome: clinical diagnosis and management. *Eur J Hum Genet*. 2007;15:724–733.

ANSWER: E

COARCTATION OF THE AORTA

" *Collateral damage?* "

Which statement about coarctation of the aorta is INCORRECT?

A. The eyes may make the diagnosis.

B. The ears may make the diagnosis.

C. The fingertips may make the diagnosis.

D. Prognosis is normal after repair.

Diagnosis of coarctation of the aorta with echocardiography requires adequate images of the aortic arch. It is important to scrutinize the aortic arch, isthmus, and descending aorta in every study that shows left ventricular hypertrophy. The femoral pulse may be delayed when compared with the right radial pulse. The ankle brachial index will be abnormal between the hypertensive RIGHT arm and the lower pressure in the legs. Consequently, someone in the vascular lab may get the glory of making the diagnosis first.

There is a loud systolic murmur in the back. It is best heard in the left interscapular region. Collaterals may be audible on auscultation as systolic or continuous murmurs. There may be notching of the ribs on the X-ray from collateral flow; this is actually a favorable prognostic sign. There may be cyanosis of the lower extremities with a pink right arm if there is an associated patent arterial duct. Hypertension may persist after repair, and life expectancy may *not* be normal.

FIGURE 13.3

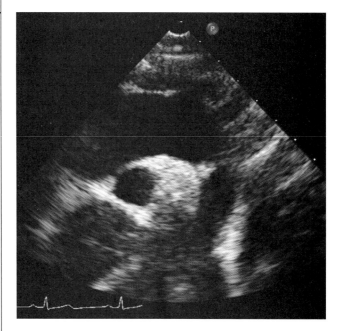

Coarctation of the aorta.

FIGURE 13.4

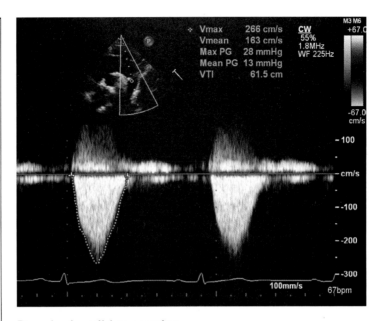

Doppler in mild coarcation.

QR 13.4: Coarctation of the aorta.

QR 13.5: Collateral flow entering the descending aorta in coarctation.

REFERENCES:

 Cohen M, Fuster V, Steele PM, et al. Coarctation of the aorta. Long-term follow-up and prediction of outcome after surgical correction. *Circulation*. 1989;80: 840–845.

 Campbell M. Natural history of coarctation of the aorta. *Br Heart J*. 1970;32: 633–640.

 Kreel L, al-Kutoubi MA. Two varieties of rib notching. *Postgrad Med J*. 1991; 67:568–570. *Rib notching is bilateral and symmetrical. The notches are small, on the inferior margin of the posterior ribs, usually in pairs. The upper six ribs are most notably affected. The notches are produced by enlarged and tortuous intercostal arteries acting as collaterals from the upper aorta that bypass the coarctation.*

 Gerbode F. A simple test to identify coarctation of the aorta. *Ann Surg*. 1976; 184:615–617. *Differences in capillary filling can be shown after relieving a constriction of the foot and hand together in patients with coarctation. On squeezing the hand and foot together for a few seconds and then suddenly releasing the compression, one will immediately notice the red flushing of the hand. This contrasts with the white marble-like appearance of the slow capillary filling of the foot.*

ANSWER: D

AORTIC ATHEROMAS

RHETORICAL QUESTION:

What is the paradox of transesophageal echo (TEE) diagnosis of aortic atheromas?

Aortic atheromas are markers of increased risk for cerebrovascular events. Yet, they are commonly found in the *descending* aorta, downstream from the head vessels. TEE is almost always necessary to make this diagnosis. Atherosclerosis of the *ascending* aorta is more difficult to image using TEE, usually due to excessive ultrasound artifacts. Direct epiaortic ultrasound of the ascending aorta is sometimes performed in the operating room prior to cannulation. It is typically done by the surgeon, forcing interruption of the usual pre-bypass routine.

FIGURE 13.5

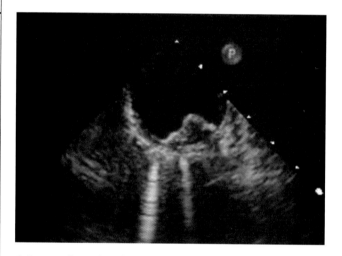

Atherosclerosis of the descending aorta.

FIGURE 13.6

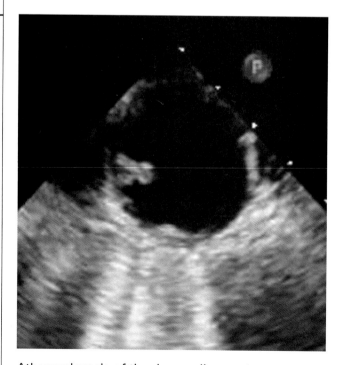

Atherosclerosis of the descending aorta.

FIGURE 13.7

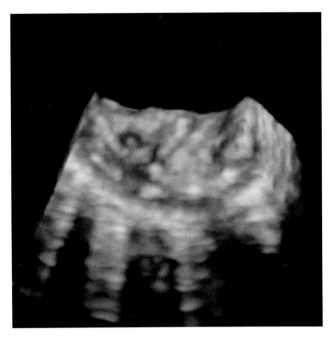

Atherosclerosis of the descending aorta.

FIGURE 13.8

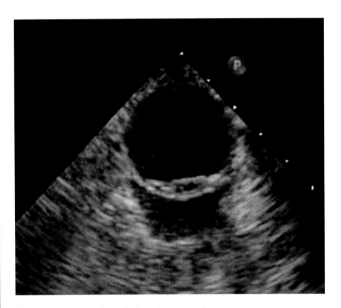

Atherosclerosis of the descending aorta.

QR 13.6: Atherosclerosis and calcification of a dilated descending aorta. The patient was a heavy smoker.

REFERENCE:

Evangelista A, Flachskampf FA, Erbel R, et al. Echocardiography in aortic diseases: EAE recommendations for clinical practice. *Eur J Echocardiogr.* 2011;11:645–58.

AORTIC DISSECTION

" *Effusion/Regurgitation/Infarction.* "

A 70-year-old hypertensive presents with new onset of ripping back pain. The echocardiogram is likely to show all of the following EXCEPT?

A. Pericardial effusion.

B. Aortic regurgitation.

C. Basal inferior left ventricular wall akinesis.

D. Annuloaortic ectasia.

The initial echocardiographic evaluation in a patient with aortic dissection may be a transthoracic study. Although this may fail to reveal the dissection flap, there may be indirect evidence of the dissection: pericardial effusion, aortic regurgitation, inferior wall motion abnormality, aortic aneurysm. The most common mode of death in acute aortic dissection is cardiac tamponade. The transthoracic study may show the presence of pericardial fluid as it begins to accumulate.

Caution! Pericardiocentesis can worsen hemodynamics and even precipitate death. Any improvement in ventricular function from relief of the tamponade may actually contribute to further propagation of the dissection. Urgent surgery remains the only lifesaving treatment in acute ascending aortic dissection. If the dissection involves the proximal ascending aorta, the coaptation of the aortic leaflets may get affected and color flow Doppler may show the presence of aortic regurgitation.

Dissection may reach a coronary artery ostium. The usual ostium is the right. As a result, wall motion abnormalities of the inferior left ventricular wall may be present. The descending aorta can be seen behind the heart in the parasternal long- and short-axis views. It may be possible to demonstrate a dissection flap in some cases. A dissection flap must be distinguished from an artifact. The proximal ascending aorta frequently has ultrasound artifacts that resemble a true flap.

FIGURE 13.9

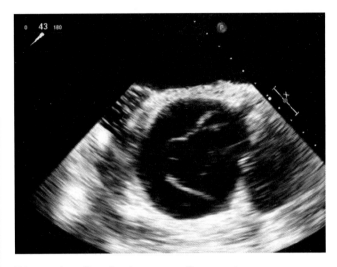

Dissection flap in the ascending aorta.

FIGURE 13.10

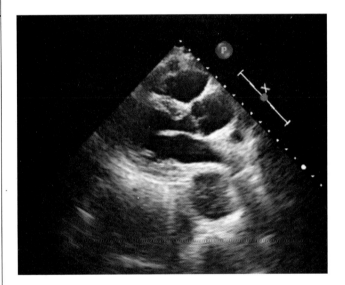

Aneurysm of the descending aorta.

QR 13.7a: Dissection of the descending aorta.

QR 13.7b: Dissection of the descending aorta.

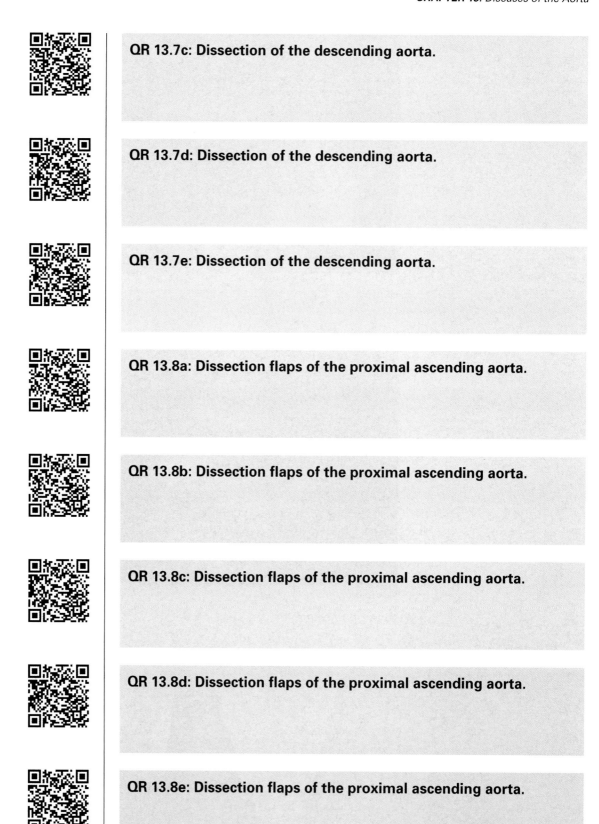

QR 13.7c: Dissection of the descending aorta.

QR 13.7d: Dissection of the descending aorta.

QR 13.7e: Dissection of the descending aorta.

QR 13.8a: Dissection flaps of the proximal ascending aorta.

QR 13.8b: Dissection flaps of the proximal ascending aorta.

QR 13.8c: Dissection flaps of the proximal ascending aorta.

QR 13.8d: Dissection flaps of the proximal ascending aorta.

QR 13.8e: Dissection flaps of the proximal ascending aorta.

QR 13.9: Mild aneurysmal dilatation of the aorta. Dissection flap close to the right coronary ostium (6 o'clock).

QR 13.10: Dissection flap close to the right coronary ostium.

QR 13.11a: Artifact in a normal ascending aorta.

QR 13.11b: Artifact in a normal ascending aorta.

REFERENCES:

Ramanath VS, Oh JK, Sundt TM 3rd, et al. Acute aortic syndromes and thoracic aortic aneurysm. *Mayo Clin Proc.* 2009;84:465–481.

Criado FJ. Aortic dissection: a 250-year perspective. *Tex Heart Inst J.* 2011;38:694–700.

ANSWER: D (see the Marfan section)

INTRAMURAL HEMATOMA

66   *A non-communicating aortic dissection.*   **99**

What is the echocardiographic feature that best distinguishes an intramural hematoma from aortic dissection?

A. Crescent shape.

B. Crescent thickness.

C. Location.

D. Lack of an intimal tear.

E. Lack of color flow in the crescent.

F. An ulcer-like appearance.

An intramural hematoma is created by hemorrhage into the medial layer of the aorta. Initially there is no communication to the true lumen. It may get bigger, rupture into the true lumen, and thus progress to aortic dissection. It may remain unchanged, or even resolve. It has a crescent shape on transesophageal echo examination. Rapidly increasing crescent thickness (on serial CT scans) may be useful to distinguish intramural hematoma from a stable atheroma in an extensively atherosclerotic aorta.

The location of an intramural hematoma can be in the ascending or in the descending thoracic aorta, just like dissection. The clinical presentation is similar to that of aortic dissection. By definition, there is no blood flow in the crescent of an intramural hematoma. The presence of blood flow within the crescent indicates that the intramural hematoma has progressed to a dissection by developing an intimal tear and a connection to the true lumen. There may still be a crescent appearance in the undissected portion.

Intramural hematoma was initially pathologically defined as a dissection *without* an intimal tear. Echocardiography may *not* detect presence or absence of an intimal tear by direct visualization of the tear. Indirect demonstration of the tear by showing blood flow in the false lumen is the best distinguishing feature.

FIGURE 13.11

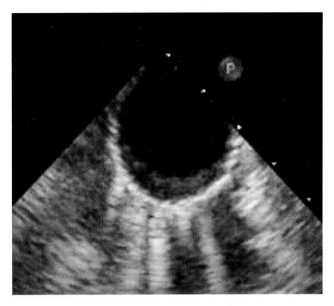

Crescent shaped intramural hematoma in the descending thoracic aorta.

FIGURE 13.12

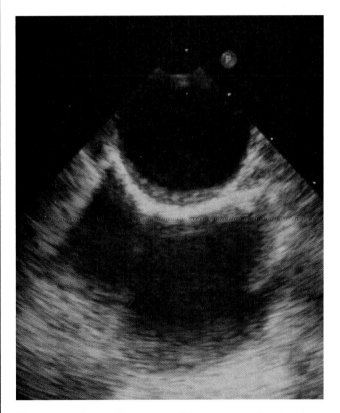

Crescent shaped intramural hematoma in the descending thoracic aorta.

PENETRATING AORTIC ULCER

A penetrating aortic ulcer refers to an atherosclerotic lesion of the aorta that penetrates into the media. It may resemble a peptic ulcer on pathological inspection, hence the name. The crater of the ulcer may be the origin of a localized descending aortic dissection. Echocardiographic diagnosis may be difficult because of the initially small size of the ulcer.

FIGURE 13.13

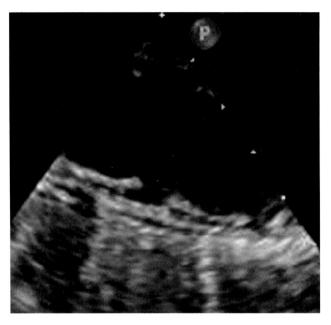

Penetrating aortic ulcer.

FIGURE 13.14

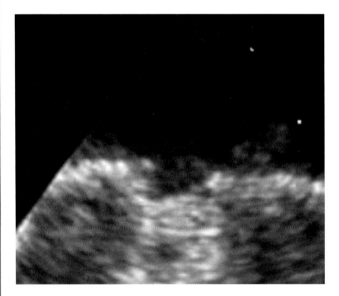

Penetrating aortic ulcer.

QR 13.12: Penetrating aortic ulcer with a mobile atheroma in the descending thoracic aorta.

REFERENCE: Sundt TM. Intramural hematoma and penetrating atherosclerotic ulcer of the aorta. *Ann Thorac Surg*. 2007;83:S835–S841.

ANSWER: E

INTRAOPERATIVE AIR IN THE AORTA

An emergency TEE is performed in the recovery room following mitral valve repair and coronary bypass. Which echocardiographic finding is likely to explain postoperative hypotension with jugular venous distension?

A. Myocardial rupture and tamponade.

B. Inferior left ventricular wall akinesis.

C. New anterior left ventricular wall akinesis.

D. New right ventricular infarction.

The right coronary sinus of Valsalva is more superiorly located in comparison to the left coronary sinus. Trapped air in the aorta will preferentially gravitate (or better said—float) to the right coronary sinus of Valsalva. When coming off bypass, air embolism to the right coronary territory is therefore more likely to occur than to the left coronary system.

The aortic ostium of a right coronary bypass graft is also situated in the superior part of the ascending aorta. Mitral valve surgery, which is frequently accompanied by a graft to the right coronary system, may thus be complicated by immediate postoperative air embolism. The resulting wall motion abnormalities are important to recognize on an emergent TEE in the recovery room. Myocardial rupture can occur if the heart is lifted by the surgeon after putting in a mechanical prosthesis.

REFERENCES:

 Draganov J, Scheeren TW. Incidental detection of paradoxical air embolism with a transoesophageal Doppler probe inserted for measuring descending aortic blood flow. *Br J Anaesth*. 2003;90:520–522.

Fathi AR, Eshtehardi P, Meier B. Patent foramen ovale and neurosurgery in sitting position: a systematic review. *Br J Anaesth*. 2009;102:588–596.

ANSWER: D

CHAPTER 14

CARDIAC TUMORS

BLOOD CYST

" *Benign mimic of ominous pathology.* "

QUESTION: **Echocardiographic mimics of blood cysts include the following, EXCEPT?**

A. Vegetations.

B. Libman–Sacks endocarditis.

C. Papillary fibroelastomas.

D. Aortic raphes.

Blood cysts are congenital, thin-walled, filled with nonorganized blood. The size ranges from microscopic to 3 mm. Occasionally, blood cysts are much larger, or multiple, making them detectable by echocardiography. In the cases where cysts are found during an echocardiographic study, their hemodynamic impact, if any, should be determined by Doppler.

They usually affect the atrioventricular valves on the endocardium, along the lines of closure. They are incidentally found during autopsy on cardiac valves in approximately 50% of infants under 2 months of age. They are rarely found on autopsy after 2 years of age. Because of their typically benign nature, they can be monitored with serial echocardiograms. Surgical resection is reserved for the very rare masses that interfere with normal cardiac function.

REFERENCES: Park MH, Jung SY, Youn HJ, et al. Blood cyst of subvalvular apparatus of the mitral valve in an adult. *J Cardiovasc Ultrasound.* 2012;20:146–149.

Agac MT, Acar Z, Turan T, et al. Blood cyst of tricuspid valve: an incidental finding in a patient with ventricular septal defect. *Eur J Echocardiogr.* 2009; 10:588–589.

ANSWER: C

TUMORS OF THE AORTA

Soft tissue sarcoma is a common malignant neoplasm of the heart, pericardium, and great vessels. Its presentation is infrequent, nonspecific, and subtle. Emboli from these tumors to the lungs or peripheral arteries may mimic thrombotic embolic disease. Angiosarcoma, the most common cardiac sarcoma, is aggressive and usually arises in the right atrium.

Kaposi sarcoma of the heart has been found in patients with AIDS and in immunosuppressed organ transplant recipients. Most primary sarcomas of the aorta and pulmonary artery (the elastic arteries) are classified as intimal sarcomas.

Leiomyosarcomas predominate in the muscular arteries and great veins. Surgical resection of any sarcoma of the vasculature, when feasible, is technically challenging but may result in cure or palliation. Adjuvant chemotherapy and radiation therapy can also relieve symptoms and prolong survival.

REFERENCES:

Raaf HN, Raaf JH. Sarcomas related to the heart and vasculature. *Semin Surg Oncol.* 1994;10:374–382.

Yasuda T, Yamamoto S, Yamaguchi S, et al. Leiomyosarcoma of the thoracic aorta. *Jpn J Thorac Cardiovasc Surg.* 1999;47:510–513. *A patient clinically suspected of dissecting aortic aneurysm underwent surgery. The descending thoracic aorta was found to be filled with a soft, yellow leiomyosarcoma.*

Lerakis S, Clements SD, Taylor WR, et al. Transesophageal echocardiography detection of an esophageal sarcoma mimicking aortic dissection. *J Am Soc Echocardiogr.* 2000; 13:619–621.

Burke AP, Virmani R. Sarcomas of the great vessels. A clinicopathologic study. *Cancer.* 1993;71:1761–1773.

 Székely E, Kulka J, Miklós I, et al. Leiomyosarcomas of great vessels. *Pathol Oncol Res.* 2000;6:233–236.

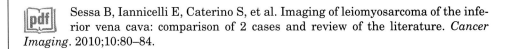 Sessa B, Iannicelli E, Caterino S, et al. Imaging of leiomyosarcoma of the inferior vena cava: comparison of 2 cases and review of the literature. *Cancer Imaging.* 2010;10:80–84.

Hsing JM, Thakkar SG, Borden EC, et al. Intimal pulmonary artery sarcoma presenting as dyspnea: case report. *Int Semin Surg Oncol.* 2007;4:14.

 Yusuf SW, Bathina JD, Qureshi S, et al. Cardiac tumors in a tertiary care cancer hospital: clinical features, echocardiographic findings, treatment and outcomes. *Heart Int.* 2012;7:e4.

VARIOUS CARDIAC TUMORS, MASSES, AND THROMBI

> " *If it is on the atrial septum—it's a tumor.* "
> *If it is on a valve—it's a vegetation.*
> *If it is in the appendage—it's a thrombus.*

FIGURE 14.1

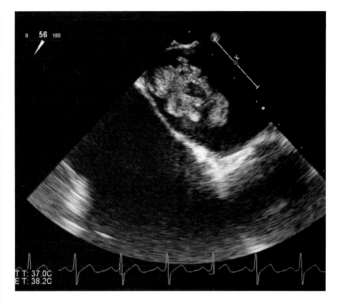

Left atrial myxoma.

QR 14.1: Left atrial myxoma.

QR 14.2a: Left atrial myxoma.

QR 14.2b: Left atrial myxoma.

QR 14.2c: Left atrial myxoma.

QR 14.2d: Left atrial myxoma.

QR 14.2e: Left atrial myxoma.

QR 14.2f: Left atrial myxoma.

QR 14.3a: Mechanical effect of atrial fibrillation on the motion of a left atrial myxoma.

QR 14.3b: Mechanical effect of atrial fibrillation on the motion of a left atrial myxoma.

QR 14.4: Left atrial myxoma and a patent foramen ovale.

QR 14.5: Left atrial myxoma extending toward the right upper pulmonary vein.

QR 14.6a: Right atrial myxoma.

QR 14.6b: Right atrial myxoma.

QR 14.6c: Right atrial myxoma.

QR 14.7: Cardiac fibroma.

QR 14.8: Metastatic breast cancer infiltrating the left ventricle. Malignant pericardial effusion.

QR 14.9: Extensive tumor infiltration of both atria by metastatic lung cancer.

QR 14.10: Mobile friable thrombus in the descending aorta of a patient with heparin, induced thrombocytopenia.

QR 14.11a: Thrombus (not a tumor) superimposed on a catheter in the superior vena cava, entering the right atrial cavity. The saline contrast is coming out of the catheter tip.

QR 14.11b: Thrombus (not a tumor) superimposed on a catheter in the superior vena cava, entering the right atrial cavity. The saline contrast is coming out of the catheter tip.

QR 14.11c: Thrombus (not a tumor) superimposed on a catheter in the superior vena cava, entering the right atrial cavity. The saline contrast is coming out of the catheter tip.

QR 14.12: Thrombus in the superior vena cava.

QR 14.13a: The normal atrial wall infolding between the left atrial appendage and the left pulmonary vein should not be mistaken for a mass.

QR 14.13b: The normal atrial wall infolding between the left atrial appendage and the left pulmonary vein should not be mistaken for a mass.

QR 14.14: Normal anatomy—no tumor. Hypertrophic left ventricular papillary muscles appear intermittently in the images. They should not be confused for masses.

QR 14.15: Submitral chordae in dilated cardiomyopathy. The (not uncommon) different degrees of mobility of these anatomical structures may wrongly suggest a tumor or a thrombus.

QR 14.16: Cardiac structures that resemble tumors. Prominent apical left ventricular trabeculation. Prominent right atrial crista terminalis.

QR 14.17a: Pulmonary vein thrombus.

QR 14.17b: Pulmonary vein thrombus.

QR 14.18: Large hiatus hernia impinging on the posterior left atrial wall. The patient was given a carbonated beverage to sip through a straw, while pulsed wave Doppler was used to "listen" for "plinks" to confirm the diagnosis.

QR 14.19: Lipomatous hypertrophy of the interatrial septum. The fatty infiltration does not extend to the membrane of the fossa ovalis, resulting in a dumbbell appearance.

QR 14.20a: Lung cancer infiltrating the atrial walls and obstructing caval inflow.

QR 14.20b: Lung cancer infiltrating the atrial walls and obstructing caval inflow.

QR 14.20c: Lung cancer infiltrating the atrial walls and obstructing caval inflow.

QR 14.20d: Lung cancer infiltrating the atrial walls and obstructing caval inflow.

QR 14.20e: Lung cancer infiltrating the atrial walls and obstructing caval inflow.

REFERENCES:

 Lee KA, Kirkpatrick JG, Moran JM, et al. Left ventricular fibroma masquerading as postinfarction myocardial rupture. *Ann Thorac Surg.* 1999;68:580–582.

Ohnishi M, Niwayama H, Miyazawa Y, et al. [Echocardiography in patients with malignant metastatic neoplasms of the heart and great vessels]. [Article in Japanese] *J Cardiol.* 1990;20:377–384.

Vidaillet HJ Jr, Seward JB, Fyke FE 3rd, et al. "Syndrome myxoma": a subset of patients with cardiac myxoma associated with pigmented skin lesions and peripheral and endocrine neoplasms. *Br Heart J.* 1987;57:247–255.

Bosi G, Lintermans JP, Pellegrino PA, et al. The natural history of cardiac rhabdomyoma with and without tuberous sclerosis. *Acta Paediatr.* 1996;85:928–931.

 Kullo IJ, Oh JK, Keeney GL, et al. Intracardiac leiomyomatosis: echocardiographic features. *Chest.* 1999;115:587–591.

 Sterns LP, Eliot RS, Varco RL, et al. Intracavitary cardiac neoplasms. A review of fifteen cases. *Br Heart J.* 1966;28:75–83.

Lam KY, Dickens P, Chan AC. Tumors of the heart. A 20-year experience with a review of 12,485 consecutive autopsies. *Arch Pathol Lab Med.* 1993;117:1027–1031.

Findings from the Department of Pathology, University of Hong Kong.

The three most common malignant neoplasms were carcinoma of the lung, esophageal carcinoma, and lymphoma. Pericardium, including epicardium, was the most common location of cardiac involvement by secondary tumors, followed by myocardium and endocardium.

For secondary tumors involving the heart (including both metastasis and local extension), important primary tumors in male subjects were carcinoma of the lung (31.7%), esophageal carcinoma (28.7%), lymphoma (11.9%), carcinoma of the liver (6.9%), leukemia (4.0%), and gastric carcinoma (4.0%), while in female subjects, carcinoma of the lung (35.9%), lymphoma (17.0%), carcinoma of the breast (7.5%), and pancreatic carcinoma (7.5%).

The study showed a higher percentage of esophageal carcinoma and carcinoma of the liver (reflecting the higher incidence of these tumors in Hong Kong Chinese), but a lower incidence of carcinoma of the breast when compared with other series. The metastatic lung tumors showed an unusual predominance of adenocarcinoma.

PAPILLARY FIBROELASTOMA

" *The improved image quality of TEE increases the sensitivity for* **"**
endocarditis but decreases the specificity.

QUESTION: **In the absence of fever and positive blood cultures, a mobile echodensity on an aortic valve can represent which one (or more) of the following?**

A. Lambl's excrescence.

B. Papillary fibroelastoma.

C. Aortic leaflet fenestration.

D. Nodule of Aranti.

E. Antiphospholipid antibody syndrome.

Valvular vegetations are said to have a "shaggy" appearance. Lambl's excrescences are histologically described as lamellar or filiform. The echocardiographic appearance is that of a strand.

Papillary fibroelastomas are histologically described as "frond like." The echocardiographic appearance is that of a "shimmering" vegetation. Antiphospholipid antibody syndrome can manifest as "kissing" vegetations. Aortic leaflet fenestration is not identifiably visualized on echo. Nodules of Aranti are easily palpated on autopsy but only rarely become thick enough to be evident on the echo of a normal aortic valve.

FIGURE 14.2

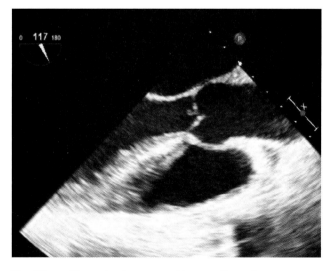

Papillary fibroelastoma on the aortic valve.

FIGURE 14.3

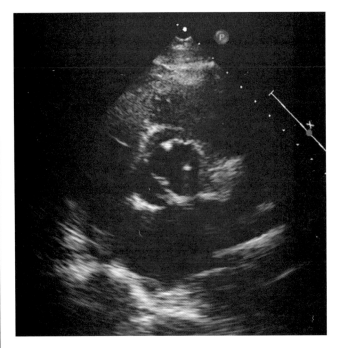

Nodules of Aranti on the aortic leaflets.

FIGURE 14.4

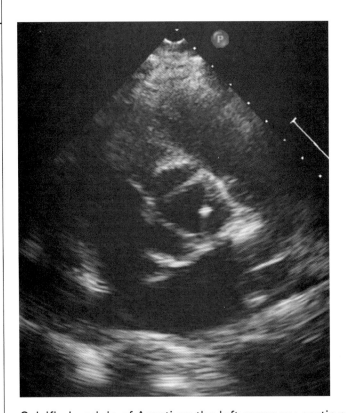

Calcified nodule of Aranti on the left coronary aortic cusp.

FIGURE 14.5

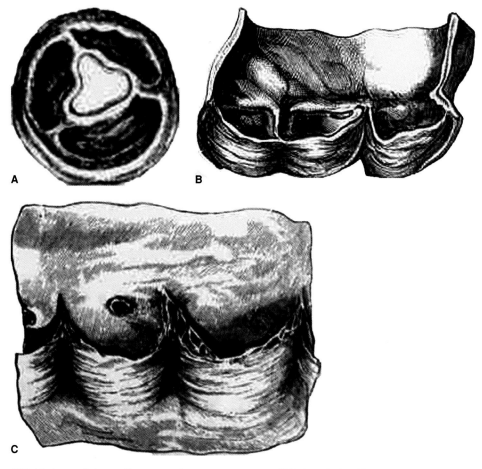

A

B

C

(A) Unicuspid semilunar valve appearance. **(B)** Aortic leaflet asymmetry. **(C)** Aortic leaflet fenestrations. (From Coats J, Sutherland LK (Eds). A manual of pathology. London: Longmans, Green and Co.; 1900.)

QR 14.21a: Lambl's excrescences on the left ventricular side of the aortic valve.

QR 14.21b: Lambl's excrescences on the left ventricular side of the aortic valve.

QR 14.21c: Lambl's excrescences on the left ventricular side of the aortic valve.

QR 14.21d: Lambl's excrescences on the left ventricular side of the aortic valve.

QR 14.21e: Lambl's excrescences on the left ventricular side of the aortic valve.

QR 14.21f: Lambl's excrescences on the left ventricular side of the aortic valve.

QR 14.21g: Lambl's excrescences on the left ventricular side of the aortic valve.

QR 14.21h: Lambl's excrescences on the left ventricular side of the aortic valve.

REFERENCES:

 Edwards FH, Hale D, Cohen A, et al. Primary cardiac valve tumors. *Ann Thorac Surg*. 1991;52:1127–1131.

 Sun JP, Asher CR, Yang XS, et al. Clinical and echocardiographic characteristics of papillary fibroelastomas: a retrospective and prospective study in 162 patients. *Circulation*. 2001;103:2687–2693.

 Colucci V, Alberti A, Bonacina E, et al. Papillary fibroelastoma of the mitral valve. A rare cause of embolic events. *Tex Heart Inst J*. 1995;22:327–331.

 Perez JE, Cordova F, Cintron G. Diastolic opening of the aortic valve in a case of aortic insufficiency due to aortic valve fenestration. *Cardiovasc Dis*. 1978; 5:254–257.

ANSWER: A, B, and E

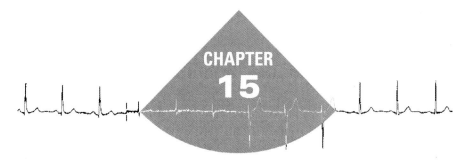

ULTRASOUND
PHYSICS

HARMONICS

You are sitting in your living room reading this book. Suddenly, there is a noise on the porch. You peer through the screen door from your *lit* room to the *unlit* porch. What is the harmonics lesson here?

A. There is an unemployed sonographer on your porch and the only way to get him off the porch is to pay him for the pizza.

B. The light from your living room has to cross the screen, reflect off our sonographer, cross the screen again, and arrive at your retina.

C. Turning *off* your room light and turning *on* the porch light will improve the information.

D. Answer B is analogous to scanning with native transducer frequencies.

E. Answer C is analogous to scanning with harmonics.

Insonating tissue with an ultrasound frequency creates new vibrations that are a multiple of the original frequency. The 2× multiple of the original frequency is the first harmonic. Insonated tissue vibrating at the first harmonic frequency sends this new frequency back to the transducer. The first harmonic ultrasound only travels from tissue to transducer (one way). The original frequency can be filtered out. There is less opportunity for artifacts if ultrasound only travels one way.

REFERENCES:

 Turner SP, Monaghan MJ. Tissue harmonic imaging for standard left ventricular measurements: fundamentally flawed? *Eur J Echocardiogr*. 2006;7:9–15.

 Boote EJ. AAPM/RSNA physics tutorial for residents: topics in US: Doppler US techniques: concepts of blood flow detection and flow dynamics. *Radiographics*. 2003;23:1315–1327.

Mitchell DG. Color Doppler imaging: principles, limitations, and artifacts. *Radiology*. 1990;177:1–10.

ANSWER: All of the above

ULTRASOUND ARTIFACTS

QUESTION: **Routine follow-up echocardiogram of a mechanical aortic prosthesis reveals spontaneous contrast on the left ventricular side of the prosthesis. What is the postulated mechanism to explain this finding?**

A. Native frequency.

B. Reverberation.

C. Hemolysis.

D. Cavitation.

The word cavitation is part of submarine lingo because it explains propeller noise. The design and manufacture of boat propellers have to be meticulously precise because of cavitation. The energy of cavitation created in the water by spinning propellers is destructive enough to affect and eventually destroy the metal of boat propellers. In similar fashion, the cavitation energy created by closure of mechanical prosthesis leaflets releases gas from the blood.

• SCANNING TIP: Cavitation artifacts are usually not seen when the native frequency is being used to scan the patient.

Harmonic imaging is needed to demonstrate their presence.

Turning harmonics on-and-off can be used to easily prove the presence of cavitation.

 QR 15.1a: Cavitation artifacts—mechanical bileaflet mitral prosthesis.

 QR 15.1b: Cavitation artifacts—mechanical bileaflet mitral prosthesis.

QR 15.2a: Reverberation artifact from a breast implant interferes with imaging.

QR 15.2b: Reverberation artifact from a breast implant interferes with imaging.

QR 15.3: Reverberation artifact from a catheter in the right ventricular outflow.

QR 15.4: Reverberation artifact from a ventricular assist device across the aortic valve.

QR 15.5: Reverberation artifact from a right atrial pacemaker wire wrongly suggests that there is something in the pericardial space. Further along the path of the same ultrasound beam, there is an attenuation artifact past the pericardial wall. There is no right atrial collapse.

QR 15.6: Apical artifact suggesting thrombus. The underlying wall motion is normal, making thrombus highly unlikely.

QR 15.7: Apical artifact. It is still possible to identify the true endocardium covered by the artifact.

QR 15.8: Artifacts that obscure apical and lateral left ventricular wall endocardial reflections.

QR 15.9a: Reverberation artifact from the tricuspid annulus that may wrongly suggest a left atrial mass.

QR 15.9b: Reverberation artifact from the tricuspid annulus that may wrongly suggest a left atrial mass.

QR 15.9c: Reverberation artifact from the tricuspid annulus that may wrongly suggest a left atrial mass.

QR 15.9d: Reverberation artifact from the tricuspid annulus that may wrongly suggest a left atrial mass.

QR 15.10: Artifactual duplication of the mitral valve.

QR 15.11: Pacemaker wire demonstrating specular reflection of ultrasound.

QR 15.12: Unusually few distracting artifacts from a pacemaker wire.

QR 15.13: Sideways artifacts from an aortic bioprosthesis.

QR 15.14: Reverberation *and* sideways artifacts from a mechanical aortic prosthesis.

QR 15.15: Mild attenuation artifact from the ring of a mitral bioprosthesis.

QR 15.16: Attenuation artifact from mitral annular calcium.

QR 15.17: Ultrasound absorption and attenuation prevents visualization of the inferior left ventricular wall.

REFERENCES:

 Russell D, Brucher R. Online automatic discrimination between solid and gaseous cerebral microemboli with the first multifrequency transcranial Doppler. *Stroke*. 2002;3:1975–1980.

Stride EP, Coussios CC. Cavitation and contrast: the use of bubbles in ultrasound imaging and therapy. *Proc Inst Mech Eng H*. 2010;224:171–191.

 de Jong N, Emmer M, van Wamel A, et al. Ultrasonic characterization of ultrasound contrast agents. *Med Biol Eng Comput*. 2009;47:861–873.

 Stewart MJ. Contrast echocardiography. *Heart*. 2003;89:342–348.

 Cosyns B, Roossens B, Hernot S, et al. Use of contrast echocardiography in intensive care and at the emergency room. *Curr Cardiol Rev*. 2011;7:157–162.

 Gillman LM, Kirkpatrick AW. Portable bedside ultrasound: the visual stethoscope of the 21st century. *Scand J Trauma Resusc Emerg Med*. 2012;20:18.

 Gargani L. Lung ultrasound: a new tool for the cardiologist. *Cardiovasc Ultrasound*. 2011;9:6.

Prabhu M, Raju D, Pauli H. Transesophageal echocardiography: instrumentation and system controls. *Ann Card Anaesth*. 2012;15:144–155.

ANSWER: D

ECHOCARDIOGRAPHIC ANATOMY

FIGURE 16.1

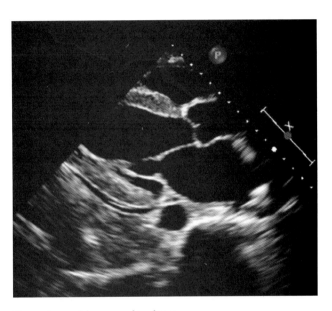

Parasternal long-axis view.

FIGURE 16.2

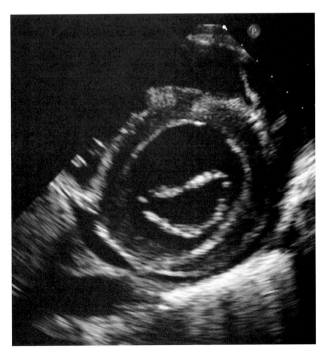

Short-axis view of the mitral valve.

FIGURE 16.3

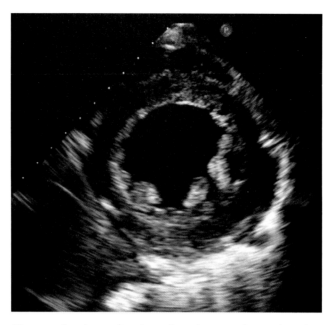

Short-axis view of trabeculated anterolateral and posteromedial papillary muscles.

FIGURE 16.4

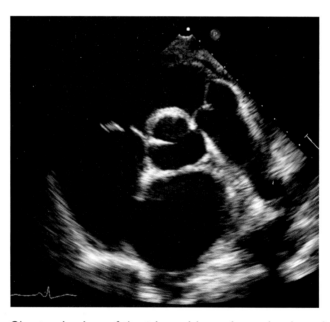

Short-axis view of the tricuspid, aortic, and pulmonic valves.

FIGURE 16.5

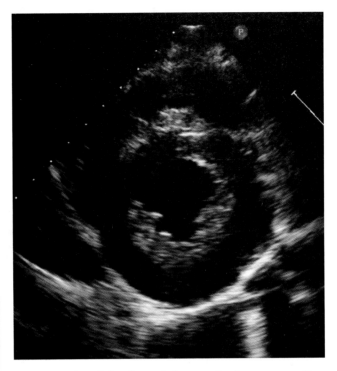

Lack of reflectivity from left ventricular myocardium due primarily to instrument settings. Ultrasound only produces images if it reflects back to the transducer. If the ultrasound is traveling through homogeneous tissue (like the ventricular myocardium in this case), very little ultrasound energy is being reflected—and the gains have to be adjusted accordingly.

FIGURE 16.6

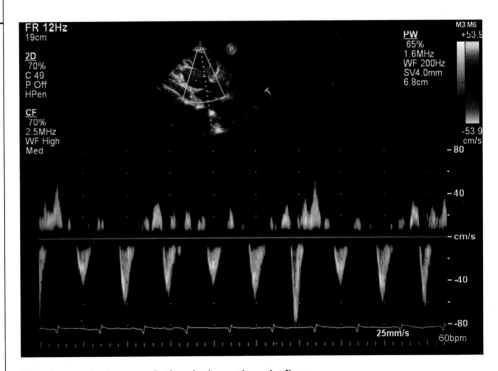

Phasic respiratory variation in hepatic vein flow.

FIGURE 16.7

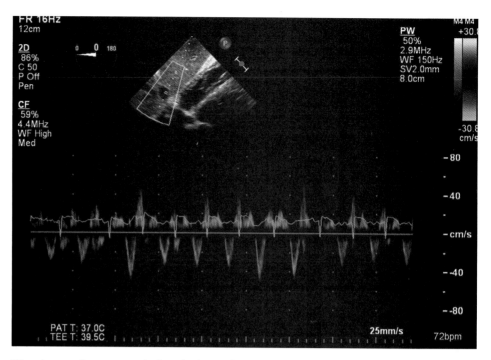

Phasic respiratory variation in hepatic vein flow.

FIGURE 16.8

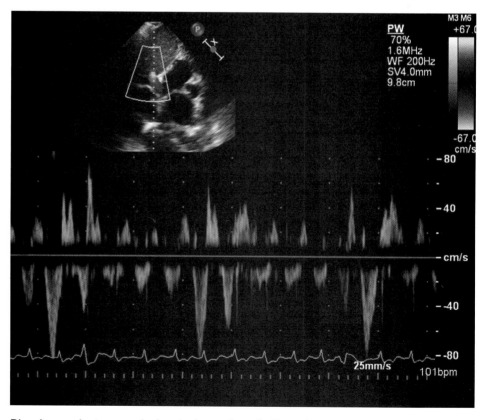

Phasic respiratory variation in hepatic vein flow. In this case, the two premature beats have less influence on flow than respiration does.

FIGURE 16.9

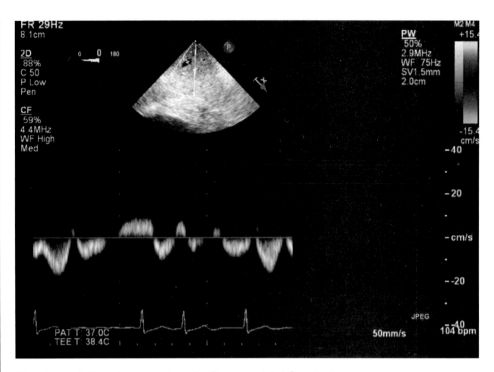

Phasic variation in hepatic vein flow in atrial fibrillation.

FIGURE 16.10

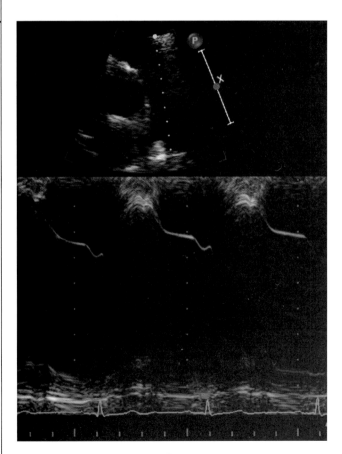

Normal pulmonic valve A wave.

FIGURE 16.11

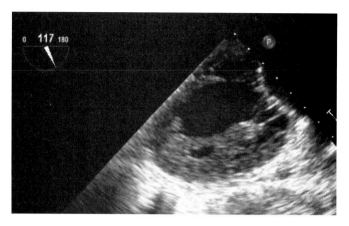

Chordal attachments from the papillary muscles to the mitral valve. Chordae that attach to the commissures are called primary. Chordae that attach to the undersurface of the leaflet body are called secondary.

FIGURE 16.12

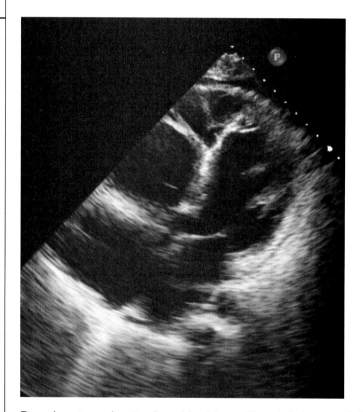

Prominent moderator band inside a dilated right ventricle.

FIGURE 16.13

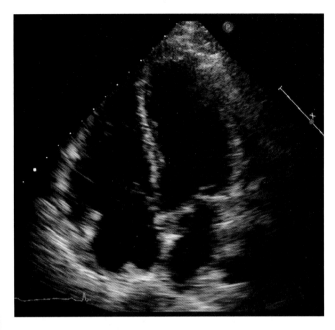

The normal anatomic features of a prominent crista terminalis in the right atrium should not be mistaken for right atrial masses.

FIGURE 16.14

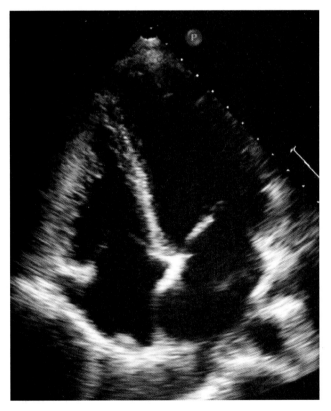

The normal anatomic features of a prominent crista terminalis in the right atrium should not be mistaken for right atrial masses.

FIGURE 16.15

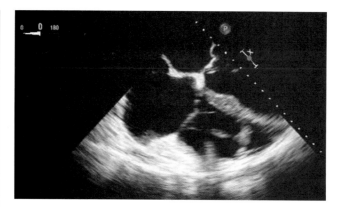

Mid esophagus view of the interatrial septum.

FIGURE 16.16

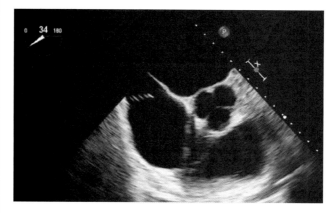

Mid esophagus view of the Eustachian valve.

FIGURE 16.17

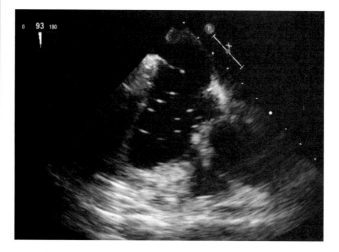

Imaging pitfall: Saline contrast in the right atrium remains primarily on one side of the Eustachian valve. The appearance should not be confused with an atrial septal defect.

FIGURE 16.18

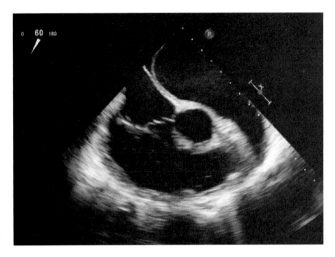

Normal Eustachian valve attaching to the atrial septum.

EUSTACHIAN VALVE ENDOCARDITIS

This rare entity broadens the differential diagnosis of endovascular infections in injection drug users. Transesophageal echocardiography is usually required to make the diagnosis.

REFERENCES:

Limacher MC, Gutgesell HP, Vick GW, et al. Echocardiographic anatomy of the eustachian valve. *Am J Cardiol*. 1986;57:363–365.

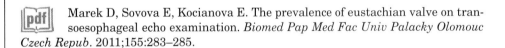 Marek D, Sovova E, Kocianova E. The prevalence of eustachian valve on transoesophageal echo examination. *Biomed Pap Med Fac Univ Palacky Olomouc Czech Repub*. 2011;155:283–285.

Alreja G, Lotfi A. Eustachian valve endocarditis: rare case reports and review of literature. *J Cardiovasc Dis Res*. 2011;2:181–5.

Bowers J, Krimsky W, Gradon JD. The pitfalls of transthoracic echocardiography. A case of eustachian valve endocarditis. *Tex Heart Inst J*. 2001;28:57–59.

James PR, Dawson D, Hardman SM. Eustachian valve endocarditis diagnosed by transesophageal echocardiography. *Heart*. 1999;81:91.

Vilacosta I, San Roman JA, Roca V. Eustachian valve endocarditis. *Br Heart J*. 1990;64:340–341.

Edwards AD, Vickers MA, Morgan CJ. Infective endocarditis affecting the eustachian valve. *Br Heart J*. 1986;56:561–562.

FIGURE 16.19

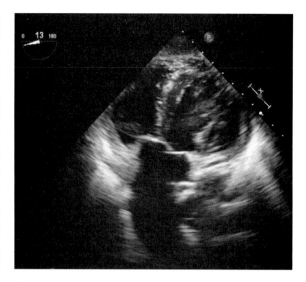

Transgastric view of the aorta.

FIGURE 16.20

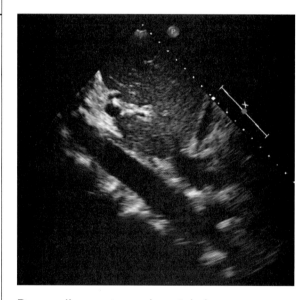

Descending aorta—subcostal view.

FIGURE 16.21

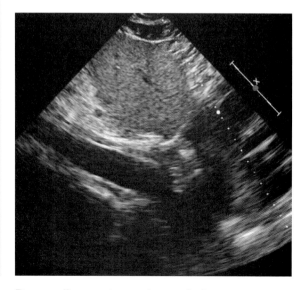

Descending aorta—subcostal view.

FIGURE 16.22

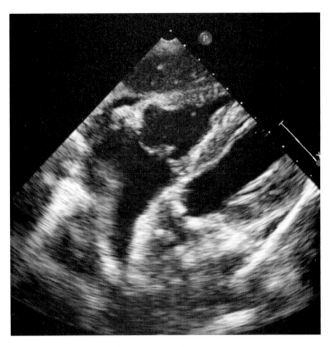

Subcostal view of the superior vena cava.

FIGURE 16.23

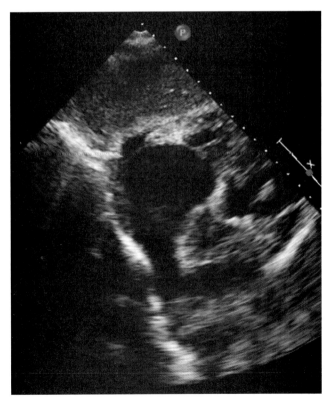

Subcostal view of the superior vena cava. Pulsed wave Doppler interrogation can be used to hone jugular venous pulse physical diagnosis skills.

QR 16.1: Normal aortic leaflets.

QR 16.2a: TEE of a normal trileaflet aortic valve.

QR 16.2b: TEE of a normal trileaflet aortic valve.

QR 16.2c: TEE of a normal trileaflet aortic valve.

QR 16.3: Normal mitral leaflets.

QR 16.4: Short-axis view of the tricuspid, aortic, and pulmonic leaflets. Small pericardial effusion.

QR 16.5: Short-axis view of the mitral valve. Moderate pericardial effusion.

QR 16.6: Both mitral leaflets are connected to the same papillary muscle in this view.

QR 16.7: Parasternal long-axis view—presence of left ventricular hypertrophy should always be confirmed in the short-axis views that follow. In some cases with an initial impression of left ventricular hypertrophy in this view, there may be a surprisingly normal wall thickness in the apical views. Classic ECG findings of left ventricular hypertrophy are always clinically useful.

QR 16.8: Normal short-axis view of the left ventricle.

QR 16.9: Minimal circumferential pericardial effusion.

QR 16.10: Normal transgastric short-axis TEE view.

QR 16.11: Short-axis view of the mitral papillary muscles. Moderate pericardial effusion.

QR 16.12: TEE of the tricuspid valve.

QR 16.13: Short-axis contrast-enhanced view of the left ventricle.

QR 16.14: Pulmonary artery bifurcation. The right pulmonary artery branch is shown on the left side of the image.

QR 16.15: Right branch of the pulmonary artery behind the aorta.

QR 16.16: High mid esophagus view of the right upper pulmonary vein, superior vena cava and aorta in cross section, and the right branch of the pulmonary artery (long section) above. Saline contrast is present in the venous vessels. The ascending aorta is mildly dilated. The superior vena cava loses the triangular shape and becomes circular when the pressures and/or size increase.

QR 16.17: Pulsatile changes in a normal size inferior vena cava indicating that the right atrial pressure is normal.

QR 16.18: Ascending aorta.

QR 16.19a: Descending thoracic aorta.

QR 16.19b: Descending thoracoabdominal aorta.

QR 16.19c: Descending thoracoabdominal aorta.

QR 16.20: Prominent systolic expansion of the aorta can be found in young people with normal aortic valve function.

QR 16.21: Subcostal view of the tricuspid, pulmonic, and aortic valves. Note the pulmonary artery bifurcation.

QR 16.22: Subcostal view of the coronary sinus. External compression of the coronary sinus by scoliosis, a hiatus hernia, or an aneurysm of the descending aorta may exaggerate the color inflow into the right atrium.

QR 16.23: Central line catheter entering the right atrium from the superior vena cava.

QR 16.24: Parasternal long-axis view in a heart transplant patient showing the suture line in the left atrium.

QR 16.25: Superior mesenteric artery on transgastric TEE of the descending aorta.

QR 16.26: Color flow in a normal aortic arch and descending aorta. Images obtained from the suprasternal notch. Red color flow (directed toward the transducer) in systole in the branch vessels from the arch. Normal brief red color flow reversal in early diastole in the descending aorta.

QR 16.27: Subcostal anatomy of right ventricular inflow and outflow.

QR 16.28: Right ventricular apex—transgastric TEE view.

QR 16.29: Right atrial crista terminalis.

QR 16.30: Coronary sinus emptying into the right atrium.

QR 16.31: Right ventricular moderator bands become more obvious with right ventricular dilatation. A moderator band is found much more frequently than a right ventricular thrombus in a dilated right ventricle.

QR 16.32a: Left ventricular false tendon.

QR 16.32b: Left ventricular false tendon.

QR 16.33a: Unusually well-demonstrated left atrial appendage on transthoracic echo.

QR 16.33b: Unusually well-demonstrated left atrial appendage on transthoracic echo.

QR 16.33c: Unusually well-demonstrated left atrial appendage on transthoracic echo.

QR 16.34: Subcostal view. Mild left atrial enlargement. The interatrial septum bulges toward the right atrium throughout the cardiac cycle.

QR 16.35: Short-axis view obtained from the subcostal window.

QR 16.36: Transgastric TEE short-axis view.

QR 16.37: Unusually well-visualized reflections from the spine—behind the left atrium.

QR 16.38: Normal short-axis subcostal view of the pulmonary artery. Some patients with lung disease may have poor quality parasternal images and excellent quality subcostal images.

QR 16.39: Vessel anatomy from the high esophagus TEE window. From left to right on the screen: Right upper pulmonary vein, superior vena cava (there is a catheter in the lumen), ascending aorta (there is a side lobe artifact in the lumen), main pulmonary artery (filled with contrast). The right branch of the pulmonary artery is on the top of the screen (it also contains contrast).

QR 16.40: Azygous vein between the descending aorta and the spine. Ignore the multiple color flow artifacts.

QR 16.41: Right atrial "floor": Coronary sinus and inferior vena cava.

QR 16.42a: Aortic arch anatomy.

QR 16.42b: Aortic arch anatomy.

QR 16.43: Aortic arch examination may show flow *toward* the transducer from the innominate or from the left carotid branches.

ANATOMY AND INTRACARDIAC ECHOCARDIOGRAPHY OF THE LEFT PUMONARY VENOUS VESTIBULE

The left pulmonary venous vestibule has four walls. There is a posterior wall, a roof, a floor, and the Marshall ridge. The Marshall ridge is the endocardial protrusion into the left atrial cavity due to the ligament of Marshall (see references). The wall of the Marshall ridge is shared by the left pulmonary venous vestibule with the left atrial appendage vestibule. The roof of the left pulmonary venous vestibule abuts the epicardial Bachmann's bundle. The posterior wall and the floor vary in their anatomic and echocardiographic characteristics.

REFERENCES:

Cabrera JA, Ho SY, Climent V, et al. The architecture of the left lateral atrial wall: a particular anatomic region with implications for ablation of atrial fibrillation. *Eur Heart J*. 2008;29:356–362.

de Oliveira IM, Scanavacca MI, Correia AT, et al. Anatomic relations of the Marshall vein: importance for catheterization of the coronary sinus in ablation procedures. *Europace*. 2007;9:915–919.

Kim DT, Lai AC, Hwang C, et al. The ligament of Marshall: a structural analysis in human hearts with implications for atrial arrhythmias. *J Am Coll Cardiol*. 2000;36:1324–1327.

CHAPTER 17

CONTRAST ECHOCARDIOGRAMS

FIGURE 17.1

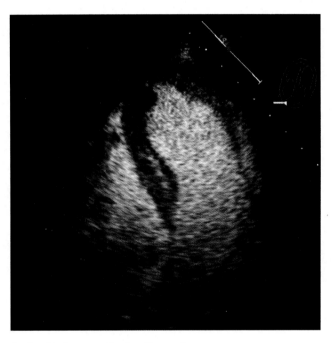

Apical left ventricular thrombus.

QR 17.1a: Normal wall motion.

QR 17.1b: Normal wall motion.

QR 17.1c: Normal wall motion.

QR 17.1d: Normal wall motion.

QR 17.2: Normal wall motion. Perfusion of the interventricular septum with contrast. Premature ventricular contraction.

QR 17.3a: Apical left ventricular trabeculations outlined by contrast.

QR 17.3b: Apical left ventricular trabeculations outlined by contrast.

QR 17.3c: Apical left ventricular trabeculations outlined by contrast.

QR 17.4a: Anteroapical left ventricular aneurysm.

QR 17.4b: Anteroapical left ventricular aneurysm.

QR 17.4c: Anteroapical left ventricular aneurysm.

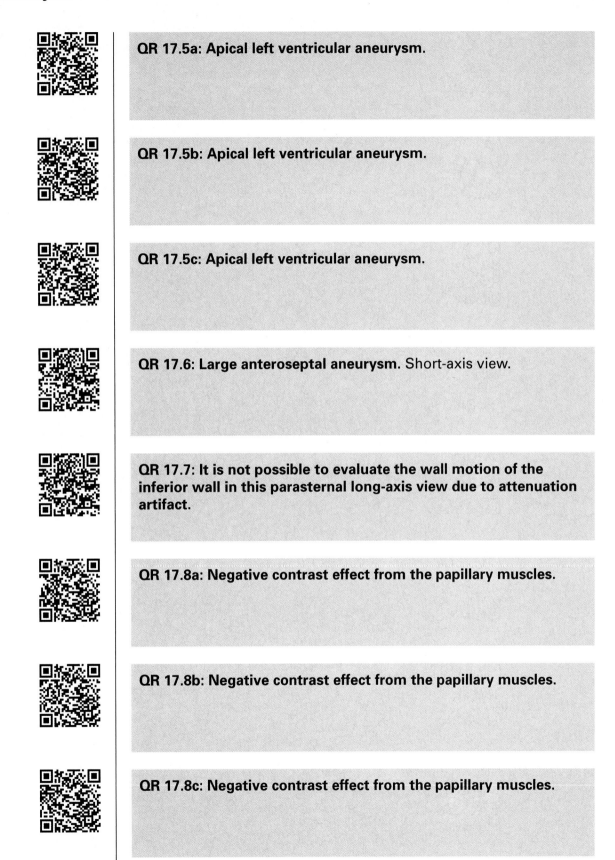

QR 17.5a: Apical left ventricular aneurysm.

QR 17.5b: Apical left ventricular aneurysm.

QR 17.5c: Apical left ventricular aneurysm.

QR 17.6: Large anteroseptal aneurysm. Short-axis view.

QR 17.7: It is not possible to evaluate the wall motion of the inferior wall in this parasternal long-axis view due to attenuation artifact.

QR 17.8a: Negative contrast effect from the papillary muscles.

QR 17.8b: Negative contrast effect from the papillary muscles.

QR 17.8c: Negative contrast effect from the papillary muscles.

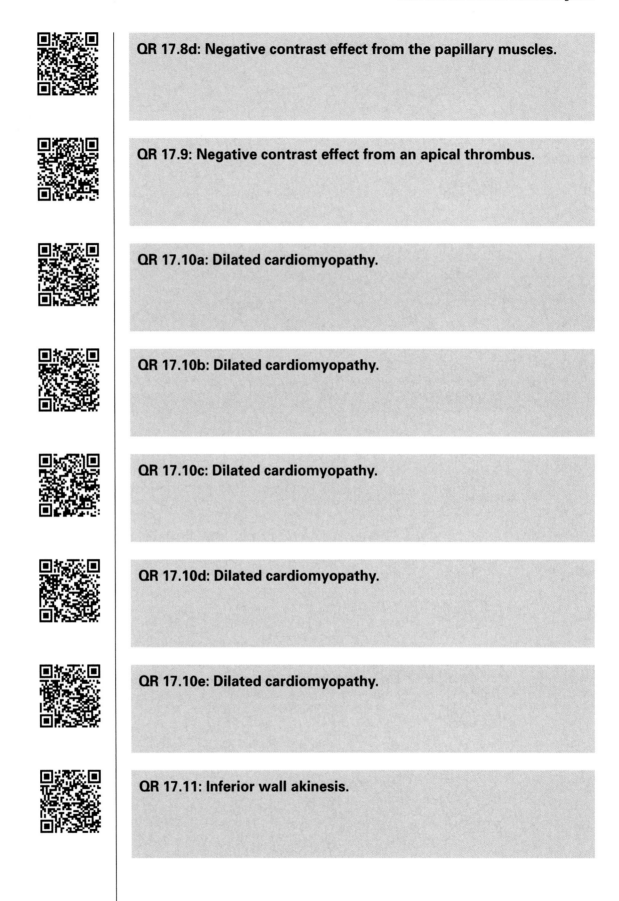

QR 17.8d: Negative contrast effect from the papillary muscles.

QR 17.9: Negative contrast effect from an apical thrombus.

QR 17.10a: Dilated cardiomyopathy.

QR 17.10b: Dilated cardiomyopathy.

QR 17.10c: Dilated cardiomyopathy.

QR 17.10d: Dilated cardiomyopathy.

QR 17.10e: Dilated cardiomyopathy.

QR 17.11: Inferior wall akinesis.

QR 17.12: Basal inferior wall akinesis. Apical tethering of the mitral valve.

QR 17.13: Mid septal thinning and akinesis.

QR 17.14a: Apical anterior akinesis. Premature ventricular contractions.

QR 17.14b: Apical anterior akinesis. Premature ventricular contractions.

QR 17.14c: Apical anterior akinesis. Premature ventricular contractions.

QR 17.15: Thinning and dyskinesis of the apical septum.

QR 17.16: Decrease in the contractility of the basal and mid interventricular septum. In comparison, the apical septum and the lateral wall contract normally.

QR 17.17a: Akinetic interventricular septum.

QR 17.17b: Akinetic interventricular septum.

QR 17.18: Paradoxical septal motion.

QR 17.19a: Normal hyperdynamic wall motion at peak stress echo.

QR 17.19b: Normal hyperdynamic wall motion at peak stress echo.

QR 17.20: Right ventricular hypertrophy—prominent right ventricular trabeculations.

QR 17.21: Short axis—normal wall motion.

QR 17.22: Short axis—abnormal lateral wall hypokinesis.

QR 17.23: Preserved myocardial thickening with a premature atrial contraction.

WALL MOTION ABNORMALITIES

WARNING: Wall motion analysis can cause elevated blood pressure. You should NOT agree with all of our segmental interpretations—locate the wall motion abnormality in the image, make up your own mind, and then find the mistakes in some of our nomenclature!

The official references are provided at the end of the chapter.

1. *We intentionally "play fast and loose" with the nomenclature of SOME of the myocardial segments—keeping it oversimplified (but perhaps, at times, more suitable for verbal communication).*
2. *"Eyeball" distinction between akinesis and hypokinesis is also subjective; and has been known to start heated arguments between different interpreters. Please feel free to disagree with our interpretations.*

Compound names in verbal communication:

Sometimes it is easier to convey wall motion verbally by being inaccurate but concise. Every user of echocardiographic imaging should understand *inferior, anterior, lateral,* and *septal.* We lose some of our audience when we sacrifice communication for accuracy. Instead of baffling them with our brilliance, we befuddle with compound and inconsistent (for them) names. The conversation (and our wall motion analysis) is different when we talk to a cardiac surgeon, coronary angiographer, medical student, family practitioner, or nurse.

Some Examples:

In the parasternal long-axis view, the *accurate* names are basal inferolateral and mid inferolateral. *Inferior* is inaccurate, but it works in getting the point across during a phone conversation. In the apical views, there are two issues. First, the accurate compound descriptions of the basal and mid wall segments *differ* from the apical segments in the apical long-axis three "chamber" view and in the four-chamber view. Second, the term *"inferior"* and *"septal"* can be inaccurate, but they work during a short conversation when echocardiographic images are not being viewed.

In the apical four-chamber view, basal and mid "*septal* and *lateral*" are inaccurate but concise.

● TECHNICAL TIP: The basal and mid wall segments of the *parasternal* long-axis view and of the *apical* long-axis view should be mentally compared for consistency before pronouncing the interpretation.

QR 18.1: Basal anteroseptal akinesis.

QR 18.2a: Mid anteroseptal akinesis.

QR 18.2b: Mid anteroseptal akinesis.

QR 18.3: Basal and mid anteroseptal akinesis. Basal and mid inferolateral hypokinesis.

QR 18.4a: Basal inferolateral akinesis. Apical tethering of mitral chordae.

QR 18.4b: Basal inferolateral akinesis. Apical tethering of mitral chordae.

QR 18.5: Basal inferolateral akinesis.

QR 18.6: Basal and mid inferolateral akinesis. Apical tethering of the mitral valve with chordal thickening and patchy calcification.

QR 18.7: Basal and mid inferolateral akinesis. Apical tethering of the mitral valve. Dilated left ventricle and left atrium.

QR 18.8: Basal and mid inferolateral hypokinesis. Mid anteroseptal hypokinesis. Dilated left ventricle. Apical tethering of the mitral valve. Preserved thickening of the basal anteroseptal segment.

QR 18.9a: Basal inferior left ventricular aneurysm with mitral regurgitation due to the wall motion abnormality.

QR 18.9b: Basal inferior left ventricular aneurysm with mitral regurgitation due to the wall motion abnormality.

QR 18.10a: Inferior hypokinesis.

QR 18.10b: Inferior hypokinesis.

QR 18.10c: Inferior hypokinesis.

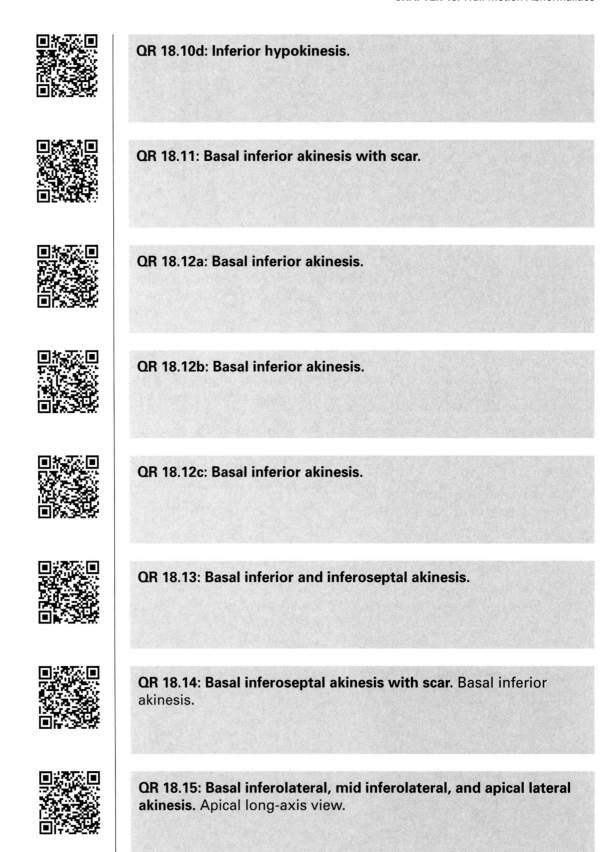

QR 18.10d: Inferior hypokinesis.

QR 18.11: Basal inferior akinesis with scar.

QR 18.12a: Basal inferior akinesis.

QR 18.12b: Basal inferior akinesis.

QR 18.12c: Basal inferior akinesis.

QR 18.13: Basal inferior and inferoseptal akinesis.

QR 18.14: Basal inferoseptal akinesis with scar. Basal inferior akinesis.

QR 18.15: Basal inferolateral, mid inferolateral, and apical lateral akinesis. Apical long-axis view.

QR 18.16: Basal inferior, mid inferior, and apical inferior akinesis. Apical two-chamber view.

QR 18.17: Basal inferior aneurysm.

QR 18.18: Basal inferoseptal akinesis.

QR 18.19: Basal inferoseptal thinning and dyskinesis.

QR 18.20: Inferior and inferoseptal mid ventricular wall akinesis and thinning, indicating scarred nonviable myocardium.

QR 18.21: Inferior and inferoseptal mid ventricular wall akinesis.

QR 18.22: Inferolateral, inferior, and inferoseptal mid ventricular wall akinesis. Note the "hinge point" at the junction of the normal anteroseptal wall with the akinetic inferoseptal wall (9 o'clock).

QR 18.23: Basal inferior, mid inferior, and apical inferior akinesis. Apical inferior thrombus. The "anterior wall" endocardium is not well visualized.

QR 18.24: Inferior dyskinesis. Transgastric view. Right ventricular assist device cannula delivering blood to the pulmonary artery.

QR 18.25: Inferior hypokinesis.

QR 18.26: Basal septal hypokinesis.

QR 18.27: Thinning, akinesis, and increased reflectivity of the interventricular septum.

QR 18.28: Basal anteroseptal akinesis. Left ventricular hypertrophy.

QR 18.29: Mid anteroseptal akinesis.

QR 18.30: Mid anteroseptal hypokinesis.

QR 18.31: Apical septal akinesis. Apical lateral hypokinesis.

QR 18.32: Apical septal akinesis.

QR 18.33: Anterior and anteroseptal akinesis. Short-axis mid ventricle.

QR 18.34: Apical akinesis.

QR 18.35a: Apical left ventricular aneurysm.

QR 18.35b: Apical left ventricular aneurysm.

QR 18.36: Apical left ventricular aneurysm. Basal inferoseptal (periinfarct) hypertrophy.

QR 18.37: Apical left ventricular aneurysm. Dyskinesis with scar of the apical lateral wall and of the apex. Akinesis of the apical septum.

QR 18.38: Mid inferoseptal akinesis. Apical septal akinesis. Apical lateral akinesis. Spontaneous contrast in the left ventricle, indicating stasis.

QR 18.39: Mid inferoseptal akinesis. Apical septal akinesis. Basal inferoseptal (periinfarct) hypertrophy. This is a foreshortened view that does not show the true apical cap. The true apical cap is thinner, or the same thickness as the adjacent apical septum and lateral wall, not thicker, like in this case. There is a pacemaker wire but the QRS is narrow, suggesting that the wall motion abnormalities are not pacemaker induced.

QR 18.40: Dilated cardiomyopathy. Diffuse wall motion abnormalities. Thinning and akinesis with scar (aneurysm) of the apical cap and apical lateral wall. Spontaneous contrast in the left ventricle, indicating stasis. Apical artifact (suggesting thrombus) is too "hazy" for an organized thrombus; and careful scrutiny shows that it continues past the apex toward the transducer.

QR 18.41: Mid inferoseptal akinesis. Apical septal akinesis. Apical lateral akinesis. Mid anterolateral akinesis. Dilated spherical left ventricle. Pacemaker wire in the right atrium.

QR 18.42: Apical septal and mid inferoseptal akinesis. Basal inferoseptal hypokinesis. Left ventricular apical false tendons manifested as triangular trabeculations. The tendons are not thick enough to reflect the ultrasound waves. Dilated right atrium.

QR 18.43: Large mid to apical aneurysm. Restraining false tendon (triangular trabeculations). Hazy apical artifact, not a thrombus.

QR 18.44: Basal and mid inferoseptal akinesis. Dilated left ventricle.

QR 18.45: Basal and mid inferoseptal aneurysm. The electronic-paced rhythm in this case does not affect or hinder the wall motion analysis.

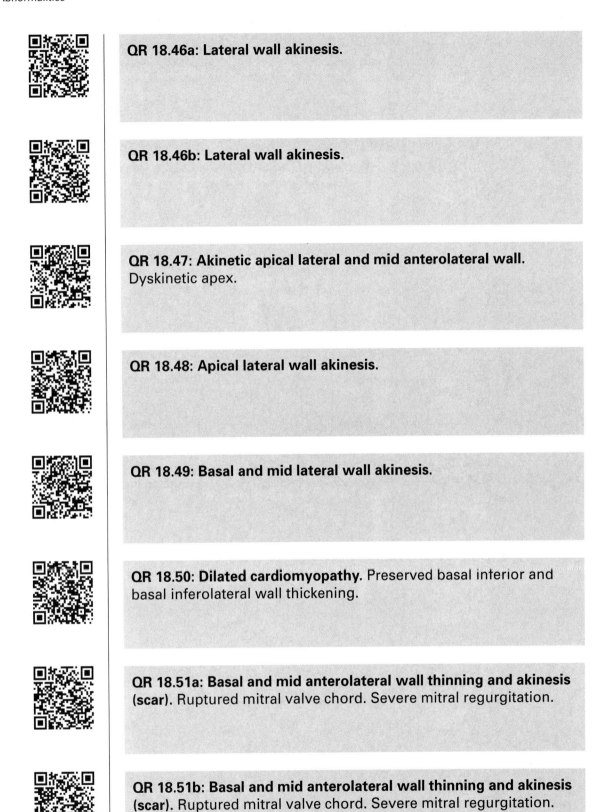

QR 18.46a: Lateral wall akinesis.

QR 18.46b: Lateral wall akinesis.

QR 18.47: Akinetic apical lateral and mid anterolateral wall. Dyskinetic apex.

QR 18.48: Apical lateral wall akinesis.

QR 18.49: Basal and mid lateral wall akinesis.

QR 18.50: Dilated cardiomyopathy. Preserved basal inferior and basal inferolateral wall thickening.

QR 18.51a: Basal and mid anterolateral wall thinning and akinesis (scar). Ruptured mitral valve chord. Severe mitral regurgitation.

QR 18.51b: Basal and mid anterolateral wall thinning and akinesis (scar). Ruptured mitral valve chord. Severe mitral regurgitation.

QR 18.51c: Basal and mid anterolateral wall thinning and akinesis (scar). Ruptured mitral valve chord. Severe mitral regurgitation.

QR 18.52a: Abnormal lateral wall motion. Suboptimal endocardial reflections of two adjacent lateral wall segments in question. Contrast is indicated.

QR 18.52b: Abnormal lateral wall motion. Suboptimal endocardial reflections of two adjacent lateral wall segments in question. Contrast is indicated.

QR 18.53: Septal scarring, thinning, and akinesis. Dilated cardiomyopathy.

QR 18.54: Basal and mid septal akinesis. Mid inferior akinesis. Right ventricular free wall akinesis.

QR 18.55a: Inferior myocardial infarction.

QR 18.55b: Inferior myocardial infarction.

QR 18.55c: Inferior myocardial infarction.

QR 18.55d: Inferior myocardial infarction.

QR 18.55e: Inferior myocardial infarction.

QR 18.55f: Inferior myocardial infarction.

QR 18.55g: Inferior myocardial infarction.

QR 18.56: Septal hypokinesis. Lateral wall akinesis.

QR 18.57: Dilated cardiomyopathy with diffuse wall motion abnormalities. Only the basal inferolateral wall is contracting. Marked thinning and akinesis of the mid anteroseptal wall.

QR 18.58: Dilated cardiomyopathy with diffuse wall motion abnormalities. The only left ventricular wall segment with preserved thickening is the basal septum.

QR 18.59: Dilated cardiomyopathy with diffuse wall motion abnormalities. The only left ventricular wall segments with preserved thickening are the anterior and anteroseptal. There is a minimal pericardial effusion, and an artifact from a right ventricular pacemaker wire.

QR 18.60: Pacing in cardiomyopathy. Akinetic septum. Hypokinetic lateral wall. The apical septum (close to the right ventricular pacemaker tip) is actually dyskinetic. The basal and mid inferoseptal walls are akinetic with negligible thickening. The apical lateral wall, the mid, and basal anterolateral walls are all hypokinetic.

QR 18.61: Scarring and akinesis of the interventricular septum. Dilated left ventricular cardiomyopathy with diffuse wall motion abnormalities. Normal right ventricular free wall motion. Pacemaker wire. Atrial flutter.

QR 18.62: Short axis. Diffuse wall motion abnormalities. The wall motion resembles a door knob turning.

QR 18.63: Preserved septal thickening. Abnormal anterior and anteroseptal wall motion due to bundle branch block.

QR 18.64: Preserved myocardial thickening. Abnormal septal wall motion due to bundle branch block.

QR 18.65: Short-axis anterolateral hypokinesis. Small pericardial effusion.

QR 18.66: Septal akinesis. Transgastric view.

QR 18.67: Exaggerated normal thickening of the basal inferolateral wall due to pericardial effusion. Hypokinetic apical anterior and mid anteroseptal wall.

QR 18.68: Akinetic right ventricular free wall. Dilated right ventricle. Respiratory displacement of the interventricular septum.

QR 18.69: Apical right ventricular free wall thinning and akinesis.

QR 18.70a: Right ventricular wall akinesis. Transgastric view.

QR 18.70b: Right ventricular wall akinesis. Transgastric view.

QR 18.71a: Effect of premature ventricular contractions on wall motion.

QR 18.71b: Effect of premature ventricular contractions on wall motion.

QR 18.71c: Effect of premature ventricular contractions on wall motion.

QR 18.71d: Effect of premature ventricular contractions on wall motion.

QR 18.71e: Effect of premature ventricular contractions on wall motion.

QR 18.72: Apical septal akinesis. Apical right ventricular AV paced rhythm. Left ventricular hypertrophy.

QR 18.73: Right ventricle being paced from the right ventricular apex.

QR 18.74: Global hypokinesis. Dilated cardiomyopathy.

QR 18.75: Global biventricular dysfunction. Small pericardial effusion.

WALL MOTION QUIZ

The following wall motion abnormalities are narrated by the author using the same informal approach (discussed above) in some cases. The video clips can be used as a quiz by first watching them with the audio turned off.

QR 18.76: Wall motion quiz 1.

QR 18.77: Wall motion quiz 2.

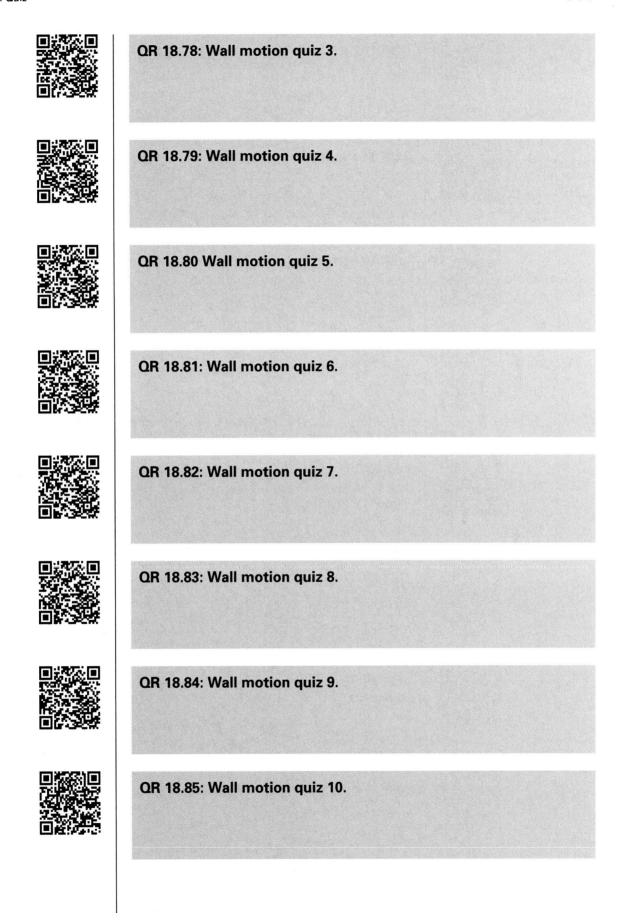

QR 18.78: Wall motion quiz 3.

QR 18.79: Wall motion quiz 4.

QR 18.80 Wall motion quiz 5.

QR 18.81: Wall motion quiz 6.

QR 18.82: Wall motion quiz 7.

QR 18.83: Wall motion quiz 8.

QR 18.84: Wall motion quiz 9.

QR 18.85: Wall motion quiz 10.

QR 18.86: Wall motion quiz 11.

QR 18.87: Wall motion quiz 12.

QR 18.88: Wall motion quiz 13.

QR 18.89: Wall motion quiz 14.

QR 18.90: Wall motion quiz 15.

QR 18.91: Wall motion quiz 16.

QR 18.92: Wall motion quiz 17.

QR 18.93: Wall motion quiz 18.

REFERENCES:

[pdf] Lang RM, Bierig M, Devereux RB, et al. American Society of Echocardiography's Nomenclature and Standards Committee; Task Force on Chamber Quantification; American College of Cardiology Echocardiography Committee; American Heart Association; European Association of Echocardiography, European Society of Cardiology. Recommendations for chamber quantification. *Eur J Echocardiogr.* 2006;7:79–108. *See Figure 8 on page 92.*

[pdf] Cerqueira MD, Weissman NJ, Dilsizian V, et al. American Heart Association Writing Group on Myocardial Segmentation and Registration for Cardiac Imaging. Standardized myocardial segmentation and nomenclature for tomographic imaging of the heart. A statement for healthcare professionals from the Cardiac Imaging Committee of the Council on Clinical Cardiology of the American Heart Association. *Circulation.* 2002;105:539–542.

Rudski LG, Lai WW, Afilalo J, et al. Guidelines for the echocardiographic assessment of the right heart in adults: a report from the American Society of Echocardiography endorsed by the European Association of Echocardiography, a registered branch of the European Society of Cardiology, and the Canadian Society of Echocardiography. *J Am Soc Echocardiogr.* 2010;23:685–713. *See Figure 1 and Figure 2.*

Web Address Index for Video/QR Codes

Below is a list of each QR code, its legend, and the Internet address where the corresponding videos or images can be found online. This is provided as a secondary way to reach the videos and images. Instead of using the QR code scanner with your mobile device, you can type the corresponding web address directly into the web browser on your mobile device, or on your desktop computer.

Chapter 1 Coronary Artery Disease

1.1: Ventricular septal rupture complicating acute myocardial infarction. Available at http://mhprofessional.com/echoatlas/index.php?VID=1_01

1.2: Large basal inferior left ventricular wall aneurysm. Available at http://mhprofessional.com/echoatlas/index.php?VID=1_02

1.3: Akinesis of the basal and mid-inferior left ventricular wall. Available at http://mhprofessional.com/echoatlas/index.php?VID=1_03

1.4: Akinesis of the basal and mid-inferior left ventricular wall. Available at http://mhprofessional.com/echoatlas/index.php?VID=1_04

1.5: Thinning, akinesis, and increased echogenicity of the interventricular septum due to an old anterior myocardial infarction. Available at http://mhprofessional.com/echoatlas/index.php?VID=1_05

1.6: Absence of myocardial thickening at the mid-portion of the interventricular septum. Available at http://mhprofessional.com/echoatlas/index.php?VID=1_06

1.7: Thinning of the apical walls. Available at http://mhprofessional.com/echoatlas/index.php?VID=1_07

1.8: Abnormal "scooped" basal inferior wall shown in the two-chamber apical view. Available at http://mhprofessional.com/echoatlas/index.php?VID=1_08

1.9: Abnormal basal inferior left ventricular wall motion. Available at http://mhprofessional.com/echoatlas/index.php?VID=1_09

1.10: Abnormal basal and mid-inferior left ventricular wall motion in a patient with known inferior myocardial infarction. Available at http://mhprofessional.com/echoatlas/index.php?VID=1_10

1.11: Basal inferior myocardial infarction that extends to the basal lateral wall. Available at http://mhprofessional.com/echoatlas/index.php?VID=1_11

1.12: Short axis—normal wall motion. Available at http://mhprofessional.com/echoatlas/index.php?VID=1_12

1.13: Dilated cardiomyopathy with left bundle branch block on the ECG and no thickening of the interventricular septum. Available at http://mhprofessional.com/echoatlas/index.php?VID=1_13

1.14: Right coronary artery—parasternal short axis view. Available at http://mhprofessional.com/echoatlas/index.php?VID=1_14

1.15: Abnormal inferior left ventricular akinesis at rest that failed to improve with stress, indicating nonviable myocardium. Available at http://mhprofessional.com/echoatlas/index.php?VID=1_15

1.16a: Distal left anterior descending (LAD) coronary artery obstruction with apical inferior and apical septal scar. Available at http://mhprofessional.com/echoatlas/index.php?VID=1_16a

1.16b: Distal left anterior descending (LAD) coronary artery obstruction with apical inferior and apical septal scar. Available at http://mhprofessional.com/echoatlas/index.php?VID=1_16b

1.17a: Dilated hypokinetic right ventricle in a patient with acute inferior myocardial infarction. Available at http://mhprofessional.com/echoatlas/index.php?VID=1_17a

1.17b: Dilated hypokinetic right ventricle in a patient with acute inferior myocardial infarction. Available at http://mhprofessional.com/echoatlas/index.php?VID=1_17b

1.18: Inferoseptal left ventricular wall hypokinesis extending to the adjacent right ventricular wall. Available at http://mhprofessional.com/echoatlas/index.php?VID=1_18

1.19: Diffuse right ventricular dysfunction with preserved wall thickness. Available at http://mhprofessional.com/echoatlas/index.php?VID=1_19

1.20: Akinetic infundibular right ventricular free wall. Available at http://mhprofessional.com/echoatlas/index.php?VID=1_20

1.21: Unusually prominent coronary artery. Available at http://mhprofessional.com/echoatlas/index.php?VID=1_21

1.22a: Normal left main. Available at http://mhprofessional.com/echoatlas/index.php?VID=1_22a

1.22b: Normal left main. Available at http://mhprofessional.com/echoatlas/index.php?VID=1_22b

1.23: Akinesis of the mid and the apical anterior left ventricular wall. Available at http://mhprofessional.com/echoatlas/index.php?VID=1_23

1.24a: Akinesis of the mid and the apical anterior left ventricular wall—extending to the apical inferior wall. Available at http://mhprofessional.com/echoatlas/index.php?VID=1_24a

1.24b: Akinesis of the mid and the apical anterior left ventricular wall—extending to the apical inferior wall. Available at http://mhprofessional.com/echoatlas/index.php?VID=1_24b

1.43: Hypertrophic cardiomyopathy. Available at http://mhprofessional.com/echoatlas/index.php?VID=1_43

Chapter 2   Pulmonary Disease

2.1a: Basal and mid right ventricular free wall akinesis. Available at http://mhprofessional.com/echoatlas/index.php?VID=2_01a

2.1b: Basal and mid right ventricular free wall akinesis. Available at http://mhprofessional.com/echoatlas/index.php?VID=2_01b

2.1c: Basal and mid right ventricular free wall akinesis. Available at http://mhprofessional.com/echoatlas/index.php?VID=2_01c

2.1d: Basal and mid right ventricular free wall akinesis. Available at http://mhprofessional.com/echoatlas/index.php?VID=2_01d

2.1e: Basal and mid right ventricular free wall akinesis. Available at http://mhprofessional.com/echoatlas/index.php?VID=2_01e

2.2: Embolus in the main pulmonary artery. Available at http://mhprofessional.com/echoatlas/index.php?VID=2_02

2.3a: Thrombus in the inferior vena cava. Available at http://mhprofessional.com/echoatlas/index.php?VID=2_03a

2.3b: Thrombus in the inferior vena cava. Available at http://mhprofessional.com/echoatlas/index.php?VID=2_03b

2.4: Loss of tricuspid leaflet opposition renders Doppler unusable for pressure estimation. Available at http://mhprofessional.com/echoatlas/index.php?VID=2_04

2.5: Right ventricular hypertrophy and dilatation in a patient with severe pulmonary hypertension. Available at http://mhprofessional.com/echoatlas/index.php?VID=2_05

2.6: Right to left displacement of the interatrial septum in pulmonary hypertension with tricuspid regurgitation. Available at http://mhprofessional.com/echoatlas/index.php?VID=2_06

2.7: Dilated right ventricle. Available at http://mhprofessional.com/echoatlas/index.php?VID=2_07

2.8: Dilated right ventricular outflow. Available at http://mhprofessional.com/echoatlas/index.php?VID=2_08

2.9: Right ventricular outflow dilatation and hypertrophy. Available at http://mhprofessional.com/echoatlas/index.php?VID=2_09

2.10a: Hypertrophy of the right ventricular free wall. Available at http://mhprofessional.com/echoatlas/index.php?VID=2_10a

2.10b: Hypertrophy of the right ventricular free wall. Available at http://mhprofessional.com/echoatlas/index.php?VID=2_10b

2.11: Right ventricular hypertrophy. Available at http://mhprofessional.com/echoatlas/index.php?VID=2_11

2.12a: Thrombus and spontaneous contrast in the inferior vena cava. Available at http://mhprofessional.com/echoatlas/index.php?VID=2_12a

2.12b: Thrombus and spontaneous contrast in the inferior vena cava. Available at http://mhprofessional.com/echoatlas/index.php?VID=2_12b

2.13a: Changes in the caliber of the inferior vena cava—indicating normal right atrial pressures. Available at http://mhprofessional.com/echoatlas/index.php?VID=2_13a

2.13b: Changes in the caliber of the inferior vena cava—indicating normal right atrial pressures. Available at http://mhprofessional.com/echoatlas/index.php?VID=2_13b

2.13c: Changes in the caliber of the inferior vena cava—indicating normal right atrial pressures. Available at http://mhprofessional.com/echoatlas/index.php?VID=2_13c

2.13d: Changes in the caliber of the inferior vena cava—indicating normal right atrial pressures. Available at http://mhprofessional.com/echoatlas/index.php?VID=2_13d

2.14: Elevated right atrial pressure—manifested as minimal collapse of the dilated inferior vena cava on inspiration. Available at http://mhprofessional.com/echoatlas/index.php?VID=2_14

2.15a: Dilated superior vena cava. Available at http://mhprofessional.com/echoatlas/index.php?VID=2_15a

2.15b: Dilated superior vena cava. Available at http://mhprofessional.com/echoatlas/index.php?VID=2_15b

2.15c: Dilated superior vena cava. Available at http://mhprofessional.com/echoatlas/index.php?VID=2_15c

2.16: Large pulmonary regurgitation color flow jet. Available at http://mhprofessional.com/echoatlas/index.php?VID=2_16

2.17: Magnified view showing loss of pulmonic leaflet coaptation. Available at http://mhprofessional.com/echoatlas/index.php?VID=2_17

2.18: Right ventricular hypertrophy. Available at http://mhprofessional.com/echoatlas/index.php?VID=2_18

Chapter 3   Valvular Disease

3.1: Aortic stenosis with delayed systolic peaking of both Doppler flow and of the stenosis murmur. Available at http://mhprofessional.com/echoatlas/index.php?VID=3_01

3.2: Aortic sclerosis: Patchy aortic leaflet calcifications appear to "hover over" mobile aortic leaflets. Available at http://mhprofessional.com/echoatlas/index.php?VID=3_02

3.3: Calcified aortic valve. Available at http://mhprofessional.com/echoatlas/index.php?VID=3_03

3.4: Patchy aortic valve calcifications. Available at http://mhprofessional.com/echoatlas/index.php?VID=3_04

3.5: Calcified aortic valve. Available at http://mhprofessional.com/echoatlas/index.php?VID=3_05

3.6: Dimensionless index. Available at http://mhprofessional.com/echoatlas/index.php?VID=3_06

3.7a: Aortic leaflet thickening. Available at http://mhprofessional.com/echoatlas/index.php?VID=3_07a

3.7b: Aortic leaflet thickening. Available at http://mhprofessional.com/echoatlas/index.php?VID=3_07b

3.8a: Bicuspid aortic valve. Available at http://mhprofessional.com/echoatlas/index.php?VID=3_08a

3.8b: Bicuspid aortic valve. Available at http://mhprofessional.com/echoatlas/index.php?VID=3_08b

3.9: Eccentric aortic regurgitation with a doming bicuspid aortic valve. Available at http://mhprofessional.com/echoatlas/index.php?VID=3_09

3.10: Artifact due to the raphe of a bicuspid aortic valve. Available at http://mhprofessional.com/echoatlas/index.php?VID=3_10

3.11: Trivial eccentric aortic regurgitation. Available at http://mhprofessional.com/echoatlas/index.php?VID=3_11

3.12: Diastolic mitral regurgitation (red color flow) is typically found in acute severe aortic regurgitation (where the left ventricular diastolic pressure rises above the left atrial pressure at end diastole). Available at http://mhprofessional.com/echoatlas/index.php?VID=3_12

3.13: Severe aortic regurgitation with loss of leaflet coaptation. Available at http://mhprofessional.com/echoatlas/index.php?VID=3_13

3.14a: Diastolic flow reversal in the descending aorta. Available at http://mhprofessional.com/echoatlas/index.php?VID=3_14a

3.14b: Diastolic flow reversal in the descending aorta. Available at http://mhprofessional.com/echoatlas/index.php?VID=3_14b

3.15: Diastolic mitral regurgitation on color M-mode—red color flow before the QRS. Available at http://mhprofessional.com/echoatlas/index.php?VID=3_15

3.16a: Continuous systolic and diastolic aortic regurgitation in a patient with a ventricular assist device, and no forward flow through the aortic valve in systole. Available at http://mhprofessional.com/echoatlas/index.php?VID=3_16a

3.16b: Continuous systolic and diastolic aortic regurgitation in a patient with a ventricular assist device, and no forward flow through the aortic valve in systole. Available at http://mhprofessional.com/echoatlas/index.php?VID=3_16b

3.17: Acute severe aortic regurgitation due to endocarditis. Available at http://mhprofessional.com/echoatlas/index.php?VID=3_17

3.18a: Color flow can be used to calculate mitral stenosis orifice area. Available at http://mhprofessional.com/echoatlas/index.php?VID=3_18a

3.18b: Color flow can be used to calculate mitral stenosis orifice area. Available at http://mhprofessional.com/echoatlas/index.php?VID=3_18b

3.18c: Color flow can be used to calculate mitral stenosis orifice area. Available at http://mhprofessional.com/echoatlas/index.php?VID=3_18c

3.19a: Anterior mitral leaflet doming in mitral stenosis. Available at http://mhprofessional.com/echoatlas/index.php?VID=3_19a

3.19b: Anterior mitral leaflet doming in mitral stenosis. Available at http://mhprofessional.com/echoatlas/index.php?VID=3_19b

3.19c: Anterior mitral leaflet doming in mitral stenosis. Available at http://mhprofessional.com/echoatlas/index.php?VID=3_19c

3.19d: Anterior mitral leaflet doming in mitral stenosis. Available at http://mhprofessional.com/echoatlas/index.php?VID=3_19d

3.20: Massively dilated left atrium in a patient with mitral stenosis. Available at http://mhprofessional.com/echoatlas/index.php?VID=3_20

3.21a: Cor triatriatum was sometimes clinically confused with mitral stenosis prior to the advent of echocardiography. Available at http://mhprofessional.com/echoatlas/index.php?VID=3_21a

3.21b: Cor triatriatum was sometimes clinically confused with mitral stenosis prior to the advent of echocardiography. Available at http://mhprofessional.com/echoatlas/index.php?VID=3_21b

3.22a: Mid-to-late systolic mitral regurgitation in mitral valve prolapse. Available at http://mhprofessional.com/echoatlas/index.php?VID=3_22a

3.22b: Mid-to-late systolic mitral regurgitation in mitral valve prolapse. Available at http://mhprofessional.com/echoatlas/index.php?VID=3_22b

3.23: Color flow of mitral regurgitation must be distinguished from pulmonary vein inflow. Available at http://mhprofessional.com/echoatlas/index.php?VID=3_23

3.24a: Posterior mitral leaflet prolapse. Available at http://mhprofessional.com/echoatlas/index.php?VID=3_24a

3.24b: Posterior mitral leaflet prolapse. Available at http://mhprofessional.com/echoatlas/index.php?VID=3_24b

3.24c: Posterior mitral leaflet prolapse. Available at http://mhprofessional.com/echoatlas/index.php?VID=3_24c

3.24d: Posterior mitral leaflet prolapse. Available at http://mhprofessional.com/echoatlas/index.php?VID=3_24d

3.24e: Posterior mitral leaflet prolapse. Available at http://mhprofessional.com/echoatlas/index.php?VID=3_24e

3.24f: Posterior mitral leaflet prolapse. Available at http://mhprofessional.com/echoatlas/index.php?VID=3_24f

3.25a: High-resolution TEE images of mitral valve prolapse. Available at http://mhprofessional.com/echoatlas/index.php?VID=3_25a

3.25b: High-resolution TEE images of mitral valve prolapse. Available at http://mhprofessional.com/echoatlas/index.php?VID=3_25b

3.26: Calcified previously prolapsing posterior mitral leaflet. Available at http://mhprofessional.com/echoatlas/index.php?VID=3_26

3.27a: Anterior mitral leaflet prolapse. Available at http://mhprofessional.com/echoatlas/index.php?VID=3_27a

3.27b: Anterior mitral leaflet prolapse. Available at http://mhprofessional.com/echoatlas/index.php?VID=3_27b

3.27c: Anterior mitral leaflet prolapse. Available at http://mhprofessional.com/echoatlas/index.php?VID=3_27c

3.28a: Flail posterior mitral leaflet chordae. Available at http://mhprofessional.com/echoatlas/index.php?VID=3_28a

3.28b: Flail posterior mitral leaflet chordae. Available at http://mhprofessional.com/echoatlas/index.php?VID=3_28b

3.28c: Flail posterior mitral leaflet chordae. Available at http://mhprofessional.com/echoatlas/index.php?VID=3_28c

3.49a: Severe tricuspid regurgitation demonstrated by reversal of saline contrast into the hepatic veins after injection into an arm vein. Available at http://mhprofessional.com/echoatlas/index.php?VID=3_49a

3.49b: Severe tricuspid regurgitation demonstrated by reversal of saline contrast into the hepatic veins after injection into an arm vein. Available at http://mhprofessional.com/echoatlas/index.php?VID=3_49b

3.50: Dilated inferior vena cava due to elevated right atrial pressure. Available at http://mhprofessional.com/echoatlas/index.php?VID=3_50

3.51a: Normal inferior vena cava oscillation in a patient with normal right atrial pressure. Available at http://mhprofessional.com/echoatlas/index.php?VID=3_51a

3.51b: Normal inferior vena cava oscillation in a patient with normal right atrial pressure. Available at http://mhprofessional.com/echoatlas/index.php?VID=3_51b

3.52: Normal brief hepatic vein flow reversal following the atrial contraction. Available at http://mhprofessional.com/echoatlas/index.php?VID=3_52

3.53: Visual exercise. Available at http://mhprofessional.com/echoatlas/index.php?VID=3_53

3.54: Normal inspiratory increase in hepatic vein flow toward the heart (blue color flow). Available at http://mhprofessional.com/echoatlas/index.php?VID=3_54

3.55: Chronic severe tricuspid regurgitation. Available at http://mhprofessional.com/echoatlas/index.php?VID=3_55

3.56: Severe tricuspid regurgitation. Available at http://mhprofessional.com/echoatlas/index.php?VID=3_56

3.57a: Severe tricuspid regurgitation with loss of leaflet coaptation. Available at http://mhprofessional.com/echoatlas/index.php?VID=3_57a

3.57b: Severe tricuspid regurgitation with loss of leaflet coaptation. Available at http://mhprofessional.com/echoatlas/index.php?VID=3_57b

3.57c: Severe tricuspid regurgitation with loss of leaflet coaptation. Available at http://mhprofessional.com/echoatlas/index.php?VID=3_57c

3.58: Tricuspid regurgitation from the mid-esophagus. Available at http://mhprofessional.com/echoatlas/index.php?VID=3_58

3.59: Tricuspid regurgitation directed toward the eustachian valve. Available at http://mhprofessional.com/echoatlas/index.php?VID=3_59

3.60a: Color flow of mild pulmonic valve regurgitation originating very close to the area where the proximal left main coronary artery can be visualized. Available at http://mhprofessional.com/echoatlas/index.php?VID=3_60a

3.60b: Color flow of mild pulmonic valve regurgitation originating very close to the area where the proximal left main coronary artery can be visualized. Available at http://mhprofessional.com/echoatlas/index.php?VID=3_60b

3.60c: Color flow of mild pulmonic valve regurgitation originating very close to the area where the proximal left main coronary artery can be visualized. Available at http://mhprofessional.com/echoatlas/index.php?VID=3_60c

3.61a: Color flow in the left main coronary artery. Available at http://mhprofessional.com/echoatlas/index.php?VID=3_61a

3.61b: Color flow in the left main coronary artery. Available at http://mhprofessional.com/echoatlas/index.php?VID=3_61b

3.61c: Color flow in the left main coronary artery. Available at http://mhprofessional.com/echoatlas/index.php?VID=3_61c

3.62: Aortic prosthesis dehiscence. Available at http://mhprofessional.com/echoatlas/index.php?VID=3_62

3.63: Abnormal bileaflet mechanical mitral prosthesis. Available at http://mhprofessional.com/echoatlas/index.php?VID=3_63

3.64a: Aortic bioprosthesis struts on TEE. Available at http://mhprofessional.com/echoatlas/index.php?VID=3_64a

3.64b: Aortic bioprosthesis struts on TEE. Available at http://mhprofessional.com/echoatlas/index.php?VID=3_64b

3.65a: Mitral bioprosthesis. Available at http://mhprofessional.com/echoatlas/index.php?VID=3_65a

3.65b: Mitral bioprosthesis. Available at http://mhprofessional.com/echoatlas/index.php?VID=3_65b

3.66: Paravalvular mitral regurgitation. Available at http://mhprofessional.com/echoatlas/index.php?VID=3_66

3.67a: Partial dehiscence of a prosthetic mitral ring. Available at http://mhprofessional.com/echoatlas/index.php?VID=3_67a

3.67b: Partial dehiscence of a prosthetic mitral ring. Available at http://mhprofessional.com/echoatlas/index.php?VID=3_67b

3.67c: Partial dehiscence of a prosthetic mitral ring. Available at http://mhprofessional.com/echoatlas/index.php?VID=3_67c

3.67d: Partial dehiscence of a prosthetic mitral ring. Available at http://mhprofessional.com/echoatlas/index.php?VID=3_67d

3.67e: Partial dehiscence of a prosthetic mitral ring. Available at http://mhprofessional.com/echoatlas/index.php?VID=3_67e

3.67f: Partial dehiscence of a prosthetic mitral ring. Available at http://mhprofessional.com/echoatlas/index.php?VID=3_67f

3.68a: Tricuspid bioprosthesis. Available at http://mhprofessional.com/echoatlas/index.php?VID=3_68a

3.68b: Tricuspid bioprosthesis. Available at http://mhprofessional.com/echoatlas/index.php?VID=3_68b

3.69: Reverberation artifact due to a mechanical aortic prosthesis. Available at http://mhprofessional.com/echoatlas/index.php?VID=3_69

3.70a: Mitral and aortic bioprosthesis. Available at http://mhprofessional.com/echoatlas/index.php?VID=3_70a

3.70b: Mitral and aortic bioprosthesis. Available at http://mhprofessional.com/echoatlas/index.php?VID=3_70b

3.71a: Fluoroscopic appearance of a mechanical mitral bileaflet prosthesis. Available at http://mhprofessional.com/echoatlas/index.php?VID=3_71a

3.71b: Fluoroscopic appearance of a mechanical mitral bileaflet prosthesis. Available at http://mhprofessional.com/echoatlas/index.php?VID=3_71b

3.72a: Fluoroscopic appearance of a ball-in-cage Starr-Edwards aortic prosthesis. Available at http://mhprofessional.com/echoatlas/index.php?VID=3_72a

3.72b: Fluoroscopic appearance of a ball-in-cage Starr-Edwards aortic prosthesis. Available at http://mhprofessional.com/echoatlas/index.php?VID=3_72b

Chapter 4 Pregnancy

4.1: Prominent pulsatility of the aorta during late pregnancy due to the increased cardiac output state. Available at http://mhprofessional.com/echoatlas/index.php?VID=4_01

Chapter 5 Murmurs

5.1a: Patent ductus arteriosus. Available at http://mhprofessional.com/echoatlas/index.php?VID=5_01a

5.1b: Patent ductus arteriosus. Available at http://mhprofessional.com/echoatlas/index.php?VID=5_01b

5.2: Overriding aorta in tetralogy of Fallot. Available at http://mhprofessional.com/echoatlas/index.php?VID=5_02

5.3: Repaired tetralogy of Fallot. Available at http://mhprofessional.com/echoatlas/index.php?VID=5_03

5.4a: Right coronary artery manifested intermittently as two parallel "railroad track" reflections. Available at http://mhprofessional.com/echoatlas/index.php?VID=5_04a

5.4b: Right coronary artery manifested intermittently as two parallel "railroad track" reflections. Available at http://mhprofessional.com/echoatlas/index.php?VID=5_04b

5.4c: Right coronary artery manifested intermittently as two parallel "railroad track" reflections. Available at http://mhprofessional.com/echoatlas/index.php?VID=5_04c

5.5: Silent patent ductus arteriosus. Available at http://mhprofessional.com/echoatlas/index.php?VID=5_05

5.6: Posteriorly directed mitral regurgitation jet. Available at http://mhprofessional.com/echoatlas/index.php?VID=5_06

Chapter 6 Endocarditis

6.1: Partial dehiscence of a prosthetic mitral ring. Available at http://mhprofessional.com/echoatlas/index.php?VID=6_01

6.2: Endocarditis with perforation of the posterior mitral leaflet. Available at http://mhprofessional.com/echoatlas/index.php?VID=6_02

6.3: Calcified vegetations on both the atrial and on the ventricular side of the mitral valve. Available at http://mhprofessional.com/echoatlas/index.php?VID=6_03

6.4a: Paravalvular mitral prosthesis regurgitation. Available at http://mhprofessional.com/echoatlas/index.php?VID=6_04a

6.4b: Paravalvular mitral prosthesis regurgitation. Available at http://mhprofessional.com/echoatlas/index.php?VID=6_04b

6.5a: Vegetation on the right atrial side of the tricuspid valve. Available at http://mhprofessional.com/echoatlas/index.php?VID=6_05a

6.5b: Vegetation on the right atrial side of the tricuspid valve. Available at http://mhprofessional.com/echoatlas/index.php?VID=6_05b

6.5c: Vegetation on the right atrial side of the tricuspid valve. Available at http://mhprofessional.com/echoatlas/index.php?VID=6_05c

6.5d: Vegetation on the right atrial side of the tricuspid valve. Available at http://mhprofessional.com/echoatlas/index.php?VID=6_05d

6.6: Vegetation on a pacemaker wire—tethered at the point of entry of the wire into the right atrium from the superior vena cava. Available at http://mhprofessional.com/echoatlas/index.php?VID=6_06

6.7: Vegetation on a pulmonic valve. Available at http://mhprofessional.com/echoatlas/index.php?VID=6_07

6.8: Aortic valve vegetation. Available at http://mhprofessional.com/echoatlas/index.php?VID=6_08

6.9: Aortic root abscess. Available at http://mhprofessional.com/echoatlas/index.php?VID=6_09

6.10: Abscess in the intervalvular fibrosa. Available at http://mhprofessional.com/echoatlas/index.php?VID=6_10

6.11: Large Lambl's excrescence on the right coronary aortic cusp. Available at http://mhprofessional.com/echoatlas/index.php?VID=6_11

6.12a: Pseudoaneurysm of the aorta in a patient with endocarditis. Available at http://mhprofessional.com/echoatlas/index.php?VID=6_12a

6.12b: Pseudoaneurysm of the aorta in a patient with endocarditis. Available at http://mhprofessional.com/echoatlas/index.php?VID=6_12b

6.13a: Pacemaker wire vegetations. Available at http://mhprofessional.com/echoatlas/index.php?VID=6_13a

6.13b: Pacemaker wire vegetations. Available at http://mhprofessional.com/echoatlas/index.php?VID=6_13b

6.14: Partial dehiscence of an aortic valve prosthesis may occur due to endocarditis. Available at http://mhprofessional.com/echoatlas/index.php?VID=6_14

6.15: Normal eustachian valve. Available at http://mhprofessional.com/echoatlas/index.php?VID=6_15

6.16a: Right atrial Chiari network should not be confused with vegetations. Available at http://mhprofessional.com/echoatlas/index.php?VID=6_16a

6.16b: Right atrial Chiari network should not be confused with vegetations. Available at http://mhprofessional.com/echoatlas/index.php?VID=6_16b

6.16c: Right atrial Chiari network should not be confused with vegetations. Available at http://mhprofessional.com/echoatlas/index.php?VID=6_16c

6.16d: Right atrial Chiari network should not be confused with vegetations. Available at http://mhprofessional.com/echoatlas/index.php?VID=6_16d

6.16e: Right atrial Chiari network should not be confused with vegetations. Available at http://mhprofessional.com/echoatlas/index.php?VID=6_16e

6.16f: Right atrial Chiari network should not be confused with vegetations. Available at http://mhprofessional.com/echoatlas/index.php?VID=6_16f

6.16g: Right atrial Chiari network should not be confused with vegetations. Available at http://mhprofessional.com/echoatlas/index.php?VID=6_19g

6.16h: Right atrial Chiari network should not be confused with vegetations. Available at http://mhprofessional.com/echoatlas/index.php?VID=6_16h

6.16i: Right atrial Chiari network should not be confused with vegetations. Available at http://mhprofessional.com/echoatlas/index.php?VID=6_16i

6.17: Systolic anterior motion of the mitral valve chordae should not be confused with vegetations. Available at http://mhprofessional.com/echoatlas/index.php?VID=6_17

Chapter 7 Hypertension and Preoperative Evaluation

7.1a: Left ventricular hypertrophy. Available at http://mhprofessional.com/echoatlas/index.php?VID=7_01a

7.1b: Left ventricular hypertrophy. Available at http://mhprofessional.com/echoatlas/index.php?VID=7_01b

7.1c: Left ventricular hypertrophy. Available at http://mhprofessional.com/echoatlas/index.php?VID=7_01c

7.1d: Left ventricular hypertrophy. Available at http://mhprofessional.com/echoatlas/index.php?VID=7_01d

7.1e: Left ventricular hypertrophy. Available at http://mhprofessional.com/echoatlas/index.php?VID=7_01e

7.1f: Left ventricular hypertrophy. Available at http://mhprofessional.com/echoatlas/index.php?VID=7_01f

7.2: Small left ventricular cavity dimensions demonstrated by color flow. Available at http://mhprofessional.com/echoatlas/index.php?VID=7_02

7.3a: Basal septal hypertrophy. Available at http://mhprofessional.com/echoatlas/index.php?VID=7_03a

7.3b: Basal septal hypertrophy. Available at http://mhprofessional.com/echoatlas/index.php?VID=7_03b

7.4: Speckled myocardial reflections in left ventricular hypertrophy. Available at http://mhprofessional.com/echoatlas/index.php?VID=7_04

7.5a: Left ventricular hypertrophy with decreased systolic function. Available at http://mhprofessional.com/echoatlas/index.php?VID=7_05a

7.5b: Left ventricular hypertrophy with decreased systolic function. Available at http://mhprofessional.com/echoatlas/index.php?VID=7_05b

7.5c: Left ventricular hypertrophy with decreased systolic function. Available at http://mhprofessional.com/echoatlas/index.php?VID=7_05c

7.6: Rim or ridge of basal left ventricular hypertrophy shown in a transgastric TEE view. Available at http://mhprofessional.com/echoatlas/index.php?VID=7_06

7.7a: Coronary artery "railroad track" reflections. Available at http://mhprofessional.com/echoatlas/index.php?VID=7_07a

7.7b: Coronary artery "railroad track" reflections. Available at http://mhprofessional.com/echoatlas/index.php?VID=7_07b

Chapter 8 Cardiomyopathies

8.1: High-velocity mitral regurgitation in hypertrophic obstructive cardiomyopathy. Available at http://mhprofessional.com/echoatlas/index.php?VID=8_01

8.2: TEE color flow Doppler of left ventricular outflow obstruction being "depressurized" by mitral regurgitation. Available at http://mhprofessional.com/echoatlas/index.php?VID=8_02

8.3a: Asymmetric septal hypertrophy. Available at http://mhprofessional.com/echoatlas/index.php?VID=8_03a

8.3b: Asymmetric septal hypertrophy. Available at http://mhprofessional.com/echoatlas/index.php?VID=8_03b

8.3c: Asymmetric septal hypertrophy. Available at http://mhprofessional.com/echoatlas/index.php?VID=8_03c

8.3d: Asymmetric septal hypertrophy. Available at http://mhprofessional.com/echoatlas/index.php?VID=8_03d

8.4a: Asymmetric septal hypertrophy—short-axis view. Available at http://mhprofessional.com/echoatlas/index.php?VID=8_04a

8.4b: Asymmetric septal hypertrophy—short-axis view. Available at http://mhprofessional.com/echoatlas/index.php?VID=8_04b

8.5a: Asymmetric septal hypertrophy. Available at http://mhprofessional.com/echoatlas/index.php?VID=8_05a

8.5b: Asymmetric septal hypertrophy. Available at http://mhprofessional.com/echoatlas/index.php?VID=8_05b

8.5c: Asymmetric septal hypertrophy. Available at http://mhprofessional.com/echoatlas/index.php?VID=8_05c

8.6a: Severe asymmetric septal hypertrophy. Available at http://mhprofessional.com/echoatlas/index.php?VID=8_06a

8.6b: Severe asymmetric septal hypertrophy. Available at http://mhprofessional.com/echoatlas/index.php?VID=8_06b

8.7: Systolic anterior mitral leaflet motion with loss of leaflet coaptation. Available at http://mhprofessional.com/echoatlas/index.php?VID=8_07

8.8: Apical left ventricular hypertrophy. Available at http://mhprofessional.com/echoatlas/index.php?VID=8_08

8.9a: Apical left ventricular hypertrophy. Available at http://mhprofessional.com/echoatlas/index.php?VID=8_09a

8.9b: Apical left ventricular hypertrophy. Available at http://mhprofessional.com/echoatlas/index.php?VID=8_09b

8.10a: Spade-shaped contrast left ventriculogram in apical hypertrophy. Available at http://mhprofessional.com/echoatlas/index.php?VID=8_10a

8.10b: Spade-shaped contrast left ventriculogram in apical hypertrophy. Available at http://mhprofessional.com/echoatlas/index.php?VID=8_10b

8.11: Concentric left ventricular hypertrophy. Available at http://mhprofessional.com/echoatlas/index.php?VID=8_11

8.12: Left ventricular hypertrophy in a hypertensive patient. Available at http://mhprofessional.com/echoatlas/index.php?VID=8_12

8.13: Pathologic left ventricular hypertrophy with decreased mitral leaflet coaptation and consequent mitral regurgitation. Available at http://mhprofessional.com/echoatlas/index.php?VID=8_13

8.14: Pathologic left ventricular hypertrophy with small left ventricular internal dimensions. Available at http://mhprofessional.com/echoatlas/index.php?VID=8_14

8.15a: Severe left ventricular hypertrophy in a patient with amyloid heart disease. Available at http://mhprofessional.com/echoatlas/index.php?VID=8_15a

8.15b: Severe left ventricular hypertrophy in a patient with amyloid heart disease. Available at http://mhprofessional.com/echoatlas/index.php?VID=8_15b

8.15c: Severe left ventricular hypertrophy in a patient with amyloid heart disease. Available at http://mhprofessional.com/echoatlas/index.php?VID=8_15c

8.16a: Amyloid heart disease: Biventricular hypertrophy, systolic dysfunction, biatrial enlargement. Available at http://mhprofessional.com/echoatlas/index.php?VID=8_16a

8.16b: Amyloid heart disease: Biventricular hypertrophy, systolic dysfunction, biatrial enlargement. Available at http://mhprofessional.com/echoatlas/index.php?VID=8_16b

8.16c: Amyloid heart disease: Biventricular hypertrophy, systolic dysfunction, biatrial enlargement. Available at http://mhprofessional.com/echoatlas/index.php?VID=8_16c

8.16d: Amyloid heart disease: Biventricular hypertrophy, systolic dysfunction, biatrial enlargement. Available at http://mhprofessional.com/echoatlas/index.php?VID=8_16d

8.17: Amyloid heart disease: Preserved tricuspid annulus systolic excursion. Available at http://mhprofessional.com/echoatlas/index.php?VID=8_17

8.18: Nondiagnostic systolic anterior motion of the mitral chordae. Available at http://mhprofessional.com/echoatlas/index.php?VID=8_18

8.19: Biatrial enlargement with severe AV valve regurgitation. Available at http://mhprofessional.com/echoatlas/index.php?VID=8_19

8.20: Early diastolic color flow propagation velocity. Available at http://mhprofessional.com/echoatlas/index.php?VID=8_20

8.21: Ventricular assist device "pushing" blood into the ascending aorta. Available at http://mhprofessional.com/echoatlas/index.php?VID=8_21

8.22a: Severely dilated, diffusely hypokinetic left ventricle. Available at http://mhprofessional.com/echoatlas/index.php?VID=8_22a

8.22b: Severely dilated, diffusely hypokinetic left ventricle. Available at http://mhprofessional.com/echoatlas/index.php?VID=8_22b

8.22c: Severely dilated, diffusely hypokinetic left ventricle. Available at http://mhprofessional.com/echoatlas/index.php?VID=8_22c

8.22d: Severely dilated, diffusely hypokinetic left ventricle. Available at http://mhprofessional.com/echoatlas/index.php?VID=8_22d

8.22e: Severely dilated, diffusely hypokinetic left ventricle. Available at http://mhprofessional.com/echoatlas/index.php?VID=8_22e

8.22f: Severely dilated, diffusely hypokinetic left ventricle. Available at http://mhprofessional.com/echoatlas/index.php?VID=8_22f

8.22g: Severely dilated, diffusely hypokinetic left ventricle. Available at http://mhprofessional.com/echoatlas/index.php?VID=8_22g

8.22h: Severely dilated, diffusely hypokinetic left ventricle. Available at http://mhprofessional.com/echoatlas/index.php?VID=8_22h

8.23: Dilated cardiomyopathy. Available at http://mhprofessional.com/echoatlas/index.php?VID=8_23

8.24: Apical left ventricular wall akinesis on TEE giving the appearance of a "door knob turning." Available at http://mhprofessional.com/echoatlas/index.php?VID=8_24

8.25: "Door knob turning" short axis view. Available at http://mhprofessional.com/echoatlas/index.php?VID=8_25

8.26: Severe dilatation, diffuse hypokinesis and akinesis, thin left ventricular walls. Available at http://mhprofessional.com/echoatlas/index.php?VID=8_26

8.27a: Apical tethering of the mitral valve in dilated cardiomyopathy. Available at http://mhprofessional.com/echoatlas/index.php?VID=8_27a

8.27b: Apical tethering of the mitral valve in dilated cardiomyopathy. Available at http://mhprofessional.com/echoatlas/index.php?VID=8_27b

8.28: Decreased aortic leaflet opening due to the decreased stroke volume. Available at http://mhprofessional.com/echoatlas/index.php?VID=8_28

8.29: Decreased biventricular function. Available at http://mhprofessional.com/echoatlas/index.php?VID=8_29

8.30: Thinning and increased reflectivity of the interventricular septum, indicating scarred, nonviable myocardium. Available at http://mhprofessional.com/echoatlas/index.php?VID=8_30

8.31: Severely decreased biventricular systolic function. Available at http://mhprofessional.com/echoatlas/index.php?VID=8_31

8.32: Mitral regurgitation in dilated cardiomyopathy. Available at http://mhprofessional.com/echoatlas/index.php?VID=8_32

8.33: Left ventricular assist device "pushing" blood from the device to the ascending aorta. Available at http://mhprofessional.com/echoatlas/index.php?VID=8_33

8.34: Right ventricular assist device "pushing" blood from the device to the pulmonary artery. Available at http://mhprofessional.com/echoatlas/index.php?VID=8_34

8.35: Impella left ventricular assist device. Available at http://mhprofessional.com/echoatlas/index.php?VID=8_35

8.36a: Impella left ventricular assist device. Available at http://mhprofessional.com/echoatlas/index.php?VID=8_36a

8.36b: Impella left ventricular assist device. Available at http://mhprofessional.com/echoatlas/index.php?VID=8_36b

8.37a: Apical left ventricular assist device. Available at http://mhprofessional.com/echoatlas/index.php?VID=8_37a

8.37b: Apical left ventricular assist device. Available at http://mhprofessional.com/echoatlas/index.php?VID=8_37b

8.38: Apical left ventricular assist device. Available at http://mhprofessional.com/echoatlas/index.php?VID=8_38

8.39a: Apical left ventricular thrombus with normal underlying left ventricular wall motion. Available at http://mhprofessional.com/echoatlas/index.php?VID=8_39a

8.39b: Apical left ventricular thrombus with normal underlying left ventricular wall motion. Available at http://mhprofessional.com/echoatlas/index.php?VID=8_39b

8.40: Apical left ventricular trabeculations may resemble a thrombus. Available at http://mhprofessional.com/echoatlas/index.php?VID=8_40

8.41: Noncompaction. Available at http://mhprofessional.com/echoatlas/index.php?VID=8_41

8.42a: Noncompaction with severely decreased systolic left ventricular function. Available at http://mhprofessional.com/echoatlas/index.php?VID=8_42a

8.42b: Noncompaction with severely decreased systolic left ventricular function. Available at http://mhprofessional.com/echoatlas/index.php?VID=8_42b

8.42c: Noncompaction with severely decreased systolic left ventricular function. Available at http://mhprofessional.com/echoatlas/index.php?VID=8_42c

8.43: Apical left ventricular thrombus in noncompaction. Available at http://mhprofessional.com/echoatlas/index.php?VID=8_43

8.44a: Cardiomyopathy with prominent trabeculations of the lateral left ventricular wall. Available at http://mhprofessional.com/echoatlas/index.php?VID=8_44a

8.44b: Cardiomyopathy with prominent trabeculations of the lateral left ventricular wall. Available at http://mhprofessional.com/echoatlas/index.php?VID=8_44b

8.45: Idiopathic cardiomyopathy with prominent biventricular trabeculations. Available at http://mhprofessional.com/echoatlas/index.php?VID=8_45

8.46: Prominent left ventricular trabeculations with preserved systolic function. Available at http://mhprofessional.com/echoatlas/index.php?VID=8_46

8.47a: Carcinoid tricuspid valve disease. Available at http://mhprofessional.com/echoatlas/index.php?VID=8_47a

8.47b: Carcinoid tricuspid valve disease. Available at http://mhprofessional.com/echoatlas/index.php?VID=8_47b

8.47c: Carcinoid pulmonic valve disease. Available at http://mhprofessional.com/echoatlas/index.php?VID=8_47c

8.48: Saline contrast in the hepatic veins following injection into an arm vein in a patient with tricuspid regurgitation. Available at http://mhprofessional.com/echoatlas/index.php?VID=8_48

Chapter 9   Pericardial Disease

9.1a: Large thrombus in the pericardial space following heart surgery. Available at http://mhprofessional.com/echoatlas/index.php?VID=9_01a

9.1b: Large thrombus in the pericardial space following heart surgery. Available at http://mhprofessional.com/echoatlas/index.php?VID=9_01b

9.2: Large pericardial effusion with partial right atrial collapse. Available at http://mhprofessional.com/echoatlas/index.php?VID=9_02

9.3: Pleural and pericardial effusion with partial right atrial collapse. Available at http://mhprofessional.com/echoatlas/index.php?VID=9_03

9.4a: Partial right atrial collapse. Available at http://mhprofessional.com/echoatlas/index.php?VID=9_04a

9.4b: Partial right atrial collapse. Available at http://mhprofessional.com/echoatlas/index.php?VID=9_04b

9.5: Partial biatrial collapse. Available at http://mhprofessional.com/echoatlas/index.php?VID=9_05

9.6: No right atrial collapse in this view. Available at http://mhprofessional.com/echoatlas/index.php?VID=9_06

9.7a: Fibrin in the pericardial space. Available at http://mhprofessional.com/echoatlas/index.php?VID=9_07a

9.7b: Fibrin in the pericardial space. Available at http://mhprofessional.com/echoatlas/index.php?VID=9_07b

9.8: Fibrin in the pericardial space. Available at http://mhprofessional.com/echoatlas/index.php?VID=9_08

9.9: Saline contrast in the pericardial space during echo-guided pericardiocentesis. Available at http://mhprofessional.com/echoatlas/index.php?VID=9_09

9.10a: Partial collapse of the right ventricular free wall. Available at http://mhprofessional.com/echoatlas/index.php?VID=9_10a

9.10b: Partial collapse of the right ventricular free wall. Available at http://mhprofessional.com/echoatlas/index.php?VID=9_10b

9.10c: Partial collapse of the right ventricular free wall. Available at http://mhprofessional.com/echoatlas/index.php?VID=9_10c

9.11: Exaggerated systolic right ventricular wall motion without diastolic inversion of the free wall. Available at http://mhprofessional.com/echoatlas/index.php?VID=9_11

9.12: Pericardial effusion in a dialysis patient. Available at http://mhprofessional.com/echoatlas/index.php?VID=9_12

9.13: Pericardial effusion in the transverse sinus between the left atrial appendage and the left upper pulmonary vein. Available at http://mhprofessional.com/echoatlas/index.php?VID=9_13

9.14a: Pericardial effusion in Dressler's syndrome following anterior myocardial infarction. Available at http://mhprofessional.com/echoatlas/index.php?VID=9_14a

9.14b: Pericardial effusion in Dressler's syndrome following anterior myocardial infarction. Available at http://mhprofessional.com/echoatlas/index.php?VID=9_14b

9.15a: Large pericardial effusion with swinging heart motion that can be responsible for an electrical alternans QRS pattern on the ECG. Available at http://mhprofessional.com/echoatlas/index.php?VID=9_15a

9.15b: Large pericardial effusion with swinging heart motion that can be responsible for an electrical alternans QRS pattern on the ECG. Available at http://mhprofessional.com/echoatlas/index.php?VID=9_15b

9.15c: Large pericardial effusion with swinging heart motion that can be responsible for an electrical alternans QRS pattern on the ECG. Available at http://mhprofessional.com/echoatlas/index.php?VID=9_15c

9.15d: Large pericardial effusion with swinging heart motion that can be responsible for an electrical alternans QRS pattern on the ECG. Available at http://mhprofessional.com/echoatlas/index.php?VID=9_15d

9.15e: Large pericardial effusion with swinging heart motion that can be responsible for an electrical alternans QRS pattern on the ECG. Available at http://mhprofessional.com/echoatlas/index.php?VID=9_15e

9.16: Pericardial effusion (not pleural) interposed between the descending aorta and the posterior left atrial wall. Available at http://mhprofessional.com/echoatlas/index.php?VID=9_16

9.17: Large pleural effusion extending behind the descending aorta. Available at http://mhprofessional.com/echoatlas/index.php?VID=9_17

9.18: Ascites on the abdominal side of the diaphragm. Available at http://mhprofessional.com/echoatlas/index.php?VID=9_18

9.19: Large pericardial effusion that extends to the transverse sinus (behind the proximal ascending aorta). Available at http://mhprofessional.com/echoatlas/index.php?VID=9_19

9.20: Pericardial fluid in the transverse sinus. Available at http://mhprofessional.com/echoatlas/index.php?VID=9_20

9.21: Exaggerated excursion of the right ventricular free wall due to pericardial fluid. Available at http://mhprofessional.com/echoatlas/index.php?VID=9_21

9.22: Questionable collapse of the basal right ventricular free wall. Available at http://mhprofessional.com/echoatlas/index.php?VID=9_22

9.23a: Fibrin in the pleural space. Available at http://mhprofessional.com/echoatlas/index.php?VID=9_23a

9.23b: Fibrin in the pleural space. Available at http://mhprofessional.com/echoatlas/index.php?VID=9_23b

9.23c: Fibrin in the pleural space. Available at http://mhprofessional.com/echoatlas/index.php?VID=9_23c

9.23d: Fibrin in the pleural space. Available at http://mhprofessional.com/echoatlas/index.php?VID=9_23d

9.24: Pleural effusion extending behind the descending aorta. Available at http://mhprofessional.com/echoatlas/index.php?VID=9_24

9.25: Ascites can be mistaken for a pericardial cyst (diverticulum). Available at http://mhprofessional.com/echoatlas/index.php?VID=9_25

9.26a: Septal "bounce" in pericardial constriction. Available at http://mhprofessional.com/echoatlas/index.php?VID=9_26a

9.26b: Septal "bounce" in pericardial constriction. Available at http://mhprofessional.com/echoatlas/index.php?VID=9_26b

9.26c: Septal "bounce" in pericardial constriction. Available at http://mhprofessional.com/echoatlas/index.php?VID=9_26c

9.27: Normal motion of the interventricular septum (no "bounce") shown for comparison. Available at http://mhprofessional.com/echoatlas/index.php?VID=9_27

9.28a: Pericardial thickness can be measured using echocardiography only when there is fluid on both sides of the pericardium. Available at http://mhprofessional.com/echoatlas/index.php?VID=9_28a

9.28b: Pericardial thickness can be measured using echocardiography only when there is fluid on both sides of the pericardium. Available at http://mhprofessional.com/echoatlas/index.php?VID=9_28b

9.28c: Pericardial thickness can be measured using echocardiography only when there is fluid on both sides of the pericardium. Available at http://mhprofessional.com/echoatlas/index.php?VID=9_28c

9.28d: Pericardial thickness can be measured using echocardiography only when there is fluid on both sides of the pericardium. Available at http://mhprofessional.com/echoatlas/index.php?VID=9_28d

9.28e: Pericardial thickness can be measured using echocardiography only when there is fluid on both sides of the pericardium. Available at http://mhprofessional.com/echoatlas/index.php?VID=9_28e

9.28f: Pericardial thickness can be measured using echocardiography only when there is fluid on both sides of the pericardium. Available at http://mhprofessional.com/echoatlas/index.php?VID=9_28f

9.29: Thick pericardium delineated by pleural and pericardial fluid. Available at http://mhprofessional.com/echoatlas/index.php?VID=9_29

9.30: Left ventricular hypertrophy with biatrial enlargement. Available at http://mhprofessional.com/echoatlas/index.php?VID=9_30

9.31a: Normal phasic decrease in the diameter of the inferior vena cava. Available at http://mhprofessional.com/echoatlas/index.php?VID=9_31a

9.31b: Normal phasic decrease in the diameter of the inferior vena cava. Available at http://mhprofessional.com/echoatlas/index.php?VID=9_31b

9.32: Dilated hepatic veins with prominent flow reversal (in blue). Available at http://mhprofessional.com/echoatlas/index.php?VID=9_32

9.33a: Fluoroscopic appearance of calcified pericardium. Available at http://mhprofessional.com/echoatlas/index.php?VID=9_33a

9.33b: Fluoroscopic appearance of calcified pericardium. Available at http://mhprofessional.com/echoatlas/index.php?VID=9_33b

9.33c: Fluoroscopic appearance of calcified pericardium. Available at http://mhprofessional.com/echoatlas/index.php?VID=9_33c

9.34: Pleuropericardial fibrin. Available at http://mhprofessional.com/echoatlas/index.php?VID=9_34

Chapter 10   Diastology

10.1a: Diastolic dominant right pulmonary vein inflow. Available at http://mhprofessional.com/echoatlas/index.php?VID=10_01a

10.1b: Diastolic dominant right pulmonary vein inflow. Available at http://mhprofessional.com/echoatlas/index.php?VID=10_01b

10.2a: Normal systolic dominant pulmonary vein inflow. Available at http://mhprofessional.com/echoatlas/index.php?VID=10_02a

10.2b: Normal systolic dominant pulmonary vein inflow. Available at http://mhprofessional.com/echoatlas/index.php?VID=10_02b

10.2c: Normal systolic dominant pulmonary vein inflow. Available at http://mhprofessional.com/echoatlas/index.php?VID=10_02c

10.3: Diastolic dominant pulmonary vein inflow pattern. Available at http://mhprofessional.com/echoatlas/index.php?VID=10_03

10.4a: Diastolic dominant pulmonary vein inflow. Available at http://mhprofessional.com/echoatlas/index.php?VID=10_04a

10.4b: Diastolic dominant pulmonary vein inflow. Available at http://mhprofessional.com/echoatlas/index.php?VID=10_04b

10.4c: Diastolic dominant pulmonary vein inflow. Available at http://mhprofessional.com/echoatlas/index.php?VID=10_04c

10.4d: Diastolic dominant pulmonary vein inflow. Available at http://mhprofessional.com/echoatlas/index.php?VID=10_04d

10.5a: Right and left pulmonary veins in the apical four chamber view. Available at http://mhprofessional.com/echoatlas/index.php?VID=10_05a

10.5b: Right and left pulmonary veins in the apical four-chamber view. Available at http://mhprofessional.com/echoatlas/index.php?VID=10_05b

10.6: Unusually well-demonstrated pulmonary vein inflow into the left atrium. Available at http://mhprofessional.com/echoatlas/index.php?VID=10_06

10.7a: Left ventricular cavity obliteration. Available at http://mhprofessional.com/echoatlas/index.php?VID=10_07a

10.7b: Left ventricular cavity obliteration. Available at http://mhprofessional.com/echoatlas/index.php?VID=10_07b

Chapter 11   Arrhythmias and Neurological Disorders

11.1: Left atrial appendage thrombus. Available at http://mhprofessional.com/echoatlas/index.php?VID=11_01

11.2: Left atrial appendage thrombus located at the far part of the appendage with "shimmering" oscillations and discrete borders. Available at http://mhprofessional.com/echoatlas/index.php?VID=11_02

11.3a: Spontaneous contrast in the left atrial appendage. Available at http://mhprofessional.com/echoatlas/index.php?VID=11_03a

11.3b: Spontaneous contrast in the left atrial appendage. Available at http://mhprofessional.com/echoatlas/index.php?VID=11_03b

11.3c: Spontaneous contrast in the left atrial appendage. Available at http://mhprofessional.com/echoatlas/index.php?VID=11_03c

11.4: Spontaneous contrast in the dilated left atrium and left atrial appendage. Available at http://mhprofessional.com/echoatlas/index.php?VID=11_04

11.5: Reverberation artifact in the left atrial appendage that can be mistaken for a thrombus. Available at http://mhprofessional.com/echoatlas/index.php?VID=11_05

11.6a: Mechanical effect of atrial flutter on the heart. Available at http://mhprofessional.com/echoatlas/index.php?VID=11_06a

11.6b: Mechanical effect of atrial flutter on the heart. Available at http://mhprofessional.com/echoatlas/index.php?VID=11_06b

11.7: Mechanical effect of atrial flutter on the heart. Available at http://mhprofessional.com/echoatlas/index.php?VID=11_07

11.8: Variable aortic leaflet opening (and variable stroke volume) in atrial flutter. Available at http://mhprofessional.com/echoatlas/index.php?VID=11_08

11.9: Triangular-shaped left atrial appendage. Available at http://mhprofessional.com/echoatlas/index.php?VID=11_09

11.10: Normal left atrial appendage contractility with prominent trabeculations and a reverberation artifact. Available at http://mhprofessional.com/echoatlas/index.php?VID=11_10

11.11a: Left atrial appendage that was sewn closed during heart surgery. Available at http://mhprofessional.com/echoatlas/index.php?VID=11_11a

11.11b: Left atrial appendage that was sewn closed during heart surgery. Available at http://mhprofessional.com/echoatlas/index.php?VID=11_11b

11.12: Left atrial appendage that was only partly closed during heart surgery. Available at http://mhprofessional.com/echoatlas/index.php?VID=11_12

11.13: Biatrial enlargement in atrial flutter. Available at http://mhprofessional.com/echoatlas/index.php?VID=11_13

11.14: Dilated cardiomyopathy with a wide QRS. Available at http://mhprofessional.com/echoatlas/index.php?VID=11_14

11.15a: Dilated cardiomyopathy with paradoxical motion of the interventricular septum due to bundle branch block. Available at http://mhprofessional.com/echoatlas/index.php?VID=11_15a

11.15b: Dilated cardiomyopathy with paradoxical motion of the interventricular septum due to bundle branch block. Available at http://mhprofessional.com/echoatlas/index.php?VID=11_15b

11.16: Pacemaker wire. Available at http://mhprofessional.com/echoatlas/index.php?VID=11_16

11.17: Pacemaker wire in the coronary sinus manifested as a reverberation artifact in the pleural effusion. Available at http://mhprofessional.com/echoatlas/index.php?VID=11_17

11.18: Chiari network in the right atrium. Available at http://mhprofessional.com/echoatlas/index.php?VID=11_18

11.19: Chiari network and a pacemaker wire in the right atrium. Available at http://mhprofessional.com/echoatlas/index.php?VID=11_19

11.20: Small left ventricular internal dimensions with systolic cavity obliteration. Available at http://mhprofessional.com/echoatlas/index.php?VID=11_20

11.21: Patent foramen ovale shown by color flow. Available at http://mhprofessional.com/echoatlas/index.php?VID=11_21

11.22a: Sometimes an unconventional view can demonstrate a patent foramen ovale with color flow. Available at http://mhprofessional.com/echoatlas/index.php?VID=11_22a

11.22b: Sometimes an unconventional view can demonstrate a patent foramen ovale with color flow. Available at http://mhprofessional.com/echoatlas/index.php?VID=11_22b

11.23a: Patent foramen ovale shown by saline contrast. Available at http://mhprofessional.com/echoatlas/index.php?VID=11_23a

11.23b: Patent foramen ovale shown by saline contrast. Available at http://mhprofessional.com/echoatlas/index.php?VID=11_23b

11.23c: Patent foramen ovale shown by saline contrast. Available at http://mhprofessional.com/echoatlas/index.php?VID=11_23c

11.23d: Patent foramen ovale shown by saline contrast. Available at http://mhprofessional.com/echoatlas/index.php?VID=11_23d

11.24: Atrial septal aneurysm. Available at http://mhprofessional.com/echoatlas/index.php?VID=11_24

11.25a: Residual interatrial communication in a patient with a stroke following attempted device closure of a patent foramen ovale. Available at http://mhprofessional.com/echoatlas/index.php?VID=11_25a

11.25b: Residual interatrial communication in a patient with a stroke following attempted device closure of a patent foramen ovale. Available at http://mhprofessional.com/echoatlas/index.php?VID=11_25b

11.26: Lambl's excrescence on the ventricular side of the aortic valve in a patient with dilated cardiomyopathy. Available at http://mhprofessional.com/echoatlas/index.php?VID=11_26

11.27a: Lambl's excrescences on the aortic valve. Available at http://mhprofessional.com/echoatlas/index.php?VID=11_27a

11.27b: Lambl's excrescences on the aortic valve. Available at http://mhprofessional.com/echoatlas/index.php?VID=11_27b

11.27c: Lambl's excrescences on the aortic valve. Available at http://mhprofessional.com/echoatlas/index.php?VID=11_27c

11.28: Papillary fibroelastoma on the aortic valve. Available at http://mhprofessional.com/echoatlas/index.php?VID=11_28

11.29: Papillary fibroelastoma in the left ventricular outflow below the aortic valve. Available at http://mhprofessional.com/echoatlas/index.php?VID=11_29

11.30a: Large serpiginous thrombus in the right atrium. Available at http://mhprofessional.com/echoatlas/index.php?VID=11_30a

11.30b: Large serpiginous thrombus in the right atrium. Available at http://mhprofessional.com/echoatlas/index.php?VID=11_30b

11.31a: Large thrombus in the left pulmonary vein of a lung cancer patient. Available at http://mhprofessional.com/echoatlas/index.php?VID=11_31a

11.31b: Large thrombus in the left pulmonary vein of a lung cancer patient. Available at http://mhprofessional.com/echoatlas/index.php?VID=11_31b

11.32a: Apical ballooning—stress induced—Takotsubo cardiomyopathy. Available at http://mhprofessional.com/echoatlas/index.php?VID=11_32a

11.32b: Apical ballooning—stress induced—Takotsubo cardiomyopathy. Available at http://mhprofessional.com/echoatlas/index.php?VID=11_32b

11.32c: Apical ballooning—stress induced—Takotsubo cardiomyopathy. Available at http://mhprofessional.com/echoatlas/index.php?VID=11_32c

11.33a: Patent foramen ovale demonstrated by intravenous agitated saline. Available at http://mhprofessional.com/echoatlas/index.php?VID=11_33a

11.33b: Patent foramen ovale demonstrated by intravenous agitated saline. Available at http://mhprofessional.com/echoatlas/index.php?VID=11_33b

11.33c: Patent foramen ovale demonstrated by intravenous agitated saline. Available at http://mhprofessional.com/echoatlas/index.php?VID=11_33c

11.33d: Patent foramen ovale demonstrated by intravenous agitated saline. Available at http://mhprofessional.com/echoatlas/index.php?VID=11_33d

11.33e: Patent foramen ovale demonstrated by intravenous agitated saline. Available at http://mhprofessional.com/echoatlas/index.php?VID=11_33e

11.33f: Patent foramen ovale demonstrated by intravenous agitated saline. Available at http://mhprofessional.com/echoatlas/index.php?VID=11_33f

11.34: Patent foramen ovale demonstrated by color flow Doppler. Available at http://mhprofessional.com/echoatlas/index.php?VID=11_34

11.35: Right atrial thrombus in a patient with patent foramen ovale and paradoxical embolism. Available at http://mhprofessional.com/echoatlas/index.php?VID=11_35

11.36a: Atrial septal aneurysm. Available at http://mhprofessional.com/echoatlas/index.php?VID=11_36a

11.36b: Atrial septal aneurysm. Available at http://mhprofessional.com/echoatlas/index.php?VID=11_36b

11.36c: Atrial septal aneurysm. Available at http://mhprofessional.com/echoatlas/index.php?VID=11_36c

11.36d: Atrial septal aneurysm. Available at http://mhprofessional.com/echoatlas/index.php?VID=11_36d

11.36e: Atrial septal aneurysm. Available at http://mhprofessional.com/echoatlas/index.php?VID=11_36e

11.36f: Atrial septal aneurysm. Available at http://mhprofessional.com/echoatlas/index.php?VID=11_36f

11.36g: Atrial septal aneurysm. Available at http://mhprofessional.com/echoatlas/index.php?VID=11_36g

11.36h: Atrial septal aneurysm. Available at http://mhprofessional.com/echoatlas/index.php?VID=11_36h

11.36i: Atrial septal aneurysm. Available at http://mhprofessional.com/echoatlas/index.php?VID=11_36i

11.37a: Atrial septal aneurysm seen intermittently, simulating a left atrial mass. Available at http://mhprofessional.com/echoatlas/index.php?VID=11_37a

11.37b: Atrial septal aneurysm seen intermittently, simulating a left atrial mass. Available at http://mhprofessional.com/echoatlas/index.php?VID=11_37b

11.37c: Atrial septal aneurysm seen intermittently, simulating a left atrial mass. Available at http://mhprofessional.com/echoatlas/index.php?VID=11_37c

11.38: Transpulmonary saline contrast shunt entering the left atrium from the left upper pulmonary vein. Available at http://mhprofessional.com/echoatlas/index.php?VID=11_38

Chapter 12   Congenital Heart Disease

12.1: Color flow Doppler pattern typically found with a restrictive perimembranous ventricular septal defect. Available at http://mhprofessional.com/echoatlas/index.php?VID=12_01

12.2: A high-velocity (4 m/s or greater) systolic flow *toward* the parasternal transducer (shown here in red) is due to a ventricular septal defect. Available at http://mhprofessional.com/echoatlas/index.php?VID=12_02

12.3: Continuous wave Doppler demonstrates that the jet is systolic, high velocity, and directed toward the transducer. Available at http://mhprofessional.com/echoatlas/index.php?VID=12_03

12.4: Normal patient. Available at http://mhprofessional.com/echoatlas/index.php?VID=12_04

12.5a: Muscular ventricular septal defect. Available at http://mhprofessional.com/echoatlas/index.php?VID=12_05a

12.5b: Muscular ventricular septal defect. Available at http://mhprofessional.com/echoatlas/index.php?VID=12_05b

12.5c: Muscular ventricular septal defect. Available at http://mhprofessional.com/echoatlas/index.php?VID=12_05c

12.5d: Muscular ventricular septal defect. Available at http://mhprofessional.com/echoatlas/index.php?VID=12_05d

12.5e: Muscular ventricular septal defect. Available at http://mhprofessional.com/echoatlas/index.php?VID=12_05e

12.5f: Muscular ventricular septal defect. Available at http://mhprofessional.com/echoatlas/index.php?VID=12_05f

12.5g: Muscular ventricular septal defect. Available at http://mhprofessional.com/echoatlas/index.php?VID=12_05g

12.6a: Perimembranous ventricular septal defect. Available at http://mhprofessional.com/echoatlas/index.php?VID=12_06a

12.6b: Perimembranous ventricular septal defect. Available at http://mhprofessional.com/echoatlas/index.php?VID=12_06b

12.6c: Perimembranous ventricular septal defect. Available at http://mhprofessional.com/echoatlas/index.php?VID=12_06c

12.7: Aneurysm created by tricuspid valve tissue in a healed ventricular septal defect. Available at http://mhprofessional.com/echoatlas/index.php?VID=12_07

12.8: Overriding aorta. Available at http://mhprofessional.com/echoatlas/index.php?VID=12_08

12.9a: Secundum atrial septal defect. Available at http://mhprofessional.com/echoatlas/index.php?VID=12_09a

12.9b: Secundum atrial septal defect. Available at http://mhprofessional.com/echoatlas/index.php?VID=12_09b

12.10: Large secundum atrial septal defect. Available at http://mhprofessional.com/echoatlas/index.php?VID=12_10

12.11: Primum atrial septal defect. Available at http://mhprofessional.com/echoatlas/index.php?VID=12_11

12.12: Negative contrast effect in the contrast-filled right atrium. Available at http://mhprofessional.com/echoatlas/index.php?VID=12_12

12.13: Intact atrial septum: Flow from the inferior vena cava into the right atrium creates a negative contrast effect. Available at http://mhprofessional.com/echoatlas/index.php?VID=12_13

12.14: Secundum atrial septal defect in a neonate. Available at http://mhprofessional.com/echoatlas/index.php?VID=12_14

12.15a: Secundum atrial septal defect. Available at http://mhprofessional.com/echoatlas/index.php?VID=12_15a

12.15b: Secundum atrial septal defect. Available at http://mhprofessional.com/echoatlas/index.php?VID=12_15b

12.15c: Secundum atrial septal defect. Available at http://mhprofessional.com/echoatlas/index.php?VID=12_15c

12.15d: Secundum atrial septal defect. Available at http://mhprofessional.com/echoatlas/index.php?VID=12_15d

12.16: Iatrogenic fenestration in the membrane of the fossa ovalis created by a previous electrophysiology procedure. Available at http://mhprofessional.com/echoatlas/index.php?VID=12_16

12.17: Increased pulmonary artery flow in a patient with a secundum atrial septal defect. Available at http://mhprofessional.com/echoatlas/index.php?VID=12_17

12.18: Intact atrial septum with negative contrast in the right atrium from inferior cava inflow. Available at http://mhprofessional.com/echoatlas/index.php?VID=12_18

12.19: Normal caval inflow may be mistaken to be an atrial septal defect. Available at http://mhprofessional.com/echoatlas/index.php?VID=12_19

12.20a: Atrial septal defect closure device. Available at http://mhprofessional.com/echoatlas/index.php?VID=12_20a

12.20b: Atrial septal defect closure device. Available at http://mhprofessional.com/echoatlas/index.php?VID=12_20b

12.21: AV canal defect. Available at http://mhprofessional.com/echoatlas/index.php?VID=12_21

12.22: AV canal defect with a dilated hypertrophic right ventricle due to severe pulmonary hypertension. Available at http://mhprofessional.com/echoatlas/index.php?VID=12_22

12.23: AV canal defect manifested as an intermittent connection of the mitral valve chordae to the interventricular septum at the left ventricular outflow. Available at http://mhprofessional.com/echoatlas/index.php?VID=12_23

12.24a: Mustard repair of D-TGA. Available at http://mhprofessional.com/echoatlas/index.php?VID=12_24a

12.24b: Mustard repair of D-TGA. Available at http://mhprofessional.com/echoatlas/index.php?VID=12_24b

12.25: Mustard procedure—severely dilated systemic ventricle. Available at http://mhprofessional.com/echoatlas/index.php?VID=12_25

12.26: Mustard procedure—Doppler inflow. Available at http://mhprofessional.com/echoatlas/index.php?VID=12_26

12.27a: Fontan operation. Available at http://mhprofessional.com/echoatlas/index.php?VID=12_27a

12.27b: Fontan operation. Available at http://mhprofessional.com/echoatlas/index.php?VID=12_27b

12.28: Congenitally corrected transposition (L-TGA) in an adult. Available at http://mhprofessional.com/echoatlas/index.php?VID=12_28

12.29: Congenitally corrected transposition (L-TGA) in an adult. Available at http://mhprofessional.com/echoatlas/index.php?VID=12_29

12.30: Lack of fibrous continuity between the systemic AV valve on the bottom of the screen (anatomic tricuspid) and the aortic valve (with coronary ostia) on the top of the screen. Available at http://mhprofessional.com/echoatlas/index.php?VID=12_30

12.31: Systemic ventricle with an infundibulum (hence the lack of fibrous continuity between the AV valve and the aortic valve). Available at http://mhprofessional.com/echoatlas/index.php?VID=12_31

12.32: Parasternal long-axis view showing a dilated coronary sinus. Available at http://mhprofessional.com/echoatlas/index.php?VID=12_32

12.33: TEE sweep from the right atrial cavity to the dilated coronary sinus. Available at http://mhprofessional.com/echoatlas/index.php?VID=12_33

12.34a: Saline contrast in the left SVC between the left pulmonary vein and the left atrial appendage. Available at http://mhprofessional.com/echoatlas/index.php?VID=12_34a

12.34b: Saline contrast in the left SVC between the left pulmonary vein and the left atrial appendage. Available at http://mhprofessional.com/echoatlas/index.php?VID=12_34b

12.34c: Saline contrast in the left SVC between the left pulmonary vein and the left atrial appendage. Available at http://mhprofessional.com/echoatlas/index.php?VID=12_34c

12.35a: Dilated coronary sinus under the mitral annulus. Available at http://mhprofessional.com/echoatlas/index.php?VID=12_35a

12.35b: Dilated coronary sinus under the mitral annulus. Available at http://mhprofessional.com/echoatlas/index.php?VID=12_35b

12.35c: Dilated coronary sinus under the mitral annulus. Available at http://mhprofessional.com/echoatlas/index.php?VID=12_35c

12.35d: Dilated coronary sinus under the mitral annulus. Available at http://mhprofessional.com/echoatlas/index.php?VID=12_35d

12.36: Dilated coronary sinus shown on a modified apical four-chamber view that scans for the coronary sinus below the posterior mitral annulus. Available at http://mhprofessional.com/echoatlas/index.php?VID=12_36

12.37: A dilated coronary sinus can easily be mistaken for a loculated pericardial effusion, or a pericardial cyst. Available at http://mhprofessional.com/echoatlas/index.php?VID=12_37

12.38: Normal coronary sinus appearance in a patient with left ventricular hypertrophy. Available at http://mhprofessional.com/echoatlas/index.php?VID=12_38

12.39: Venous flow *towards* the heart on the *left* side of the chest. Available at http://mhprofessional.com/echoatlas/index.php?VID=12_39

12.40a: Ebstein's abnormality of the tricuspid valve. Available at http://mhprofessional.com/echoatlas/index.php?VID=12_40a

12.40b: Ebstein's abnormality of the tricuspid valve. Available at http://mhprofessional.com/echoatlas/index.php?VID=12_40b

Chapter 13 Diseases of the Aorta

13.1: Mildly dilated sinus of Valsalva with stretching of the aortic leaflets. Available at http://mhprofessional.com/echoatlas/index.php?VID=13_01

13.2a: Aneurysm of the proximal ascending aorta. Available at http://mhprofessional.com/echoatlas/index.php?VID=13_02a

13.2b: Aneurysm of the proximal ascending aorta. Available at http://mhprofessional.com/echoatlas/index.php?VID=13_02b

13.2c: Aneurysm of the proximal ascending aorta. Available at http://mhprofessional.com/echoatlas/index.php?VID=13_02c

13.2d: Aneurysm of the proximal ascending aorta. Available at http://mhprofessional.com/echoatlas/index.php?VID=13_02d

13.3: Aneurysm of the descending aorta. Available at http://mhprofessional.com/echoatlas/index.php?VID=13_03

13.4: Coarctation of the aorta. Available at http://mhprofessional.com/echoatlas/index.php?VID=13_04

13.5: Collateral flow entering the descending aorta in coarctation. Available at http://mhprofessional.com/echoatlas/index.php?VID=13_05

13.6: Atherosclerosis and calcification of a dilated descending aorta. Available at http://mhprofessional.com/echoatlas/index.php?VID=13_06

13.7a: Dissection of the descending aorta. Available at http://mhprofessional.com/echoatlas/index.php?VID=13_07a

13.7b: Dissection of the descending aorta. Available at http://mhprofessional.com/echoatlas/index.php?VID=13_07b

13.7c: Dissection of the descending aorta. Available at http://mhprofessional.com/echoatlas/index.php?VID=13_07c

13.7d: Dissection of the descending aorta. Available at http://mhprofessional.com/echoatlas/index.php?VID=13_07d

13.7e: Dissection of the descending aorta. Available at http://mhprofessional.com/echoatlas/index. php?VID=13_07e

13.8a: Dissection flaps of the proximal ascending aorta. Available at http://mhprofessional.com/echoatlas/index. php?VID=13_08a

13.8b: Dissection flaps of the proximal ascending aorta. Available at http://mhprofessional.com/echoatlas/index. php?VID=13_08b

13.8c: Dissection flaps of the proximal ascending aorta. Available at http://mhprofessional.com/echoatlas/index. php?VID=13_08c

13.8d: Dissection flaps of the proximal ascending aorta. Available at http://mhprofessional.com/echoatlas/index. php?VID=13_08d

13.8e: Dissection flaps of the proximal ascending aorta. Available at http://mhprofessional.com/echoatlas/index. php?VID=13_08e

13.9: Mild aneurysmal dilatation of the aorta. Available at http://mhprofessional.com/echoatlas/index.php?VID=13_09

13.10: Dissection flap close to the right coronary ostium. Available at http://mhprofessional.com/echoatlas/index. php?VID=13_10

13.11a: Artifact in a normal ascending aorta. Available at http://mhprofessional.com/echoatlas/index.php?VID=13_11a

13.11b: Artifact in a normal ascending aorta. Available at http://mhprofessional.com/echoatlas/index. php?VID=13_11b

13.12: Penetrating aortic ulcer with a mobile atheroma in the descending thoracic aorta. Available at http://mhprofessional.com/echoatlas/index.php?VID=13_12

Chapter 14   Cardiac Tumors

14.1: Left atrial myxoma. Available at http://mhprofessional.com/echoatlas/index.php?VID=14_01

14.2a: Left atrial myxoma. Available at http://mhprofessional.com/echoatlas/index.php?VID=14_02a

14.2b: Left atrial myxoma. Available at http://mhprofessional.com/echoatlas/index.php?VID=14_02b

14.2c: Left atrial myxoma. Available at http://mhprofessional.com/echoatlas/index.php?VID=14_02c

14.2d: Left atrial myxoma. Available at http://mhprofessional.com/echoatlas/index.php?VID=14_02d

14.2e: Left atrial myxoma. Available at http://mhprofessional.com/echoatlas/index.php?VID=14_02e

14.2f: Left atrial myxoma. Available at http://mhprofessional.com/echoatlas/index.php?VID=14_02f

14.3a: Mechanical effect of atrial fibrillation on the motion of a left atrial myxoma. Available at http://mhprofessional. com/echoatlas/index.php?VID=14_03a

14.3b: Mechanical effect of atrial fibrillation on the motion of a left atrial myxoma. Available at http://mhprofessional. com/echoatlas/index.php?VID=14_03b

14.4: Left atrial myxoma and a patent foramen ovale. Available at http://mhprofessional.com/echoatlas/index. php?VID=14_04

14.5: Left atrial myxoma extending toward the right upper pulmonary vein. Available at http://mhprofessional.com/echoatlas/index.php?VID=14_05

14.6a: Right atrial myxoma. Available at http://mhprofessional.com/echoatlas/index.php?VID=14_06a

14.6b: Right atrial myxoma. Available at http://mhprofessional.com/echoatlas/index.php?VID=14_06b

14.6c: Right atrial myxoma. Available at http://mhprofessional.com/echoatlas/index.php?VID=14_06c

14.7: Cardiac fibroma. Available at http://mhprofessional.com/echoatlas/index.php?VID=14_07

14.8: Metastatic breast cancer infiltrating the left ventricle. Available at http://mhprofessional.com/echoatlas/index.php?VID=14_08

14.9: Extensive tumor infiltration of both atria by metastatic lung cancer. Available at http://mhprofessional.com/echoatlas/index.php?VID=14_09

14.10: Mobile friable thrombus in the descending aorta of a patient with heparin, induced thrombocytopenia. Available at http://mhprofessional.com/echoatlas/index. php?VID=14_10

14.11a: Thrombus (not a tumor) superimposed on a catheter in the superior vena cava, entering the right atrial cavity. Available at http://mhprofessional.com/echoatlas/index.php?VID=14_11a

14.11b: Thrombus (not a tumor) superimposed on a catheter in the superior vena cava, entering the right atrial cavity. Available at http://mhprofessional.com/echoatlas/index.php?VID=14_11b

14.11c: Thrombus (not a tumor) superimposed on a catheter in the superior vena cava, entering the right atrial cavity. Available at http://mhprofessional.com/echoatlas/index.php?VID=14_11c

14.12: Thrombus in the superior vena cava. Available at http://mhprofessional.com/echoatlas/index.php? VID=14_12

14.13a: The normal atrial wall infolding between the left atrial appendage and the left pulmonary vein should not be mistaken for a mass. Available at http://mhprofessional. com/echoatlas/index.php?VID=14_13a

14.13b: The normal atrial wall infolding between the left atrial appendage and the left pulmonary vein should not be mistaken for a mass. Available at http://mhprofessional. com/echoatlas/index.php?VID=14_13b

14.14: Normal anatomy—no tumor. Available at http://mhprofessional.com/echoatlas/index.php?VID=14_14

14.15: Submitral chordae in dilated cardiomyopathy. Available at http://mhprofessional.com/echoatlas/index. php?VID=14_15

14.16: Cardiac structures that resemble tumors. Available at http://mhprofessional.com/echoatlas/index. php?VID=14_16

14.17a: Pulmonary vein thrombus. Available at http://mhprofessional.com/echoatlas/index.php?VID=14_17a

14.17b: Pulmonary vein thrombus. Available at http://mhprofessional.com/echoatlas/index.php? VID=14_17b

14.18: Large hiatus hernia impinging on the posterior left atrial wall. Available at http://mhprofessional.com/echoatlas/index.php?VID=14_18

14.19: Lipomatous hypertrophy of the interatrial septum. Available at http://mhprofessional.com/echoatlas/index.php?VID=14_19

14.20a: Lung cancer infiltrating the atrial walls and obstructing caval inflow. Available at http://mhprofessional.com/echoatlas/index.php?VID=14_20a

14.20b: Lung cancer infiltrating the atrial walls and obstructing caval inflow. Available at http://mhprofessional.com/echoatlas/index.php?VID=14_20b

14.20c: Lung cancer infiltrating the atrial walls and obstructing caval inflow. Available at http://mhprofessional.com/echoatlas/index.php?VID=14_20c

14.20d: Lung cancer infiltrating the atrial walls and obstructing caval inflow. Available at http://mhprofessional.com/echoatlas/index.php?VID=14_20d

14.20e: Lung cancer infiltrating the atrial walls and obstructing caval inflow. Available at http://mhprofessional.com/echoatlas/index.php?VID=14_20e

14.21a: Lambl's excrescences on the left ventricular side of the aortic valve. Available at http://mhprofessional.com/echoatlas/index.php?VID=14_21a

14.21b: Lambl's excrescences on the left ventricular side of the aortic valve. Available at http://mhprofessional.com/echoatlas/index.php?VID=14_21b

14.21c: Lambl's excrescences on the left ventricular side of the aortic valve. Available at http://mhprofessional.com/echoatlas/index.php?VID=14_21c

14.21d: Lambl's excrescences on the left ventricular side of the aortic valve. Available at http://mhprofessional.com/echoatlas/index.php?VID=14_21d

14.21e: Lambl's excrescences on the left ventricular side of the aortic valve. Available at http://mhprofessional.com/echoatlas/index.php?VID=14_21e

14.21f: Lambl's excrescences on the left ventricular side of the aortic valve. Available at http://mhprofessional.com/echoatlas/index.php?VID=14_21f

14.21g: Lambl's excrescences on the left ventricular side of the aortic valve. Available at http://mhprofessional.com/echoatlas/index.php?VID=14_21g

14.21h: Lambl's excrescences on the left ventricular side of the aortic valve. Available at http://mhprofessional.com/echoatlas/index.php?VID=14_21h

Chapter 15   Ultrasound Physics

15.1a: Cavitation artifacts—mechanical bileaflet mitral prosthesis. Available at http://mhprofessional.com/echoatlas/index.php?VID=15_01a

15.1b: Cavitation artifacts—mechanical bileaflet mitral prosthesis. Available at http://mhprofessional.com/echoatlas/index.php?VID=15_01b

15.2a: Reverberation artifact from a breast implant interferes with imaging. Available at http://mhprofessional.com/echoatlas/index.php?VID=15_02a

15.2b: Reverberation artifact from a breast implant interferes with imaging. Available at http://mhprofessional.com/echoatlas/index.php?VID=15_02b

15.3: Reverberation artifact from a catheter in the right ventricular outflow. Available at http://mhprofessional.com/echoatlas/index.php?VID=15_03

15.4: Reverberation artifact from a ventricular assist device across the aortic valve. Available at http://mhprofessional.com/echoatlas/index.php?VID=15_04

15.5: Reverberation artifact from a right atrial pacemaker wire wrongly suggests that there is something in the pericardial space. Available at http://mhprofessional.com/echoatlas/index.php?VID=15_05

15.6: Apical artifact suggesting thrombus. Available at http://mhprofessional.com/echoatlas/index.php?VID=15_06

15.7: Apical artifact. Available at http://mhprofessional.com/echoatlas/index.php?VID=15_07

15.8: Artifacts that obscure apical and lateral left ventricular wall endocardial reflections. Available at http://mhprofessional.com/echoatlas/index.php?VID=15_08

15.9a: Reverberation artifact from the tricuspid annulus that may wrongly suggest a left atrial mass. Available at http://mhprofessional.com/echoatlas/index.php?VID=15_09a

15.9b: Reverberation artifact from the tricuspid annulus that may wrongly suggest a left atrial mass. Available at http://mhprofessional.com/echoatlas/index.php?VID=15_09b

15.9c: Reverberation artifact from the tricuspid annulus that may wrongly suggest a left atrial mass. Available at http://mhprofessional.com/echoatlas/index.php?VID=15_09c

15.9d: Reverberation artifact from the tricuspid annulus that may wrongly suggest a left atrial mass. Available at http://mhprofessional.com/echoatlas/index.php?VID=15_09d

15.10: Artifactual duplication of the mitral valve. Available at http://mhprofessional.com/echoatlas/index.php?VID=15_10

15.11: Pacemaker wire demonstrating specular reflection of ultrasound. Available at http://mhprofessional.com/echoatlas/index.php?VID=15_11

15.12: Unusually few distracting artifacts from a pacemaker wire. Available at http://mhprofessional.com/echoatlas/index.php?VID=15_12

15.13: Sideways artifacts from an aortic bioprosthesis. Available at http://mhprofessional.com/echoatlas/index.php?VID=15_13

15.14: Reverberation *and* sideways artifacts from a mechanical aortic prosthesis. Available at http://mhprofessional.com/echoatlas/index.php?VID=15_14

15.15: Mild attenuation artifact from the ring of a mitral bioprosthesis. Available at http://mhprofessional.com/echoatlas/index.php?VID=15_15

15.16: Attenuation artifact from mitral annular calcium. Available at http://mhprofessional.com/echoatlas/index.php?VID=15_16

15.17: Ultrasound absorption and attenuation prevents visualization of the inferior left ventricular wall. Available at http://mhprofessional.com/echoatlas/index.php?VID=15_17

Chapter 16   Echocardiographic Anatomy

16.1: Normal aortic leaflets. Available at http://mhprofessional.com/echoatlas/index.php?VID=16_01

16.2a: TEE of a normal trileaflet aortic valve. Available at http://mhprofessional.com/echoatlas/index.php?VID=16_02a

16.2b: TEE of a normal trileaflet aortic valve. Available at http://mhprofessional.com/echoatlas/index.php?VID=16_02b

16.2c: TEE of a normal trileaflet aortic valve. Available at http://mhprofessional.com/echoatlas/index.php?VID=16_02c

16.3: Normal mitral leaflets. Available at http://mhprofessional.com/echoatlas/index.php?VID=16_03

16.4: Short-axis view of the tricuspid, aortic, and pulmonic leaflets. Available at http://mhprofessional.com/echoatlas/index.php?VID=16_04

16.5: Short-axis view of the mitral valve. Available at http://mhprofessional.com/echoatlas/index.php?VID=16_05

16.6: Both mitral leaflets are connected to the same papillary muscle in this view. Available at http://mhprofessional.com/echoatlas/index.php?VID=16_06

16.7: Parasternal long-axis view—presence of left ventricular hypertrophy should always be confirmed in the short-axis views that follow. Available at http://mhprofessional.com/echoatlas/index.php?VID=16_07

16.8: Normal short-axis view of the left ventricle. Available at http://mhprofessional.com/echoatlas/index.php?VID=16_08

16.9: Minimal circumferential pericardial effusion. Available at http://mhprofessional.com/echoatlas/index.php?VID=16_09

16.10: Normal transgastric short-axis TEE view. Available at http://mhprofessional.com/echoatlas/index.php?VID=16_10

16.11: Short-axis view of the mitral papillary muscles. Available at http://mhprofessional.com/echoatlas/index.php?VID=16_11

16.12: TEE of the tricuspid valve. Available at http://mhprofessional.com/echoatlas/index.php?VID=16_12

16.13: Short-axis contrast-enhanced view of the left ventricle. Available at http://mhprofessional.com/echoatlas/index.php?VID=16_13

16.14: Pulmonary artery bifurcation. Available at http://mhprofessional.com/echoatlas/index.php?VID=16_14

16.15: Right branch of the pulmonary artery behind the aorta. Available at http://mhprofessional.com/echoatlas/index.php?VID=16_15

16.16: High mid esophagus view of the right upper pulmonary vein, superior vena cava and aorta in cross section, and the right branch of the pulmonary artery (long section) above. Available at http://mhprofessional.com/echoatlas/index.php?VID=16_16

16.17: Pulsatile changes in a normal size inferior vena cava indicating that the right atrial pressure is normal. Available at http://mhprofessional.com/echoatlas/index.php?VID=16_17

16.18: Ascending aorta. Available at http://mhprofessional.com/echoatlas/index.php?VID=16_18

16.19a: Descending thoracic aorta. Available at http://mhprofessional.com/echoatlas/index.php?VID=16_19a

16.19b: Descending thoracoabdominal aorta. Available at http://mhprofessional.com/echoatlas/index.php?VID=16_19b

16.19c: Descending thoracoabdominal aorta. Available at http://mhprofessional.com/echoatlas/index.php?VID=16_19c

16.20: Prominent systolic expansion of the aorta can be found in young people with normal aortic valve function. Available at http://mhprofessional.com/echoatlas/index.php?VID=16_20

16.21: Subcostal view of the tricuspid, pulmonic, and aortic valves. Available at http://mhprofessional.com/echoatlas/index.php?VID=16_21

16.22: Subcostal view of the coronary sinus. Available at http://mhprofessional.com/echoatlas/index.php?VID=16_22

16.23: Central line catheter entering the right atrium from the superior vena cava. Available at http://mhprofessional.com/echoatlas/index.php?VID=16_23

16.24: Parasternal long-axis view in a heart transplant patient showing the suture line in the left atrium. Available at http://mhprofessional.com/echoatlas/index.php?VID=16_24

16.25: Superior mesenteric artery on transgastric TEE of the descending aorta. Available at http://mhprofessional.com/echoatlas/index.php?VID=16_25

16.26: Color flow in a normal aortic arch and descending aorta. Available at http://mhprofessional.com/echoatlas/index.php?VID=16_26

16.27: Subcostal anatomy of right ventricular inflow and outflow. Available at http://mhprofessional.com/echoatlas/index.php?VID=16_27

16.28: Right ventricular apex—transgastric TEE view. Available at http://mhprofessional.com/echoatlas/index.php?VID=16_28

16.29: Right atrial crista terminalis. Available at http://mhprofessional.com/echoatlas/index.php?VID=16_29

16.30: Coronary sinus emptying into the right atrium. Available at http://mhprofessional.com/echoatlas/index.php?VID=16_30

16.31: Right ventricular moderator bands become more obvious with right ventricular dilatation. Available at http://mhprofessional.com/echoatlas/index.php?VID=16_31

16.32a: Left ventricular false tendon. Available at http://mhprofessional.com/echoatlas/index.php?VID=16_32a

16.32b: Left ventricular false tendon. Available at http://mhprofessional.com/echoatlas/index.php?VID=16_32b

16.33a: Unusually well-demonstrated left atrial appendage on transthoracic echo. Available at http://mhprofessional.com/echoatlas/index.php?VID=16_33a

16.33b: Unusually well-demonstrated left atrial appendage on transthoracic echo. Available at http://mhprofessional.com/echoatlas/index.php?VID=16_33b

16.33c: Unusually well-demonstrated left atrial appendage on transthoracic echo. Available at http://mhprofessional.com/echoatlas/index.php?VID=16_33c

16.34: Subcostal view. Available at http://mhprofessional.com/echoatlas/index.php?VID=16_34

16.35: Short-axis view obtained from the subcostal window. Available at http://mhprofessional.com/echoatlas/index.php?VID=16_35

16.36: Transgastric TEE short-axis view. Available at http://mhprofessional.com/echoatlas/index.php?VID=16_36

16.37: Unusually well-visualized reflections from the spine—behind the left atrium. Available at http://mhprofessional.com/echoatlas/index.php?VID=16_37

16.38: Normal short-axis subcostal view of the pulmonary artery. Available at http://mhprofessional.com/echoatlas/index.php?VID=16_38

16.39: Vessel anatomy from the high esophagus TEE window. Available at http://mhprofessional.com/echoatlas/index.php?VID=16_39

16.40: Azygous vein between the descending aorta and the spine. Available at http://mhprofessional.com/echoatlas/index.php?VID=16_40

16.41: Right atrial "floor": Coronary sinus and inferior vena cava. Available at http://mhprofessional.com/echoatlas/index.php?VID=16_41

16.42a: Aortic arch anatomy. Available at http://mhprofessional.com/echoatlas/index.php?VID=16_42a

16.42b: Aortic arch anatomy. Available at http://mhprofessional.com/echoatlas/index.php?VID=16_42b

16.43: Aortic arch examination may show flow *toward* the transducer from the innominate or from the left carotid branches. Available at http://mhprofessional.com/echoatlas/index.php?VID=16_43

Chapter 17 Contrast Echocardiograms

17.1a: Normal wall motion. Available at http://mhprofessional.com/echoatlas/index.php?VID=17_01a

17.1b: Normal wall motion. Available at http://mhprofessional.com/echoatlas/index.php?VID=17_01b

17.1c: Normal wall motion. Available at http://mhprofessional.com/echoatlas/index.php?VID=17_01c

17.1d: Normal wall motion. Available at http://mhprofessional.com/echoatlas/index.php?VID=17_01d

17.2: Normal wall motion. Available at http://mhprofessional.com/echoatlas/index.php?VID=17_02

17.3a: Apical left ventricular trabeculations outlined by contrast. Available at http://mhprofessional.com/echoatlas/index.php?VID=17_03a

17.3b: Apical left ventricular trabeculations outlined by contrast. Available at http://mhprofessional.com/echoatlas/index.php?VID=17_03b

17.3c: Apical left ventricular trabeculations outlined by contrast. Available at http://mhprofessional.com/echoatlas/index.php?VID=17_03c

17.4a: Anteroapical left ventricular aneurysm. Available at http://mhprofessional.com/echoatlas/index.php?VID=17_04a

17.4b: Anteroapical left ventricular aneurysm. Available at http://mhprofessional.com/echoatlas/index.php?VID=17_04b

17.4c: Anteroapical left ventricular aneurysm. Available at http://mhprofessional.com/echoatlas/index.php?VID=17_04c

17.5a: Apical left ventricular aneurysm. Available at http://mhprofessional.com/echoatlas/index.php?VID=17_05a

17.5b: Apical left ventricular aneurysm. Available at http://mhprofessional.com/echoatlas/index.php?VID=17_05b

17.5c: Apical left ventricular aneurysm. Available at http://mhprofessional.com/echoatlas/index.php?VID=17_05c

17.6: Large anteroseptal aneurysm. Available at http://mhprofessional.com/echoatlas/index.php?VID=17_06

17.7: It is not possible to evaluate the wall motion of the inferior wall in this parasternal long-axis view due to attenuation artifact. Available at http://mhprofessional.com/echoatlas/index.php?VID=17_07

17.8a: Negative contrast effect from the papillary muscles. Available at http://mhprofessional.com/echoatlas/index.php?VID=17_08a

17.8b: Negative contrast effect from the papillary muscles. Available at http://mhprofessional.com/echoatlas/index.php?VID=17_08b

17.8c: Negative contrast effect from the papillary muscles. Available at http://mhprofessional.com/echoatlas/index.php?VID=17_08c

17.8d: Negative contrast effect from the papillary muscles. Available at http://mhprofessional.com/echoatlas/index.php?VID=17_08d

17.9: Negative contrast effect from an apical thrombus. Available at http://mhprofessional.com/echoatlas/index.php?VID=17_09

17.10a: Dilated cardiomyopathy. Available at http://mhprofessional.com/echoatlas/index.php?VID=17_10a

17.10b: Dilated cardiomyopathy. Available at http://mhprofessional.com/echoatlas/index.php?VID=17_10b

17.10c: Dilated cardiomyopathy. Available at http://mhprofessional.com/echoatlas/index.php?VID=17_10c

17.10d: Dilated cardiomyopathy. Available at http://mhprofessional.com/echoatlas/index.php?VID=17_10d

17.10e: Dilated cardiomyopathy. Available at http://mhprofessional.com/echoatlas/index.php?VID=17_10e

17.11: Inferior wall akinesis. Available at http://mhprofessional.com/echoatlas/index.php?VID=17_11

17.12: Basal inferior wall akinesis. Available at http://mhprofessional.com/echoatlas/index.php?VID=17_12

17.13: Mid septal thinning and akinesis. Available at http://mhprofessional.com/echoatlas/index.php?VID=17_13

17.14a: Apical anterior akinesis. Available at http://mhprofessional.com/echoatlas/index.php?VID=17_14a

17.14b: Apical anterior akinesis. Available at http://mhprofessional.com/echoatlas/index.php?VID=17_14b

17.14c: Apical anterior akinesis. Available at http://mhprofessional.com/echoatlas/index.php?VID=17_14c

17.15: Thinning and dyskinesis of the apical septum. Available at http://mhprofessional.com/echoatlas/index.php?VID=17_15

17.16: Decrease in the contractility of the basal and mid interventricular septum. Available at http://mhprofessional.com/echoatlas/index.php?VID=17_16

17.17a: Akinetic interventricular septum. Available at http://mhprofessional.com/echoatlas/index.php?VID=17_17a

17.17b: Akinetic interventricular septum. Available at http://mhprofessional.com/echoatlas/index.php?VID=17_17b

17.18: Paradoxical septal motion. Available at http://mhprofessional.com/echoatlas/index.php?VID=17_18

17.19a: Normal hyperdynamic wall motion at peak stress echo. Available at http://mhprofessional.com/echoatlas/index.php?VID=17_19a

17.19b: Normal hyperdynamic wall motion at peak stress echo. Available at http://mhprofessional.com/echoatlas/index.php?VID=17_19b

17.20: Right ventricular hypertrophy—prominent right ventricular trabeculations. Available at http://mhprofessional.com/echoatlas/index.php?VID=17_20

17.21: Short axis—normal wall motion. Available at http://mhprofessional.com/echoatlas/index.php?VID=17_21

17.22: Short axis—abnormal lateral wall hypokinesis. Available at http://mhprofessional.com/echoatlas/index.php?VID=17_22

17.23: Preserved myocardial thickening with a premature atrial contraction. Available at http://mhprofessional.com/echoatlas/index.php?VID=17_23

Chapter 18 Wall Motion Abnormalities

18.1: Basal anteroseptal akinesis. Available at http://mhprofessional.com/echoatlas/index.php?VID=18_01

18.2a: Mid anteroseptal akinesis. Available at http://mhprofessional.com/echoatlas/index.php?VID=18_02a

18.2b: Mid anteroseptal akinesis. Available at http://mhprofessional.com/echoatlas/index.php?VID=18_02b

18.3: Basal and mid anteroseptal akinesis. Available at http://mhprofessional.com/echoatlas/index.php?VID=18_03

18.4a: Basal inferolateral akinesis. Available at http://mhprofessional.com/echoatlas/index.php?VID=18_04a

18.4b: Basal inferolateral akinesis. Available at http://mhprofessional.com/echoatlas/index.php?VID=18_04b

18.5: Basal inferolateral akinesis. Available at http://mhprofessional.com/echoatlas/index.php?VID=18_05

18.6: Basal and mid inferolateral akinesis. Available at http://mhprofessional.com/echoatlas/index.php?VID=18_06

18.7: Basal and mid inferolateral akinesis. Available at http://mhprofessional.com/echoatlas/index.php?VID=18_07

18.8: Basal and mid inferolateral hypokinesis. Available at http://mhprofessional.com/echoatlas/index.php?VID=18_08

18.9a: Basal inferior left ventricular aneurysm with mitral regurgitation due to the wall motion abnormality. Available at http://mhprofessional.com/echoatlas/index.php?VID=18_09a

18.9b: Basal inferior left ventricular aneurysm with mitral regurgitation due to the wall motion abnormality. Available at http://mhprofessional.com/echoatlas/index.php?VID=18_09b

18.10a: Inferior hypokinesis. Available at http://mhprofessional.com/echoatlas/index.php?VID=18_10a

18.10b: Inferior hypokinesis. Available at http://mhprofessional.com/echoatlas/index.php?VID=18_10b

18.10c: Inferior hypokinesis. Available at http://mhprofessional.com/echoatlas/index.php?VID=18_10c

18.10d: Inferior hypokinesis. Available at http://mhprofessional.com/echoatlas/index.php?VID=18_10d

18.11: Basal inferior akinesis with scar. Available at http://mhprofessional.com/echoatlas/index.php?VID=18_11

18.12a: Basal inferior akinesis. Available at http://mhprofessional.com/echoatlas/index.php?VID=18_12a

18.12b: Basal inferior akinesis. Available at http://mhprofessional.com/echoatlas/index.php?VID=18_12b

18.12c: Basal inferior akinesis. Available at http://mhprofessional.com/echoatlas/index.php?VID=18_12c

18.13: Basal inferior and inferoseptal akinesis. Available at http://mhprofessional.com/echoatlas/index.php?VID=18_13

18.14: Basal inferoseptal akinesis with scar. Available at http://mhprofessional.com/echoatlas/index.php?VID=18_14

18.15: Basal inferolateral, mid inferolateral, and apical lateral akinesis. Available at http://mhprofessional.com/echoatlas/index.php?VID=18_15

18.16: Basal inferior, mid inferior, and apical inferior akinesis. Available at http://mhprofessional.com/echoatlas/index.php?VID=18_16

18.17: Basal inferior aneurysm. Available at http://mhprofessional.com/echoatlas/index.php?VID=18_17

18.18: Basal inferoseptal akinesis. Available at http://mhprofessional.com/echoatlas/index.php?VID=18_18

18.19: Basal inferoseptal thinning and dyskinesis. Available at http://mhprofessional.com/echoatlas/index.php?VID=18_19

18.20: Inferior and inferoseptal mid ventricular wall akinesis and thinning, indicating scarred nonviable myocardium. Available at http://mhprofessional.com/echoatlas/index.php?VID=18_20

18.21: Inferior and inferoseptal mid ventricular wall akinesis. Available at http://mhprofessional.com/echoatlas/index.php?VID=18_21

18.22: Inferolateral, inferior, and inferoseptal mid ventricular wall akinesis. Available at http://mhprofessional.com/echoatlas/index.php?VID=18_22

18.23: Basal inferior, mid inferior, and apical inferior akinesis. Available at http://mhprofessional.com/echoatlas/index.php?VID=18_23

18.24: Inferior dyskinesis. Available at http://mhprofessional.com/echoatlas/index.php?VID=18_24

18.25: Inferior hypokinesis. Available at http://mhprofessional.com/echoatlas/index.php?VID=18_25

18.26: Basal septal hypokinesis. Available at http://mhprofessional.com/echoatlas/index.php?VID=18_26

18.27: Thinning, akinesis, and increased reflectivity of the interventricular septum. Available at http://mhprofessional.com/echoatlas/index.php?VID=18_27

18.28: Basal anteroseptal akinesis. Available at http://mhprofessional.com/echoatlas/index.php?VID=18_28

18.29: Mid anteroseptal akinesis. Available at http://mhprofessional.com/echoatlas/index.php?VID=18_29

18.30: Mid anteroseptal hypokinesis. Available at http://mhprofessional.com/echoatlas/index.php?VID=18_30

18.31: Apical septal akinesis. Available at http://mhprofessional.com/echoatlas/index.php?VID=18_31

18.32: Apical septal akinesis. Available at http://mhprofessional.com/echoatlas/index.php?VID=18_32

18.33: Anterior and anteroseptal akinesis. Available at http://mhprofessional.com/echoatlas/index.php?VID=18_33

18.34: Apical akinesis. Available at http://mhprofessional.com/echoatlas/index.php?VID=18_34

18.35a: Apical left ventricular aneurysm. Available at http://mhprofessional.com/echoatlas/index.php?VID=18_35a

18.35b: Apical left ventricular aneurysm. Available at http://mhprofessional.com/echoatlas/index.php?VID=18_35b

18.36: Apical left ventricular aneurysm. Available at http://mhprofessional.com/echoatlas/index.php?VID=18_36

18.37: Apical left ventricular aneurysm. Available at http://mhprofessional.com/echoatlas/index.php?VID=18_37

18.38: Mid inferoseptal akinesis. Available at http://mhprofessional.com/echoatlas/index.php?VID=18_38

18.39: Mid inferoseptal akinesis. Available at http://mhprofessional.com/echoatlas/index.php?VID=18_39

18.40: Dilated cardiomyopathy. Available at http://mhprofessional.com/echoatlas/index.php?VID=18_40

18.41: Mid inferoseptal akinesis. Available at http://mhprofessional.com/echoatlas/index.php?VID=18_41

18.42: Apical septal and mid inferoseptal akinesis. Available at http://mhprofessional.com/echoatlas/index.php?VID=18_42

18.43: Large mid to apical aneurysm. Available at http://mhprofessional.com/echoatlas/index.php?VID=18_43

18.44: Basal and mid inferoseptal akinesis. Available at http://mhprofessional.com/echoatlas/index.php?VID=18_44

18.45: Basal and mid inferoseptal aneurysm. Available at http://mhprofessional.com/echoatlas/index.php?VID=18_45

18.46a: Lateral wall akinesis. Available at http://mhprofessional.com/echoatlas/index.php?VID=18_46a

18.46b: Lateral wall akinesis. Available at http://mhprofessional.com/echoatlas/index.php?VID=18_46b

18.47: Akinetic apical lateral and mid anterolateral wall. Available at http://mhprofessional.com/echoatlas/index.php?VID=18_47

18.48: Apical lateral wall akinesis. Available at http://mhprofessional.com/echoatlas/index.php?VID=18_48

18.49: Basal and mid lateral wall akinesis. Available at http://mhprofessional.com/echoatlas/index.php?VID=18_49

18.50: Dilated cardiomyopathy. Available at http://mhprofessional.com/echoatlas/index.php?VID=18_50

18.51a: Basal and mid anterolateral wall thinning and akinesis (scar). Available at http://mhprofessional.com/echoatlas/index.php?VID=18_51a

18.51b: Basal and mid anterolateral wall thinning and akinesis (scar). Available at http://mhprofessional.com/echoatlas/index.php?VID=18_51b

18.51c: Basal and mid anterolateral wall thinning and akinesis (scar). Available at http://mhprofessional.com/echoatlas/index.php?VID=18_51c

18.52a: Abnormal lateral wall motion. Available at http://mhprofessional.com/echoatlas/index.php?VID=18_52a

18.52b: Abnormal lateral wall motion. Available at http://mhprofessional.com/echoatlas/index.php?VID=18_52b

18.53: Septal scarring, thinning, and akinesis. Available at http://mhprofessional.com/echoatlas/index.php?VID=18_53

18.54: Basal and mid septal akinesis. Available at http://mhprofessional.com/echoatlas/index.php?VID=18_54

18.55a: Inferior myocardial infarction. Available at http://mhprofessional.com/echoatlas/index.php?VID=18_55a

18.55b: Inferior myocardial infarction. Available at http://mhprofessional.com/echoatlas/index.php?VID=18_55b

18.55c: Inferior myocardial infarction. Available at http://mhprofessional.com/echoatlas/index.php?VID=18_55c

18.55d: Inferior myocardial infarction. Available at http://mhprofessional.com/echoatlas/index.php?VID=18_55d

18.55e: Inferior myocardial infarction. Available at http://mhprofessional.com/echoatlas/index.php?VID=18_55e

18.55f: Inferior myocardial infarction. Available at http://mhprofessional.com/echoatlas/index.php?VID=18_55f

18.55g: Inferior myocardial infarction. Available at http://mhprofessional.com/echoatlas/index.php?VID=18_55g

18.56: Septal hypokinesis. Lateral wall akinesis. Available at http://mhprofessional.com/echoatlas/index.php?VID=18_56

18.57: Dilated cardiomyopathy with diffuse wall motion abnormalities. Available at http://mhprofessional.com/echoatlas/index.php?VID=18_57

18.58: Dilated cardiomyopathy with diffuse wall motion abnormalities. Available at http://mhprofessional.com/echoatlas/index.php?VID=18_58

18.59: Dilated cardiomyopathy with diffuse wall motion abnormalities. Available at http://mhprofessional.com/echoatlas/index.php?VID=18_59

18.60: Pacing in cardiomyopathy. Available at http://mhprofessional.com/echoatlas/index.php?VID=18_60

18.61: Scarring and akinesis of the interventricular septum. Available at http://mhprofessional.com/echoatlas/index.php?VID=18_61

18.62: Short axis. Available at http://mhprofessional.com/echoatlas/index.php?VID=18_62

18.63: Preserved septal thickening. Available at http://mhprofessional.com/echoatlas/index.php?VID=18_63

18.64: Preserved myocardial thickening. Available at http://mhprofessional.com/echoatlas/index.php?VID=18_64

18.65: Short-axis anterolateral hypokinesis. Available at http://mhprofessional.com/echoatlas/index.php?VID=18_65

18.66: Septal akinesis. Available at http://mhprofessional.com/echoatlas/index.php?VID=18_66

18.67: Exaggerated normal thickening of the basal inferolateral wall due to pericardial effusion. Available at http://mhprofessional.com/echoatlas/index.php?VID=18_67

18.68: Akinetic right ventricular free wall. Dilated right ventricle. Available at http://mhprofessional.com/echoatlas/index.php?VID=18_68

18.69: Apical right ventricular free wall thinning and akinesis. Available at http://mhprofessional.com/echoatlas/index.php?VID=18_69

18.70a: Right ventricular wall akinesis. Available at http://mhprofessional.com/echoatlas/index.php?VID=18_70a

18.70b: Right ventricular wall akinesis. Available at http://mhprofessional.com/echoatlas/index.php?VID=18_70b

18.71a: Effect of premature ventricular contractions on wall motion. Available at http://mhprofessional.com/echoatlas/index.php?VID=18_71a

18.71b: Effect of premature ventricular contractions on wall motion. Available at http://mhprofessional.com/echoatlas/index.php?VID=18_71b

18.71c: Effect of premature ventricular contractions on wall motion. Available at http://mhprofessional.com/echoatlas/index.php?VID=18_71c

18.71d: Effect of premature ventricular contractions on wall motion. Available at http://mhprofessional.com/echoatlas/index.php?VID=18_71d

18.71e: Effect of premature ventricular contractions on wall motion. Available at http://mhprofessional.com/echoatlas/index.php?VID=18_71e

18.72: Apical septal akinesis. Available at http://mhprofessional.com/echoatlas/index.php?VID=18_72

18.73: Right ventricle being paced from the right ventricular apex. Available at http://mhprofessional.com/echoatlas/index.php?VID=18_73

18.74: Global hypokinesis. Dilated cardiomyopathy. Available at http://mhprofessional.com/echoatlas/index.php?VID=18_74

18.75: Global biventricular dysfunction. Available at http://mhprofessional.com/echoatlas/index.php?VID=18_75

18.76: Wall motion quiz 1. Available at http://mhprofessional.com/echoatlas/index.php?VID=18_76

18.77: Wall motion quiz 2. Available at http://mhprofessional.com/echoatlas/index.php?VID=18_77

18.78: Wall motion quiz 3. Available at http://mhprofessional.com/echoatlas/index.php?VID=18_78

18.79: Wall motion quiz 4. Available at http://mhprofessional.com/echoatlas/index.php?VID=18_79

18.80: Wall motion quiz 5. Available at http://mhprofessional.com/echoatlas/index.php?VID=18_80

18.81: Wall motion quiz 6. Available at http://mhprofessional.com/echoatlas/index.php?VID=18_81

18.82: Wall motion quiz 7. Available at http://mhprofessional.com/echoatlas/index.php?VID=18_82

18.83: Wall motion quiz 8. Available at http://mhprofessional.com/echoatlas/index.php?VID=18_83

18.84: Wall motion quiz 9. Available at http://mhprofessional.com/echoatlas/index.php?VID=18_84

18.85: Wall motion quiz 10. Available at http://mhprofessional.com/echoatlas/index.php?VID=18_85

18.86: Wall motion quiz 11. Available at http://mhprofessional.com/echoatlas/index.php?VID=18_86

18.87: Wall motion quiz 12. Available at http://mhprofessional.com/echoatlas/index.php?VID=18_87

18.88: Wall motion quiz 13. Available at http://mhprofessional.com/echoatlas/index.php?VID=18_88

18.89: Wall motion quiz 14. Available at http://mhprofessional.com/echoatlas/index.php?VID=18_89

18.90: Wall motion quiz 15. Available at http://mhprofessional.com/echoatlas/index.php?VID=18_90

18.91: Wall motion quiz 16. Available at http://mhprofessional.com/echoatlas/index.php?VID=18_91

18.92: Wall motion quiz 17. Available at http://mhprofessional.com/echoatlas/index.php?VID=18_92

18.93: Wall motion quiz 18. Available at http://mhprofessional.com/echoatlas/index.php?VID=18_93

INDEX

Note: Page number followed by *f*, indicates figure.

NOTES

NOTES

NOTES

NOTES

NOTES

NOTES

NOTES

NOTES

NOTES